Radiographic Imaging for the Dental Team

Radiographic Imaging for the Dental Team

Fourth Edition

Dale A. Miles BA, DDS, MS, FRCD(C), Dip. ABOM, Dip. ABOMR
Adjunct Professor
University of Texas Health Science Center at San Antonio
San Antonio, Texas
Adjunct Professor
Arizona School of Dentistry and Oral Health
Mesa, Arizona
CEO, Digital Radiographic Solutions
Fountain Hills, Arizona

Margot L. Van Dis, DDS, MS, Dip. ABOMR
Professor
Department of Oral Pathology, Medicine and Radiology
Indiana University School of Dentistry
Indianapolis, Indiana

Gail F. Williamson, RDH, MS
Professor
Department of Oral Pathology, Medicine and Radiology
Indiana University School of Dentistry
Indianapolis, Indiana

Catherine W. Jensen, RDH, MHE
Carbondale, Illinois

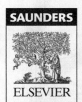

SAUNDERS

ELSEVIER

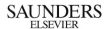

SAUNDERS
ELSEVIER

11830 Westline Industrial Drive
St. Louis, Missouri 63146

RADIOGRAPHIC IMAGING FOR THE DENTAL TEAM   ISBN: 978-1-4160-6004-8

Library of Congress Cataloging-in-Publication Data
Radiographic imaging for the dental team / Dale A. Miles ... [et al.]. -- 4th ed.   p. ; cm.
  Rev. ed. of: Radiographic imaging for dental auxiliaries / Dale A. Miles ... [et al.]. 3rd ed. c1999.
  Includes bibliographical references and index.
  ISBN 978-1-4160-6004-8 (pbk. : alk. paper) 1. Teeth--Radiography. 2. Dental auxiliary personnel.
I. Miles, Dale A. II. Radiographic imaging for dental auxiliaries.
  [DNLM: 1. Radiography, Dental--methods. 2. Dental Auxiliaries. WN 230 R1289 2009]

  RK309.M384 2009
  617.6'07572--dc22   2008038973

Vice President and Publisher: Linda Duncan
Senior Editor: John Dolan
Senior Developmental Editor: Courtney Sprehe
Publishing Services Manager: Julie Eddy
Senior Project Manager: Laura Loveall
Design Direction: Amy Buxton

Printed in Canada

Last digit is the print number: 9 8 7 6 5 4 3 2 1

Preface

It has been nearly twenty years since the first edition of this book was published and nearly ten years since the third edition was released. We are grateful to the loyal instructors who have continued to use the book throughout the years, and we appreciate the helpful suggestions for improvements that have been made by its users. It's certainly rewarding to see that good instruction can stand the test of time!

Despite a great deal of change in the field of oral and maxillofacial radiology over the past ten years, the basic principles of x-ray production, image geometry, film processing, and image receptor placement remain relatively constant. Fortunately, because of the constancy of this information, concepts for teaching the subject matter remain pertinent to today's instructor and student.

NEW TO THIS EDITION

We are delighted to welcome Gail F. Williamson to the author team for the fourth edition. Gail is a nationally recognized oral and maxillofacial radiology faculty member for dental assisting and dental hygiene students at Indiana University and an active member of the American Academy of Oral and Maxillofacial Radiology. Because of her expertise in educational methodology, she has been especially helpful in developing materials for the new Evolve site (discussed later).

One of the main goals of this new edition is to help better prepare students to obtain and evaluate a variety of diagnostic images. To that end, some of the updates include:

- Chapter 1: Intraoral Imaging Technique and Chapter 8: Panoramic Imaging—the addition of information on digital imaging and "image receptors"
- Chapter 5: Radiation Biology and Protection—the latest information from The National Council on Radiation Protection (NCRP) report, *Radiation Protection in Dentistry*
- Chapter 11: Extraoral, Specialized, and Implant Imaging—updated information on imaging for implant placement and volumetric imaging
- Chapter 12: Basics of Interpretation—reorganization and expansion of the chapter to provide better examples of common dental diseases, such as caries and alveolar bone loss, as well as some of the more unusual conditions seen in patients

EVOLVE

The innovative Evolve site, which is new to this edition, offers a variety of supplemental materials for both instructors and students.

For instructors, it allows you to supplement your own materials with additional teaching tools such as, an image collection containing every image in the book, teaching tips, and PowerPoint lectures slides for each chapter.

For students, it offers you a variety of self-study tools including: two interactive practice exams; six drag-and-drop identification exercises that test on topics such as, exposure and processing errors, interpretation of dental disease and anomalies, panoramic errors, technical errors, interpretation of radiographic anatomy, and mounting; and a variety of weblinks.

Plus, the **Answers to the Chapter Study Questions** are now found on the Evolve site.

NOTE FROM THE AUTHORS

If this is the first time you, as an instructor, have selected this text for use in your course, we hope you find it easy to use, presented in a manner that closely parallels how radiology is taught to dental assisting and dental hygiene students, and complementary to your own teaching materials.

To the students, we hope you enjoy using this text, that you find it easy to read and understand, and that you will take full advantage of the study materials within the text and on the Evolve site. We have done our best to provide you with an excellent educational aid to help you master the art and science of oral and maxillofacial radiology.

It has been our pleasure to restructure and re-engergize the book for you.

DAM

MLV

GFW

CWJ

Acknowledgments

This fourth edition would not have been possible without the efforts of Mr. John Dolan, our senior editor at Elsevier, who thought that yes, indeed, it was time for a new edition; Ms. Courtney Sprehe, our developmental editor, who joined us midway through the project but helped us keep track of all the details; Ms. Laura Loveall, our project manager, who made sure the book was as attractive as possible; and Cindy Ahlheim, who helped in the creation of the Evolve site.

We would also like to thank our Indianapolis photographer, Mr. Terry L. Wilson, Jr., and our new models, Ms. Aja Nichols, Ms. Rehka Chaudhari, Mr. Shadraq Gonqueh, and Ms. Ankita Shah for their willingness to share their spare time to help us obtain some additional illustrations. We would also like to thank the folks at Laserwords in Burlington, Ontario, Canada for their assistance in updating many of the line drawings in the text.

Contents

CHAPTER 8

Panoramic Imaging, 153

CHAPTER 9

Trouble-Shooting Technique and Processing Errors, 173

CHAPTER 10

Accessory Radiographic Techniques and Patient Management, 203

CHAPTER 11

Extraoral, Specialized, and Implant Imaging, 225

CHAPTER 12

Basics of Interpretation: Normal versus Abnormal and Common Radiographic Presentation of Lesions, 251

Radiographic Imaging for the Dental Team

Intraoral Radiographic Technique

BEFORE YOU BEGIN

Radiation, what you will be using to produce radiographs (x-ray films) or digital images, is biologically damaging. Any exposure, no matter how insignificant it may seem, has the potential to damage living tissues—yours or your patient's. You need to begin your radiologic education by practicing techniques and skills and by acquiring habits that will protect both you and your patient. The beginning of this chapter gives you enough practical guidelines to complete laboratory exercises safely on a phantom, manikin, or skull. For those who begin practice on patients early in the program, a summary of patient protection procedures is also included. An in-depth discussion of radiation biology and protection procedures is presented in Chapter 5.

Practical Guidelines

1. Never do anything to your patient that you would not like to have done to you.
2. It is easier to do it right the first time than to explain why you did it wrong.

These basic rules are the foundation for most of the safety and protection procedures.

Before you set foot in a radiographic operatory, you should be familiar with the equipment. To use the equipment properly, you need to be able to select the exposure settings correctly. These exposure settings may vary for different units. The correct exposure settings for your unit will have been determined in advance; your responsibility is to know the correct settings and how to change the settings if they are incorrect. A chart showing settings for time (seconds or impulses), kilovolt peak (kVp), and milliamperage (mA) for commonly used techniques should be posted close to the control panel of each x-ray unit. Check with your instructor about the location of this chart (Fig. 1-1).

Operator Protection

One of your additional responsibilities is to learn and practice some basic rules of *operator protection* relating to your laboratory experience.

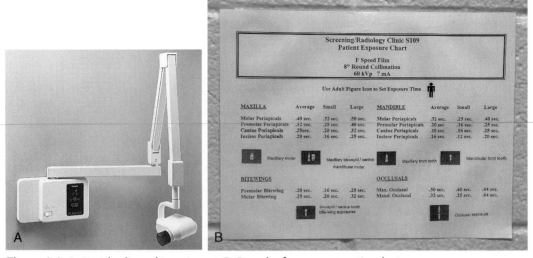

Figure 1-1 **A,** Dental radiographic equipment. **B,** Example of an exposure setting chart.

1. *Never* stand in direct line of the primary beam (the open end of the cylinder, where the radiation exits the unit). It is best to stand behind a lead barrier (Fig. 1-2). If you cannot place an acceptable barrier between you and the beam, stand at right angles to the beam (Fig. 1-3) at a distance of 6 feet or greater.
2. *Never* hold the film or image receptor in a patient's mouth or in any radiographic training phantom. If the patient cannot hold the film without help, use alternative placement methods or obtain assistance from your instructor.
3. *Never* stand closer than 6 feet to the x-ray unit during an exposure unless you are behind an acceptable barrier.
4. *Never* use equipment that is faulty or that you suspect is faulty. For example, if the x-ray tubehead drifts (moves) after it is positioned, the unit should be repaired before further use. If unusual noises come from the unit or if the unit fails to make an audible and visible sound during exposure, the unit should not be used until it is repaired. *Anything out of the ordinary should be reported to the appropriate person before the equipment is used.*

Patient Protection

Radiographic practice on clinical patients should not begin until a reasonable level of competence is achieved in a closely supervised laboratory environment. Principles of *patient protection* must be understood before exposing patients to x rays.

1. Radiographic images should never be made of a patient unless they offer a benefit to the patient that outweighs the risk of the radiation exposure.
2. Each patient should be protected from unnecessary exposure to radiation as much as possible. Protection should include a *leaded thyroid shield* for all intraoral exposures. The amount of radiation reaching the abdomen during dental radiographic procedures is negligible, and the most recent radiation guidelines[*] say that use of a **leaded apron** in adults is not considered

---

[*]National Council on Radiation Protection and Measurements (NCRP), *Radiation protection in dentistry,* Bethesda, Md., 2003, NCRP, Report No. 145.

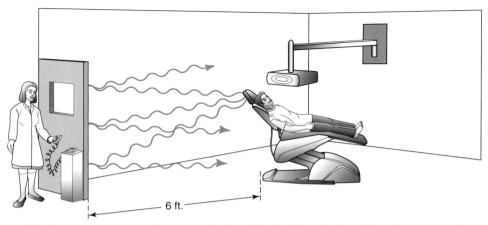

Figure 1-2 The operator stands behind a protective leaded barrier. The patient is visible to the operator throughout the procedure.

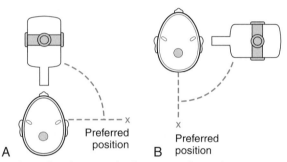

Figure 1-3 **A,** The *X* shows the preferred position for the operator during the x-ray exposure of an anterior image (90° to the primary beam). **B,** The preferred position for a posterior exposure.

mandatory *if* all other appropriate steps are taken to keep patient exposure to a minimum (see Chapter 5 for more details on patient protection). However, use of the leaded apron is essential for children and women who are pregnant or who might be pregnant.

3. The **paralleling technique** for intraoral films is recommended by the American Dental Association and the American Academy of Oral and Maxillofacial Radiology unless circumstances or anatomy dictate the use of other techniques. The paralleling technique not only produces better images with less distortion and greater accuracy but also significantly reduces the patient radiation dose.

4. Proper exposure and processing techniques should be employed to produce the most diagnostically useful images possible. Minimizing retakes necessitated by improper exposure or processing may be the single most effective method for reducing radiation exposure to patients.

Patient and Operator Protection

1. *Always* review the patient's medical history for medical problems that may complicate radiography and, in the case of female patients of childbearing years, for pregnancy. Some clinicians prefer to postpone nonemergency images until the patient is past the first trimester of pregnancy, and in some instances, elective radiographic procedures may be postponed until after delivery of the child.

2. *Always* wear clean gloves, a mask, a gown, and protective eyewear when performing radiographic procedures. Universal infection control precautions as advised by the Centers for Disease Control and Prevention (CDC) should be followed during radiographic procedures for all patients. Infection control guidelines appear at the end of this chapter.

INTRAORAL RADIOGRAPHIC TECHNIQUES

Radiographic images are two-dimensional images of three-dimensional objects. The objects that are imaged have length, width, and depth, yet the image on the film or screen is a representation that has only length and width. The depth, or thickness, of the object cannot be determined on the image unless specialized three-dimensional imaging systems are used. The images produced on a radiographic film or with a digital imaging receptor represent a number of the patient's anatomic structures superimposed over each other. The images afford the clinician an opportunity to "look inside" and "see" internal structures as if they were transparent (Fig. 1-4). The patient's anatomic structures need to be reconstructed in the mind's eye. Simply looking at the image may not tell the viewer whether structures are facial (outside the dental arch), lingual (inside the dental arch, toward the tongue in the mandible), or palatal (inside the dental arch toward the palate in the maxilla).

Throughout this chapter there are many references to "films" and "film packets." If you are using digital radiography, the digital image receptor is analogous to x-ray film, and the concepts that pertain to intraoral image acquisition are true for digital imaging as well as film-based imaging. Digital receptors may be solid-state sensors or phosphor plates that yield a digital image after they are scanned by an image or plate reader.

Intraoral Film Types

Dental radiographs may be intraoral or extraoral. **Intraoral radiographs** are made by placing the x-ray film or image receptor inside the mouth and projecting x rays from a source outside the face, through the anatomic structures of interest (the

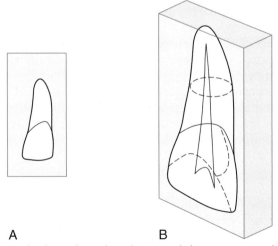

A   B

Figure 1-4 **A,** Two-dimensional radiograph. **B,** Three-dimensional object or structure that was radiographed. We "see" internal structures; in reality, these structures are superimposed over each other, each stopping a different number of x rays.

object being imaged), and onto the film or image receptor. **Extraoral radiographs,** discussed in a later chapter, are made by placing the film or image receptor outside the oral cavity.

There are three types of intraoral images: (1) periapical, (2) bitewing, and (3) occlusal. Periapical and bitewing images are the most commonly used intraoral projections in dentistry (Figs. 1-5 through 1-7).

Periapical radiographs record images of the teeth (outlines, positions, dimensions) and supporting structures such as alveolar bone, lamina dura, and periodontal membrane space. Each film usually contains an image of a group of teeth in one area of the dental arch at a time. Periapical images are used to interpret normal anatomy and pathologic conditions in the root area and in the surrounding bony structures. *It is critical to obtain an image that includes the entire length of the teeth of interest plus 3 to 4 mm of supporting tissue beyond the root apex* (Fig. 1-8). It is permissible to occasionally sacrifice the incisal or occlusal edges of the teeth to record the apical information. The incisal or occlusal surfaces may always be seen clinically. A "retake" or repeated exposure is seldom required because the biting surface information is missing. Additional exposure to the patient to obtain a "perfect" image is inappropriate.

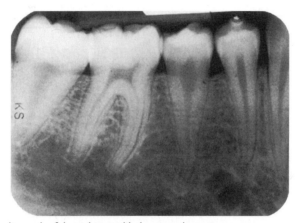

Figure 1-5   Periapical radiograph of the right mandibular premolar region.

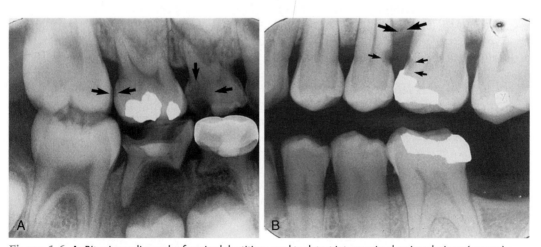

Figure 1-6   **A,** Bitewing radiograph of a mixed dentition, used to detect interproximal carious lesions *(arrows).* **B,** Adult bitewing radiograph demonstrating both root caries *(small arrows)* and bone loss *(large arrows).*

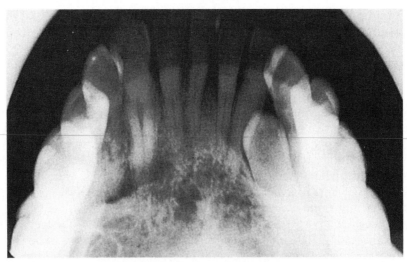

Figure 1-7   Typical topographic mandibular occlusal radiograph (see Chapter 10 on accessory techniques). Note the impacted canine. *(From Miles DA, Van Dis ML, Razmus TF: Basic principles of oral and maxillofacial radiology, ed 1, Philadelphia, 1992, Saunders).*

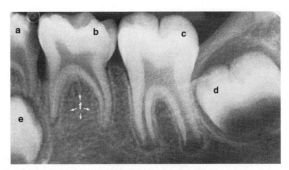

Figure 1-8   Periapical radiograph of a 7- to 8-year-old child, showing the erupted primary and the developing permanent teeth in the mandibular left quadrant; *a,* primary first molar; *b,* primary second molar; *c,* permanent first molar; *d,* developing permanent first bicuspid; *e,* developing permanent first premolar; *f,* region of the permanent second premolar that failed to develop.

Bitewing radiographs record images of the crowns and interproximal regions of the maxillary and mandibular teeth on the same film (Figs. 1-9 and 1-10). Film placement in this technique generally produces a more anatomically and dimensionally accurate image than that seen in a periapical view. However, the image is limited to the coronal one third of the teeth and related structures. This type of image is used to reveal interproximal carious lesions (cavities), recurrent decay in the interproximal areas, faulty restorations (overhangs, for example), the presence of calculus, crestal bone levels, pulp chamber shapes, and occlusal relationships. Bitewing images offer a diagnostic aid for detecting enamel caries (incipient lesions) that may not be detectable by any other clinical methods. Bitewing images also provide the most accurate assessment of interproximal alveolar crestal bone levels. The use of bitewings for incipient cavity detection will become even more important as the use of sealants and other preventive materials increases. The identification of incipient lesions may allow the clinician to implement methods that lead to cavity remineralization or arrest.

Occlusal radiographs record images of a large portion of a dental arch on one film. There are several useful projections for occlusal images (Figs. 1-11 and 1-12).

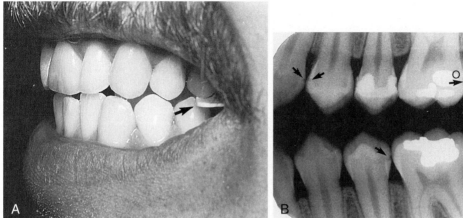
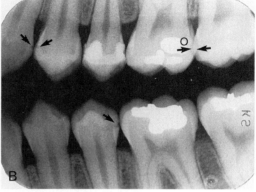

Figure 1-9 **A,** This clinical photograph shows the difficulty in visualizing the film placement when the patient has closed on the bite tab, a cardboard loop used to hold the film. If the film is centered in the holder, then the tab *(black arrow)* should be centered at the second premolar/first molar contact, as illustrated. **B,** This premolar bitewing view shows the correct positioning of the teeth. All contacts between the teeth are "open," and the distal half of each canine is included on the film. Carious lesions are then visible with no overlap between the enamel of adjacent teeth *(arrows).* Overlap is, however, seen between the maxillary first and second molars *(o).*

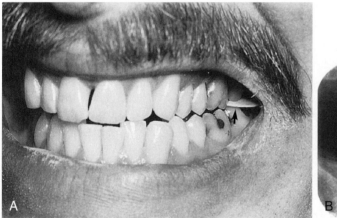
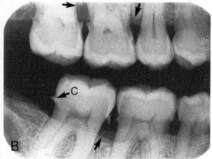

Figure 1-10 **A,** This is the correct position of the bite tab between the maxillary and mandibular second molars *(arrow).* This placement will ensure "open" contacts in the molar region. **B,** The resultant molar bitewing views, showing bone loss *(arrows)* and interproximal calculus, seen as white "spikes" between the teeth in this view *(c).*

The technique, purpose, and interpretation of occlusal films are discussed in more detail in Chapter 10.

TYPES OF RADIOGRAPHIC SURVEYS

Two common dental radiographic surveys are the bitewing survey (BWS) and the **complete mouth radiographic survey (CMRS),** or full mouth x-ray series (FMX). The BWS normally consists of two or four posterior films with molars grouped together and premolars grouped together. Both left and right sides of the patient's mouth are imaged (Figs. 1-13 and 1-14).

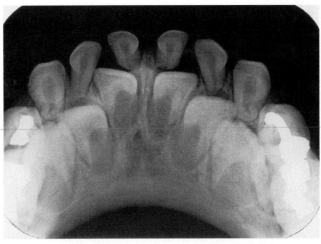

Figure 1-11   Mandibular occlusal radiograph of the primary dentition of a child about 4 years old.

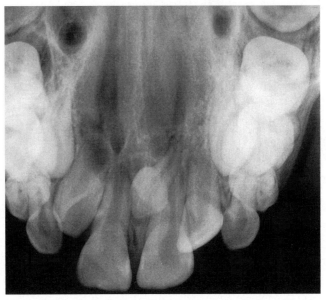

Figure 1-12   Maxillary occlusal radiograph of the same child as in Figure 1-11. Note the extra toothlike structure between the central incisors. This is called a *mesiodens*. (See also Chapter 12).

The CMRS, or FMX, is composed of a number of periapical images and usually bitewing images as well. The survey must include every tooth, every apex, 3 to 4 mm of supporting structures beyond the apices, every contact area, and all tooth-bearing areas (even if edentulous) at least once somewhere on the survey. To obtain images of all of these structures, an operator may take as few as 10 or as many as 18 periapical images plus whichever bitewing images are indicated. The number and size of film used in a CMRS depend on the number of teeth present, the size of the oral cavity, the anatomic structures within the mouth, the age of the patient, the technique used, and the level of patient cooperation (Fig. 1-15).

CMRSs may be performed with the use of either a paralleling or a bisecting-angle technique. The American Dental Association and the American Academy of Oral and Maxillofacial Radiology recommend the use of the paralleling technique for periapical exposures; in accordance with these recommendations, the remainder

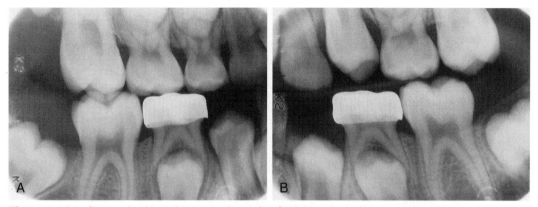

Figure 1-13   Left **(A)** and right **(B)** bitewing radiographs of a child. Only two bitewing views are required.

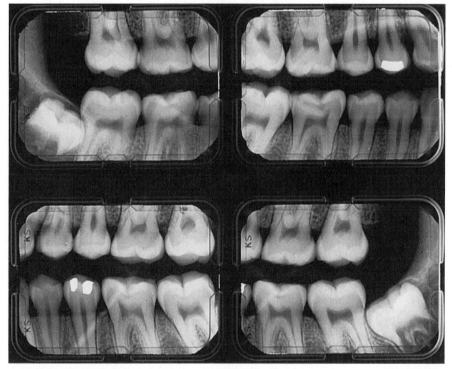

Figure 1-14   Left *(bottom)* and right *(top)* bitewing radiographs of an adult. Four bitewing films are needed to ensure that all contacts are "open."

of this book considers paralleling as the standard technique. Paralleling is also the most appropriate technique for digital image acquisition. This is discussed more fully in Chapter 7. Nevertheless, the bisecting-angle technique remains a valuable accessory technique and, as such, is included in Chapter 10.

Film Sizes for Complete Mouth Radiographic Survey

X-ray film is the current imaging medium that is most commonly used to record anatomic images; however, more and more practitioners are adopting digital imaging techniques. When film is used, there are five sizes from which to select, shown

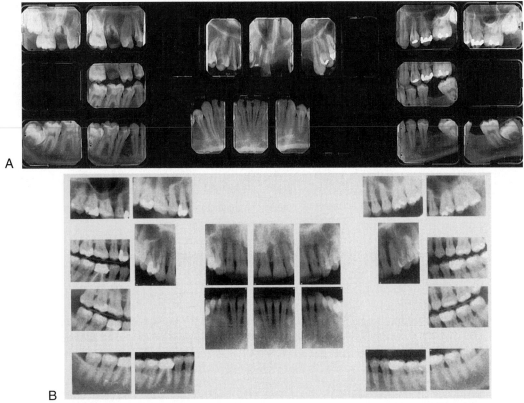

Figure 1-15 **A,** Typical complete mouth radiographic series with size no. 1 and size no. 2 film. **B,** Full mouth survey with size no. 2 direct digital imaging sensor. *(B: From Razmus TF, Williamson GF:* Current oral and maxillofacial imaging, *ed 1, Philadelphia, 1996, Saunders.)*

in Fig. 1-16. CMRSs for adults normally use film sizes no. 1 and no. 2. Adult bitewing surveys normally use no. 2 size film. Smaller film (no. 0) may be used for children younger than 3 years old. Note that films for anterior teeth are placed with the longest dimension vertically oriented, and posterior films are placed horizontally (Fig. 1-17).

The Need for Each Image Type

A common misconception among beginning radiography students is that areas that have no teeth (edentulous areas) do not need to be imaged. The purpose of imaging edentulous regions is to aid in diagnosing problems that cannot be seen clinically. Such problems may include more than just the tooth-related ones. The appearance of supporting structures, such as bone and soft tissues, may reflect health or disease. Changes in trabecular patterns, the presence or absence of structures, and other radiographic alterations may provide information regarding a patient's health status. Therefore periapical films of areas where teeth are not clinically present should also be included in the CMRS or FMX if the dentist has so prescribed. However, desired information in edentulous areas can be captured in a film-based or a digital panoramic image. The resolution (detail) in a digital panoramic image is sufficient to be an acceptable alternative to the CMRS in instances in which intraoral images cannot be obtained.

The need for bitewing images is different. Bitewings are needed only in areas where teeth have interproximal contact with other teeth, obstructing a clinical view

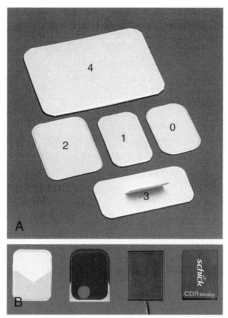

Figure 1-16   A, Photograph of the five sizes of intraoral radiographic films. Film size no. 0 is used for children with primary dentition; no. 1 is used for mixed dentition radiographs, and in many cases, for anterior views in adult dentition; no. 2 is used for both vertical and horizontal positions for periapicals and bitewings, mainly in adult dentition; no. 3 is a longer version of the no. 2 size film and is used for interproximal bitewing radiographs; no. 4 is used for occlusal radiographs. **B,** Examples of digital imaging sensors. *(B: From White SC, Pharoah MJ:* Oral radiology, principles and interpretation, *ed 6, St Louis, 2009, Mosby.)*

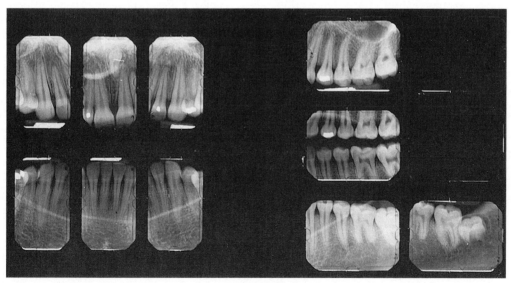

Figure 1-17   Photograph of six anterior and four posterior films. The anterior views are size no. 1. All are in the vertical position. The molar views are size no. 2, used in a horizontal position. The maxillary molar periapical view and the molar bitewing view were not necessary, and two exposed, processed *(black)* films are placed in the mount to block extraneous light.

of the mesial and distal surfaces. The primary use of bitewing images is to detect interproximal carious lesions (see Figs. 1-6 and 1-9). If interproximal spaces can be examined clinically, a particular bitewing image may not be needed.

Because the anterior teeth are thinner than the posterior teeth in a facial-to-lingual dimension, it may be much easier to see the interproximal spaces with direct vision and transillumination. These procedures eliminate the need for anterior bitewings in most cases. However, because the levels of the alveolar bone crests are also imaged in bitewings, these projections may be used to evaluate periodontal health or disease. In some instances, bone levels may be apical enough to require positioning a bitewing in a vertical rather than horizontal position, and the dentist may prescribe anterior bitewings to evaluate bone rather than interproximal contacts.

INTRAORAL RADIOGRAPHY: BASIC PRINCIPLES

Paralleling Periapical Technique

The paralleling periapical technique is used in dental imaging to minimize shape distortion of the image and to reduce the radiation on dose from x rays to the patient's head and neck. The geometric principle of this technique is to place the film or image receptor parallel to the long axes of the teeth to be imaged while aiming the central x ray (central ray, CR, or x-ray beam) perpendicular to both. The following basic principles must be understood when periapical intraoral radiographic techniques are practiced: (1) anatomic considerations, (2) x-ray beam angulation, (3) point of entry, and (4) film or image receptor placement.

Anatomic Considerations

Location of the Long Axes of the Teeth. Most root apices in the maxilla tilt inward toward the palate. The flatter or more shallow the palatal vault of the maxilla is, the greater the tendency for the apices to tilt inward. The crowns of the six anterior teeth usually tilt outward (Fig. 1-18).

The mandibular premolars are more nearly vertical (Fig. 1-19). Mandibular molars tilt inward slightly. Although the crowns of the teeth appear to tilt one way, the entire structure actually tilts another; you cannot assume that roots are perfectly vertical just because the crowns appear to be so.

This concept is important because the film or image receptor is placed parallel to the long axis of the *whole tooth* in the paralleling technique, not just parallel to the crown. In addition, anatomic structures such as the palate or the floor of the mouth may influence the extent to which the film can parallel the long axes of the teeth. The anatomy of a patient's mouth may dictate the use of an alternative technique or modification of the paralleling principle.

Location of the Apices and Respective Head Positions. The apical region of the maxillary teeth is located on an imaginary line drawn from the ala of the nose to the tragus of the ear (Fig. 1-20). It may be helpful to have the ala–tragus line parallel to the floor when you make a radiograph of the maxillary teeth. This also makes the maxillary occlusal plane parallel to the floor. The correct head position is your starting point.

The paralleling technique requires the use of a film-holding device. Many of the film-holding devices have an extraoral marker of some sort; it is usually a locator ring to help you position the x-ray tube exactly over the film (Fig. 1-21). When using these devices, you may place the patient in almost any position you choose and still produce quality images. The most important point to remember is to place the patient in a position that will make the procedure successful and the patient comfortable.

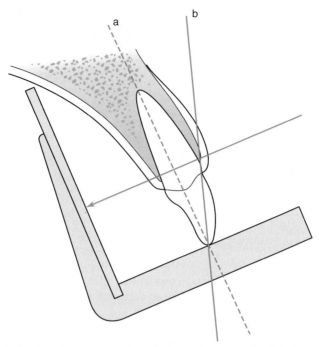

Figure 1-18 Schematic drawing of tilting of maxillary anterior teeth. The film parallels the long axis *(dotted line a)*; however, the operator sees only the crowns, and the inclination of the crown seems more vertically oriented *(solid line b)*.

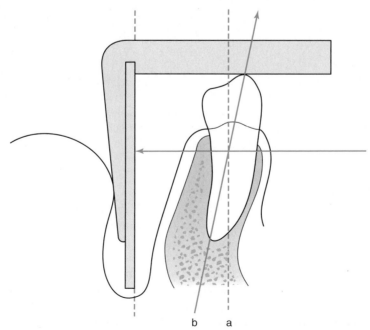

Figure 1-19 The long axis *(solid line b)* of this premolar is less vertical than one would expect from looking at the teeth clinically *(dotted line a)*.

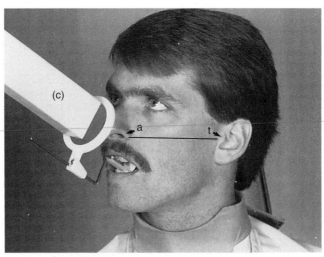

Figure 1-20 Ala–tragus line. The ala *(a)* is the side of the nose. The tragus (the cartilaginous projection just anterior to the opening of the ear) is labeled *t*. This line closely parallels the tips of the maxillary teeth from canine to third molar; it is easier to visualize than the occlusal plane when the patient has closed. Pictured here is a typical rectangular "cone" or "cylinder," labeled *(c)*.

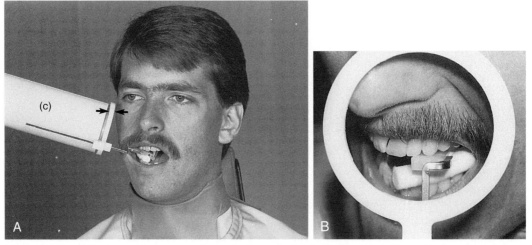

Figure 1-21 A, The locator ring *(arrows)* is attached to a metal rod, which in turn holds the film or receptor. The cylinder *(c)* is aligned precisely with the locator ring and the metal rod in both horizontal and vertical directions. **B,** The tooth of interest, the canine, is centered in the ring.

X-Ray Beam Angulation

Vertical Angulation. The x-ray tube has two directional positions that must be adjusted during an exposure. The **vertical angulation** is the movement of the tubehead up and down, similar to someone nodding his or her head yes. If the x-ray tubehead is pointing down, the angulation is positive. If the x-ray tubehead is pointing up, the angulation is negative. Some x-ray units have dials on the arms that indicate the positive or negative angulation by degrees. If the tubehead is parallel to the floor, its vertical angulation is zero degrees (0°). If the tubehead is pointing straight down at the floor, the vertical angulation is positive 90 degrees (+90°); if the tubehead is pointing straight upward, the vertical angulation is negative 90 degrees (–90°). This concept is illustrated in Figure 1-22. In the paralleling technique, the vertical angle

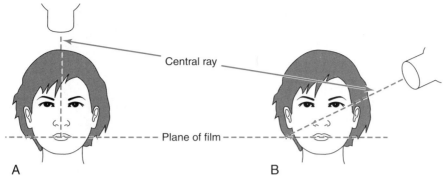

Figure 1-22 **A,** Positive 90 degrees (+90°). **B,** Positive vertical angulation.

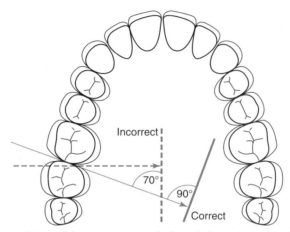

Figure 1-23 In this diagram the parallel x rays pass precisely through the contact areas of the teeth because the tubehead cylinder is angled at 90 degrees to the film plane. If the film is angled less than 90 degrees to the x rays, overlap of the enamel areas will occur. (See Chapter 9 for a more thorough explanation of horizontal angulation errors.)

of the x-ray beam must be perpendicular to both the film or image receptor and to the long axes of the teeth.

Horizontal Angulation. The **horizontal angulation** is the position of the x-ray tubehead in the same direction as the horizon. Horizontal angulation movement may be compared with someone shaking his or her head no. The horizontal angles rotate around the patient's head 360 degrees, as if the head were the center of a circle. Imagine someone standing behind a tree. If you look directly at the front of the tree, you cannot see any part of the person behind it. If you move in a wide circle around the tree, you will begin to see the person behind the tree because you are changing the horizontal angle of your vision. Keep this example in mind when you think of horizontal angulation. The horizontal angulation of the x-ray beam should be directed through the contacts of the teeth, as perpendicular to the horizontal plane of the film or image receptor as possible (Fig. 1-23).

Point of Entry

The point of entry of the x-ray beam should be directed through the center of the region being radiographed. The objective is to completely cover the film with the beam of radiation. If this is not done, a "cone cut," or partial image, will be seen in the resulting image (Fig. 1-24). The use of film-holding devices that have extraoral markers can reduce the problem with cone-cut images. A detailed discussion of errors such as these comes later.

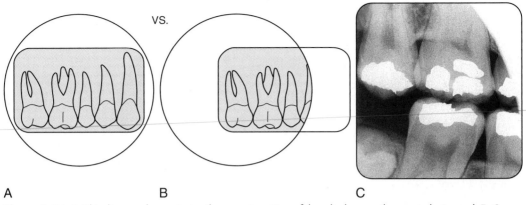

A   B   C

Figure 1-24 **A,** This diagram demonstrates the correct position of the cylinder over the area to be imaged. **B,** Cone positioned so far distally that the anterior portion of the film receives no exposure. **C,** The resultant radiographic image.

Film Packet or Image Receptor Placement

Vertical Placement

Maxillary Arch. The film or image receptor should be placed so that it parallels the long axis of the tooth being imaged. This is accomplished by placing it toward the midline of the palate. If the film packet or image receptor is placed directly against the lingual side of the teeth, one of three things will happen:

1. The film will not be parallel to the long axes of the teeth, producing an image that is foreshortened, looking as if it were squashed (Fig. 1-25).
2. The film will not be high enough in the palate to capture the image of the apices, resulting in an image with a large empty margin at the occlusal or incisal edge of the image and incomplete coverage of the apices ("cut off" apices) (Fig. 1-26).
3. The film will bend beyond the end of the bite block, producing a distorted image that looks as if the top of it slid off or was pulled off the end of the film (Fig. 1-27).

Mandibular Arch. The mandible has a much different shape than the maxilla. The floor of the mouth is occupied by musculature, including the tongue. Because it is muscular, the floor of the mouth can be flexible or rigid. When tensed, it is almost as firm as the hard palate. The apices of the mandibular teeth do not tilt as far inward as those of the maxillary arch; hence, film packet or image receptor placement should not tilt as much. To keep the film packet or image receptor from tilting, one must place it down low into the floor of the mouth, actually displacing the tissues. If the patient tenses the muscles of the floor of the mouth, the procedure may be painful, especially if the film packet or image receptor is placed too close to the mylohyoid ridge, and the patient may not fully close on the bite block.

It is rare that anyone has such a shallow floor of the mouth that the film or image receptor will not fit. More often the procedure is unsuccessful because the patient is apprehensive, sensitive, or both and tenses the muscles of the floor of the mouth. It is imperative that the floor of the mouth stay relaxed. One method of film placement is to angle the lower edge away from the teeth initially and then bring the bite block into contact with the incisal edges. Ask the patient to *slowly close,* then rotate the instrument upward as the patient closes, bringing the film more parallel to the teeth. The patient's floor of the mouth will stay more relaxed, and the procedure will be more comfortable.

The second problem is managing the patient's tongue, which may seem to have a mind of its own. Asking the patient to do something with the tongue usually makes

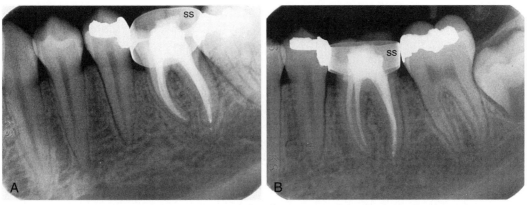

Figure 1-25   **A,** The radiographic image that results if the film is not parallel to long axes of teeth. **B,** The correct image; note that the stainless steel crown *(ss)* appears more anatomically correct than the one in *A.*

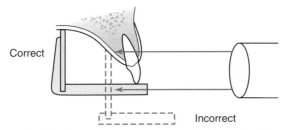

Figure 1-26   Film contacts palate, but the instrument is *not* contacting the teeth of interest. The apices will *not* be recorded, and a large black area will be seen below the occlusal edges of the teeth in the resultant image, providing no useful information (see Fig. 1-28).

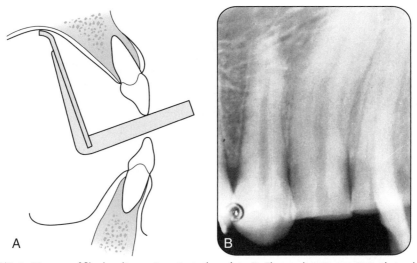

Figure 1-27   **A,** Diagram of film bending as it contacts the palate. **B,** The resultant image. Note that only the apical areas are blurred and distorted unlike the case of motion artifact, in which the whole image is blurred.

the tongue more active and difficult to work around; relaxation techniques and psychology work better. The tongue acts as a physical barrier to the center of the mouth. Obviously, the mandibular films will have to be placed between the tongue and the lingual side of the teeth.

Common problems associated with mandibular film placement are as follows:

1. The film or image receptor may be placed too close to the lingual side of the teeth (either because the tongue pushed it there or the operator placed it there). This placement may cause one of two problems:
    a. The film may not be parallel with the long axes of the teeth because of the inclined plane of the lingual alveolar ridge, resulting in a foreshortened image.
    b. The film may not reach into the floor of the mouth, resulting in an image with a wide black (empty) area above the crowns and apices that are cut off (Fig. 1-28).
2. The tongue may be trapped under the bottom edge of the film packet or image receptor, resulting in any of the following three problems:
    a. The film may bend because of the pressure of the tongue, producing a blurred, unsharp image.
    b. The film or image receptor may not reach the floor of the mouth, producing a distorted occlusal image with cut off apices.
    c. The film or image receptor may have proper position and angulation, but the image of the tongue may appear on the processed image. As long as this image can be identified as the shadow of the tongue and as long as the teeth are clearly represented, this technique error is minor (Fig. 1-29).

The following technique will help you avoid the previously discussed problems: Position the film packet or image receptor in the desired posterior region but do not force it into the floor of the mouth. A variety of placement techniques will work well for different people under different circumstances. The following example will increase the likelihood of success with mandibular films in many instances.

Tilt the film away from the mylohyoid ridge as you place it in the mouth, making an inverted **V**, or tent; the bite block should be over the occlusal surfaces. Place your index finger in the patient's mouth so that it is between the film or image receptor and the mylohyoid ridge. When you rock or slide the film into position on the floor

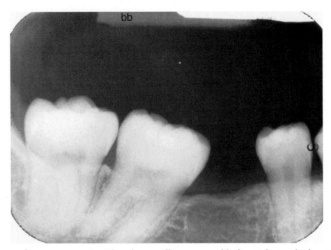

Figure 1-28 This type of image occurs in either the maxillary or mandibular arch, in which patient anatomy or poor film placement prevents imaging of the apices of the teeth of interest. The bite block *(bb)* can be seen far above the teeth in this mandibular view.

of the mouth, your finger will keep the film or image receptor from scraping the alveolar mucosa. The film or receptor can then be positioned for proper mesial/ distal placement and correct horizontal angulation.

Horizontal Placement: Maxillary or Mandibular. The horizontal placement of the film packet or receptor is the critical factor in avoiding overlapped images owing to the incorrect horizontal angulation and in avoiding loss of visualization of anatomic structures owing to incorrect anteroposterior placement of the film or receptor. The placement of the film packet or image receptor (by virtue of the placement of the bite block) will determine correct horizontal angulation and correct anteroposterior placement at the same time.

The film must be placed in a well-defined anteroposterior position (the distance forward or backward in the mouth) to afford a view of the correct anatomy. These guidelines are described later in this chapter under the heading "Anatomic Structures in Each Image."

The horizontal angulation is determined by selecting a contact point through which to direct the **x-ray beam** (sometimes called the *direction of the central ray*). Figure 1-30 illustrates examples of this principle. Correct positioning is crucial to obtaining an "open contact" and clear view of the interproximal areas of interest.

Bitewing or Interproximal Techniques

Horizontal Placement. Correct angulation in the horizontal placement of the film packet or image receptor for a bitewing radiograph is crucial to the diagnostic value of the image. Even a slight amount of overlap may lead to a misdiagnosis (Fig. 1-31). The goal is to obtain bitewings with no overlapping. Extra films may be required because of anatomic deviations and rotated or misaligned teeth.

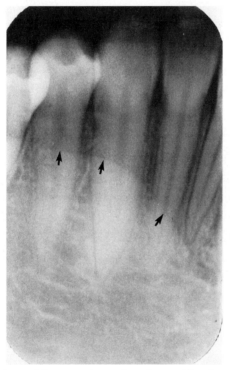

Figure 1-29 Image of the soft tissue of the tongue is seen here *(arrows)* but does not interfere significantly with interpretation.

Vertical Placement. Whether you are using a cardboard tab or a film- or receptor-holding instrument, it is important that the film or image receptor not be forced into an inaccurate position by the maxillary teeth. The operator can avoid this problem by allowing the film packet or receptor to move slightly to the lingual as the patient closes. The film or receptor should then move into the proper vertical position as the teeth occlude with the tab or bite block.

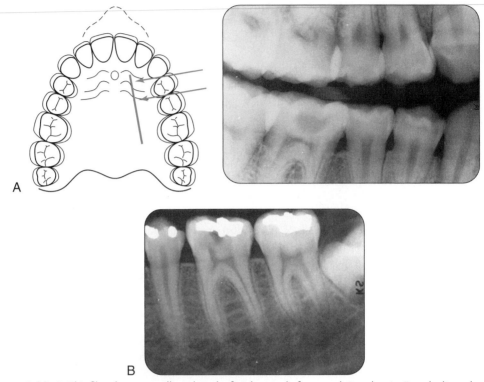

Figure 1-30 **A,** This film placement will result in the facial enamel of one tooth "overlapping" on the lingual enamel of the adjacent tooth. **B,** Correct horizontal angulation is seen in this periapical view.

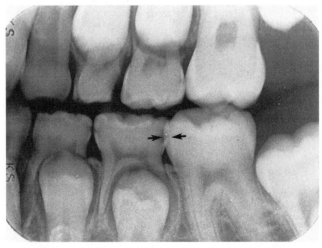

Figure 1-31 Overlap *(arrows)* between the mandibular primary second molar and permanent first molar obscures detection of the carious lesion on the primary molar.

Anteroposterior Placement. A good basic setup on molar bitewing views is to place the middle of the tab or bite block over the contact between the first and second molars. This technique ensures room on the film for all molars, including the contact between the second and third molars, if present. The premolar bitewing view should include the contacts between the canines and the premolars in both arches; therefore, if the distal half of the mandibular canine is included in the image, the maxillary canine–premolar contact will also be included because the mandibular canine is normally positioned more anteriorly than the maxillary canine. Precise anteroposterior placement in bitewing imaging is absolutely critical, not only to get the appropriate anatomic structures on the image but also to avoid placement errors resulting from a patient's individual anatomic variations.

Here is one final thought about the importance of open contacts on bitewings: Because the primary purpose of a bitewing is to obtain a clear view of the contact areas and interproximal spaces, overlapping on a bitewing is a critical error. An overlapped image on periapical images is considered a technical error, but they are not as serious as those on bitewing views, because the purpose of a periapical view is to image the periapical areas rather than the interproximal areas.

PARALLELING TECHNIQUE

Paralleling Instruments: Film- or Receptor-Holding Devices

Paralleling techniques require the use of film- or receptor-holding devices. One of the most commonly used types is the Dentsply Rinn XCP* (extension cone paralleling) instrument. The technique descriptions that follow are for use with the Rinn XCP technique, but the basic principles of placement and paralleling are similar no matter which film- or receptor-holding device is used.

Advantages

The extraoral marker or locator ring on the holder makes it easier to set the position of the x-ray unit cylinder without risk of cone-cut (misaligned) images, which is a definite advantage over the use of tabs or holders without rings (see Fig. 1-21). If you correctly assemble the XCP instrument and look through the ring, the bite block and the film or image receptor should be centered in the ring (Fig. 1-32). As you look through the ring at a film packet, you should see only the white (front) side of the film. The embossed dot on the film packet is commonly placed into the slot of the bite block. The bar or rod connecting the bite block with the ring can be compared with the line between the contacts to help determine horizontal angulation. Most holders also keep the film or receptor more stable, holding it in position. A *disadvantage* to using a film or receptor holder is the possibility of patient discomfort.

Film or Image Receptor Placement

The following pages outline the techniques for periapical and bitewing imaging using paralleling principles and a conventional holding device. Correct film or receptor placement will be illustrated for each view.

Anatomic Structures in Each Image

A typical CMRS using the paralleling technique consists of 14 to 16 periapical projections and four bitewing projections (Fig. 1-33). Each film or receptor must be placed so that it covers the appropriate anatomic structures, as described in the following section.

Dentsply Rinn Corporation, Elgin, Ill.

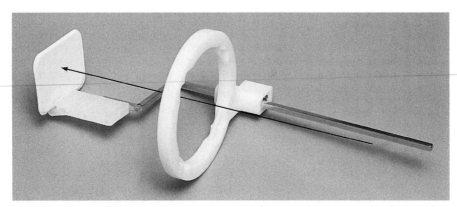

Figure 1-32 Correctly assembled positioning instrument, with film in bite block centered in the ring. The arrow indicates the central ray of the x-ray beam.

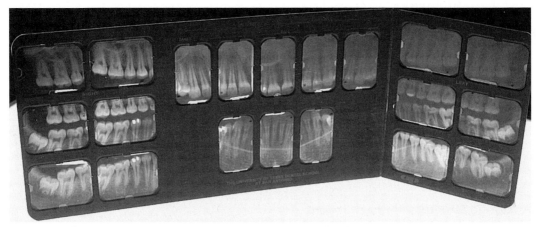

Figure 1-33 Typical complete mouth radiographic survey using the paralleling technique.

PROCEDURE *Box* **1-1**

Paralleling Technique

Maxillary central incisor region. The shaded area shows the ideal placement for anatomic coverage of the maxillary central incisor region.

In this view the maxillary central incisors are centered on the bite block (see also diagram on the next page). If you use a size no. 2 film, the apices and crowns of all four incisors should be visible on the image. Slightly less anatomic coverage is demonstrated with the size no. 1 film used here.

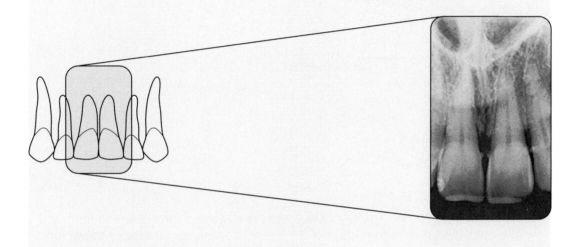

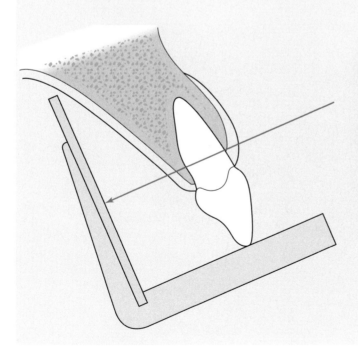

The plastic bite block contacts the palate and the teeth of interest and is parallel to the long axis of the tooth. The film should never be placed against the teeth; rather, as much of the bite block as possible should be used to place the film near the center of the palate. The central ray is directed perpendicular (at 90°) to the film plane.

Continued

PROCEDURE *Box* 1-1—cont'd

Paralleling Technique

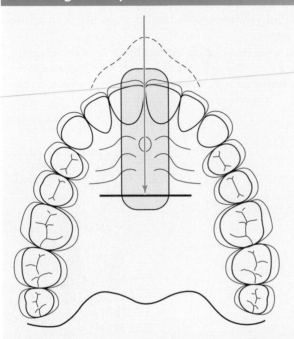

The diagram shows that the central incisors are centered, and the film is positioned well into the oral cavity.

Final positioning of film and instrument. The patient is asked to close slowly and firmly on the bite block. Note that the lower edge of the cylinder parallels the metallic indicating rod. The cylinder is brought to within ½ inch or less from the plastic ring. The exposure is made. Operators often struggle with making the last little cylinder adjustments. Often it is easier to move the patient's head a little bit than to struggle with the tubehead and cylinder.

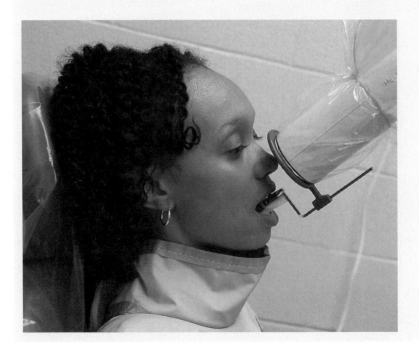

PROCEDURE *Box* **1-1—cont'd**

Paralleling Technique

Maxillary lateral incisor region. The shaded area shows the ideal placement for anatomic coverage of the lateral incisor region. Size no. 1 film is used in a vertical orientation.

In this view the lateral incisor is centered on the bite block. The apices of the central incisor and the cuspid area are also visible.

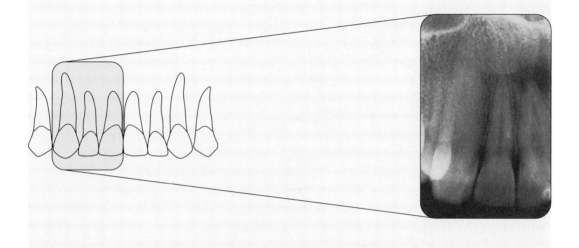

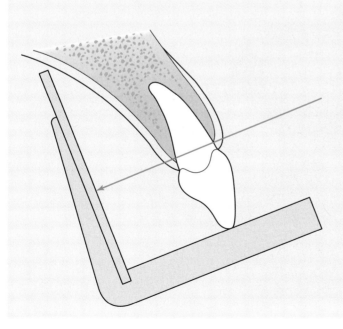

This diagram and the one on the next page show the positioning of the film near the center of the palate. The central ray is directed perpendicular to the film plane.

Continued

PROCEDURE *Box* **1-1—cont'd**

Paralleling Technique

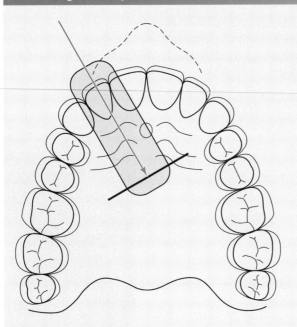

This diagram shows the lateral incisor centered, and the film is placed well into the oral cavity.

Final positioning of film and instrument. Note that the instrument contacts the tooth of interest and that the opposing teeth also contact the bite block.

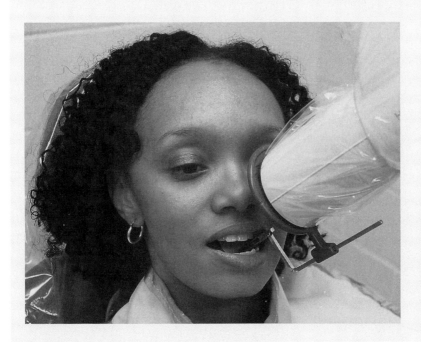

PROCEDURE *Box* 1-1—cont'd

Paralleling Technique

Maxillary canine region. The shaded area shows the ideal placement for anatomic coverage of the canine region.

In this view the canine is centered on the bite block. Note that the lingual cusp of the first premolar is superimposed on the distal surface of the cuspid. This superimposition is almost unavoidable because of the maxillary arch curvature, but it should be minimized as much as possible by trying to open the distal contact more than the mesial. This contact area must be "opened" on the next view, the premolar region, seen on the following pages.

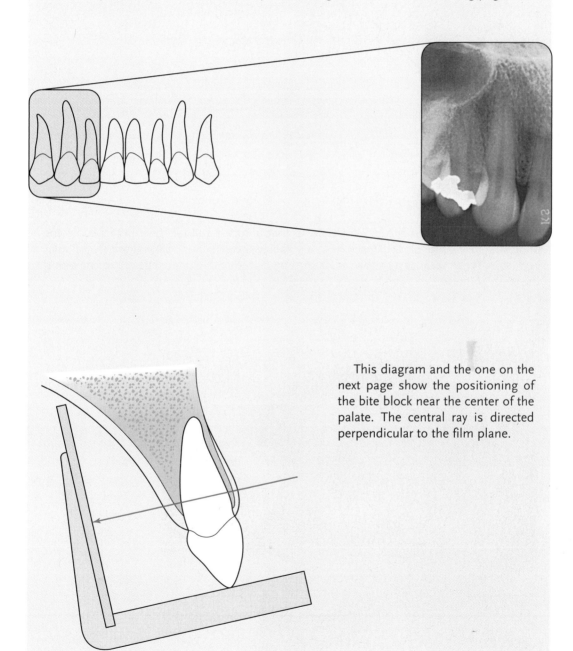

This diagram and the one on the next page show the positioning of the bite block near the center of the palate. The central ray is directed perpendicular to the film plane.

Continued

PROCEDURE *Box* **1-1—cont'd**

Paralleling Technique

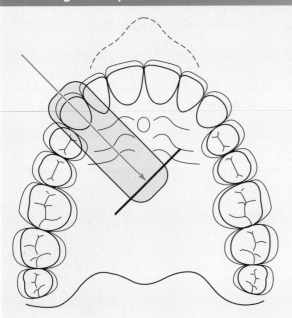

This diagram shows the canine centered, and the bite block is placed well into the oral cavity.

Final positioning of film and instrument. Note that a cotton roll has been attached to the underside of the bite block. This serves to stabilize the bite block against the mandibular occlusion. When you use a cotton roll, it *must* be placed on the underside of the bite block; the teeth of interest *must* be in direct contact with the bite block.

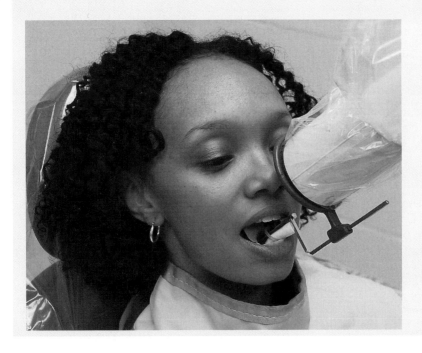

PROCEDURE *Box* 1-1—cont'd

Paralleling Technique

Maxillary premolar region. The shaded area shows the ideal placement for anatomic coverage of the premolar and first molar region. Note here that the distal half of the cuspid is visible without overlap, as seen in a typical cuspid view. Size no. 2 film is used in a horizontal orientation.

In this view the contact between the second premolar and first molar is centered on the film.

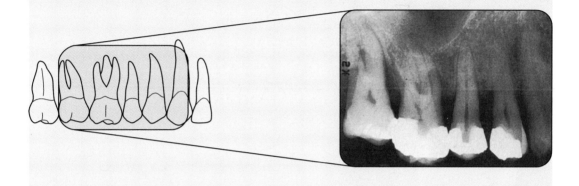

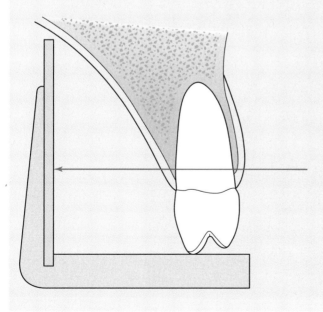

This diagram and the one on the next page show the positioning of the film near the center of the palate. The central ray is directed perpendicular to the film plane.

Continued

PROCEDURE *Box* **1-1—cont'd**

Paralleling Technique

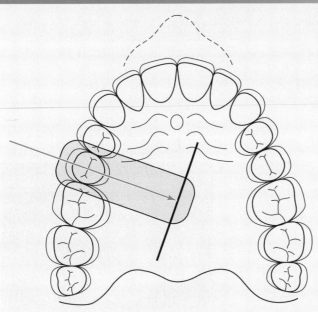

This diagram shows the second premolar being centered on the bite block. The contact between the first molar and the second premolar may also be the centering point.

Final positioning of film and bite block. The patient is asked to close slowly and firmly on the bite block.

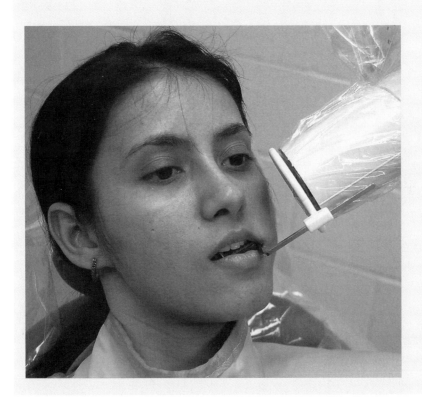

PROCEDURE *Box* **1-1—cont'd**

Paralleling Technique

Maxillary molar region. The shaded area shows the ideal placement for anatomic coverage of the molar region. It is important to include *all of the third molar region* in this view.

In this view the second molar is centered on the film. This technique usually ensures complete coverage of the third molar region regardless of whether the tooth is present.

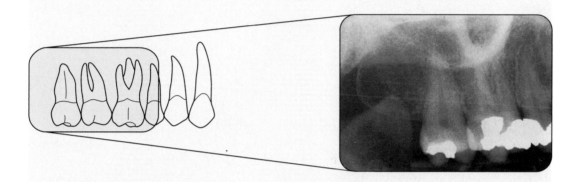

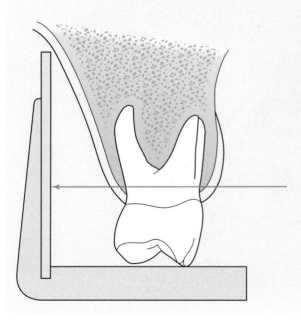

This diagram and the one on the next page show the positioning of the film near the center of the oral cavity. The central ray is directed perpendicular to the film plane.

Continued

PROCEDURE *Box* **1-1—cont'd**

Paralleling Technique

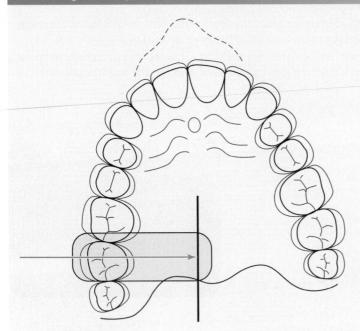

This view shows the second molar centered on the bite block and on the film.

Final positioning of film and bite block. The patient is asked to close slowly and firmly on the bite block. Compare the cylinder position here with that of the maxillary premolar view shown on the previous pages. Note that the cylinder has been placed only slightly more posteriorly for this region.

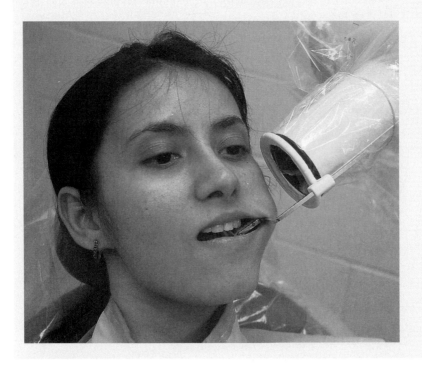

PROCEDURE *Box* 1-1—cont'd

Paralleling Technique

Mandibular central incisor region. In this view the mandibular incisors are centered on the bite block. The contact point between the two central incisors would ideally be centered on the bite block; however, sometimes the patient's anatomy dictates a slightly different alignment. Nevertheless, in this case it is only a minor positioning error, and a retake is not warranted because all of the periapical anatomy of the four incisors is visible.

The shaded area shows the ideal placement for anatomic coverage of the mandibular incisors. Because of their smaller size, all four mandibular incisors can be imaged on a size no. 1 film in a vertical orientation.

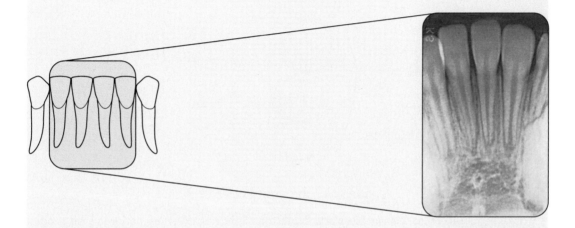

This diagram and the one on the next page show the film centered on the teeth of interest and contacting the floor of the mouth. The tongue has been slightly displaced by the operator with the film to ensure that the film reaches the floor of the mouth. The central ray is directed perpendicular to the film plane.

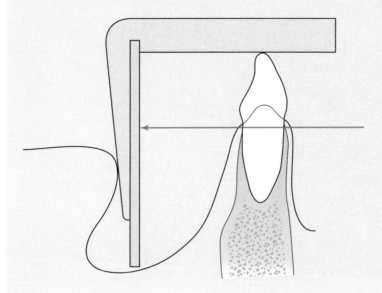

Continued

PROCEDURE *Box* **1-1—cont'd**

Paralleling Technique

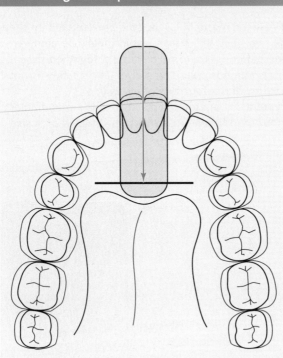

The film is placed as far into the oral cavity as the patient's anatomy will allow. Except in a patient with unusually wide arches, correct positioning rarely results in the film touching or even being close to the lingual surfaces of the teeth.

Final positioning of the film and bite block. Note the slight negative angulation of the tubehead. The cylinder still parallels the metallic indicating rod, as in the maxillary views.

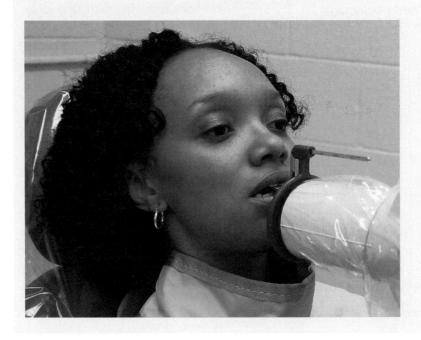

PROCEDURE *Box* **1-1—cont'd**

Paralleling Technique

Mandibular canine region. The shaded area shows the ideal film placement for anatomic coverage of the lower canine region. Again, size no. 1 film is used in a vertical orientation. In this view the mandibular canine is centered.

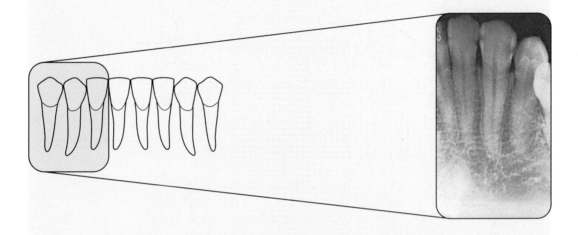

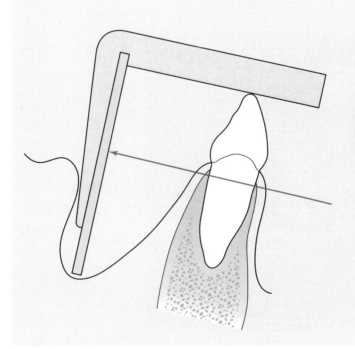

This diagram and the one on the next page show the cuspid centered on the bite block and the tongue mildly displaced to allow the film to contact the floor of the mouth. The central ray is directed perpendicular to the film plane.

Continued

PROCEDURE *Box* **1-1—cont'd**

Paralleling Technique

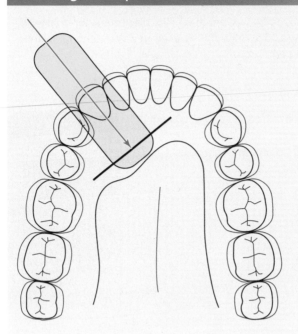

The film is again placed as far into the oral cavity as the patient's anatomy will allow.

Final positioning of film and bite block. The patient is asked to close slowly and firmly so that the teeth being imaged are in contact with the bite block.

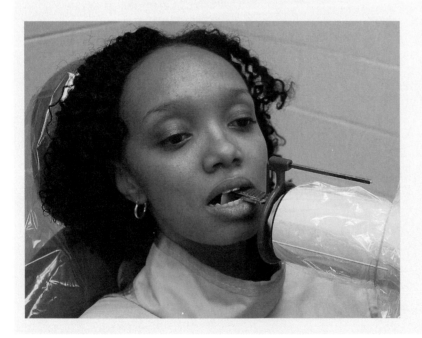

PROCEDURE *Box* **1-1—cont'd**

Paralleling Technique

Mandibular premolar region. The shaded area shows the ideal film placement for anatomic coverage of the premolar/first molar region. Size no. 2 film is used in a horizontal orientation. As with the maxillary premolar view, it is important to show the distal half of the cuspid in this view.

In this view the contact point between the second premolar and the first molar should be centered.

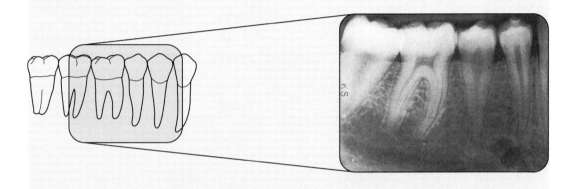

This diagram and the one on the next page show the bite block centered on the teeth of interest and the film touching the floor of the mouth.

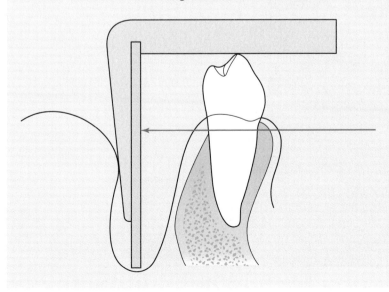

Continued

PROCEDURE *Box* **1-1—cont'd**

Paralleling Technique

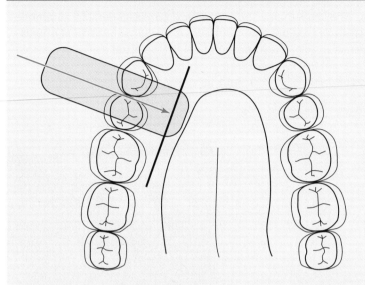

The film is placed as far into the oral cavity as the patient's anatomy will allow. It is important for patient comfort to keep the film *away* from the lingual surfaces of the teeth. Placing the film farther toward the tongue will allow the film to rest in the deeper portions of the floor of the mouth and away from the area where the mylohyoid muscle attaches to the lingual aspect of the mandible.

Final positioning of the film and bite block. The patient is asked to close slowly and firmly on the bite block.

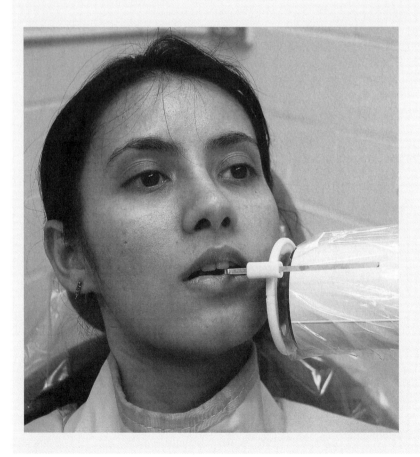

PROCEDURE *Box* **1-1—cont'd**

Paralleling Technique

Mandibular molar region. The shaded area shows the ideal film placement for anatomic coverage of the molar region. It is essential to position the film to show *all of the third molar region.*

In this view the second molar has been centered on the film, which allows enough film to be positioned in the third molar region to capture all of that tooth.

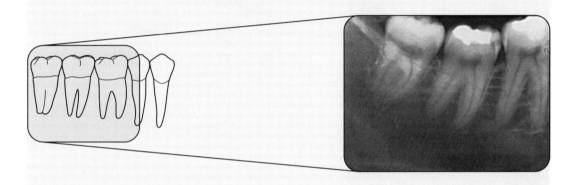

This diagram and the one on the next page show the bite block centered on the teeth of interest and the film touching the floor of the mouth. Often more room exists in the floor of the mouth in this region than in the premolar area because of attachments of the mylohyoid muscle.

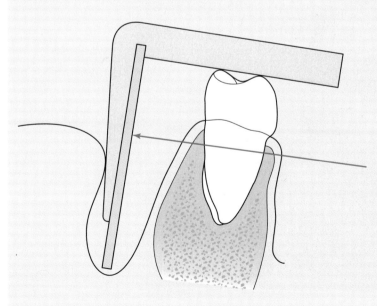

Continued

PROCEDURE *Box* **1-1—cont'd**

Paralleling Technique

This film is often placed closer to the teeth for the molar view than for premolar or anterior views. The tongue is more difficult to displace in the molar region, and space is sufficient for the inferior portion of the film to extend into the floor of the mouth.

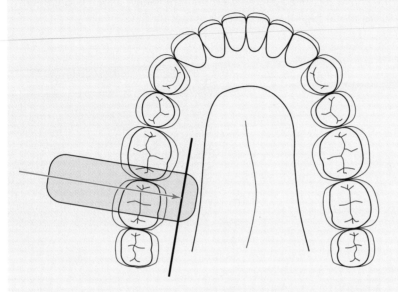

Final positioning of the film and bite block. The patient is asked to close slowly and firmly on the bite block.

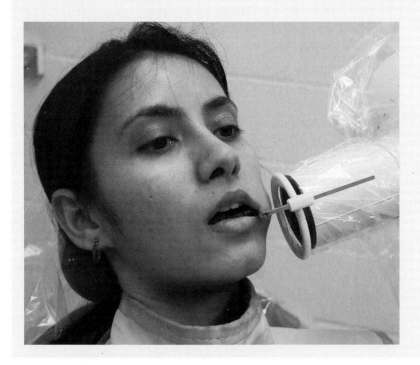

HELPFUL HINTS FOR INTRAORAL IMAGING

Patient Position

Position the chair high enough so that you can see the occlusal surfaces of the maxillary teeth when doing maxillary views and so that you will not have to bend over to reach your patient. Lower the chair slightly when doing mandibular views. Look at the teeth you are going to image. Adjusting the patient's head position is simpler when using indicator rings for alignment. You will not disturb your correct film or receptor placement, and the horizontal and vertical angulation of the beam will be guided by the holding device.

Opening Contacts

Before placing anything in the patient's mouth, take a good look at the teeth you are going to image. The teeth may be rotated or deviated from the normal occlusal pattern in countless ways. Without knowing what the contact lines between the teeth look like, you cannot be assured of obtaining open contacts on your films. Never guess! If you are going to look at the occlusal surfaces of the teeth to try to see the lines made by the contact areas, do not look at them while standing in front of the patient; your view is distorted from that angle. The only way you can obtain a clear view is to stand *beside* the patient and position yourself so that your eyes are in the same plane that the x-ray beam will be coming from (Fig. 1-34). Pretend you are the central ray.

If you are looking for mandibular occlusal surfaces, retract the cheek with your finger and look down. If you are looking for the maxillary surfaces, *you cannot see them unless you position your eyes lower than the maxillary occlusal surface and then look straight up.* This means that you are going to have to bend your knees and squat down briefly as you are looking up.

Getting the Film or Receptor Inside the Mouth

Holding the instrument by the bite block or the ring, place the film packet or receptor inside the mouth. For *maxillary films*, tilt the top portion of the film packet toward the center of the mouth, making a V shape with the bite block (Fig. 1-35). This technique keeps you from scraping the film or receptor across the oral tissues. The more you

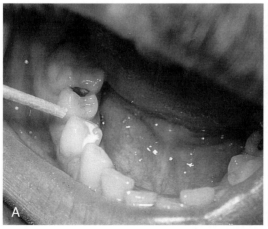
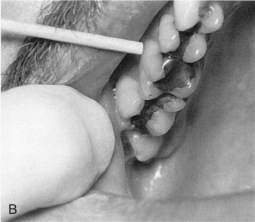

Figure 1-34 **A,** Operator examining contacts of mandibular teeth. **B,** Operator has bent down and is looking up to determine contacts of maxillary teeth. Patient has been asked to tip his head back to assist the operator.

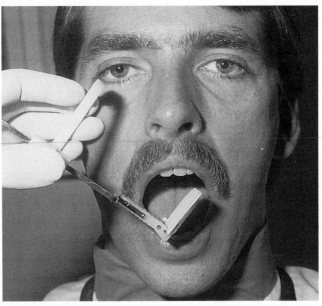

Figure 1-35 The large black arrow points to the V shape of the instrument as it is placed into the mouth. Keeping this angle, the operator guides the bite block up to contact the tooth of interest.

can keep the film or receptor from scraping the palate or alveolar ridges, the better your patient will cooperate.

For *mandibular films or bitewings,* you need to move the tongue out of the way with your index finger so that the lower border of the film packet or receptor can slide into place between the tongue and the lingual side of the teeth. Keep the film packet or receptor about ¼ inch away from the lingual surface of the teeth. *Do not place the film packet or receptor in direct contact with the lingual surface of the teeth.* If you do, you will be inclined to make several technical errors on your image that you will not see until it is processed. Keeping your finger between the film packet or receptor and the alveolar ridge ensures that only the soft pad of your finger, not the edge of the film or receptor, will touch sensitive mucosa as you place the holder in the mouth.

Keeping the Film or Receptor in Place

When you are ready for the patient to bring his or her teeth together on the bite block, use this phrase: "*Slowly* close, please." Putting the word *slowly* first, with emphasis, and saying "close" instead of "bite" will give you a chance to keep the film or receptor where you placed it and to remove your fingers before the teeth close on the bite block; it will also help the patient maintain a more relaxed state. Clenching the teeth around the bite block increases the chance of film displacement or patient discomfort. Saying "bite" to a child patient often results in chewing motions from the child, increasing the chances of injury to you and inadequate images.

Maintaining Patient Cooperation

Place and expose the film as quickly as possible. Remember to turn the unit on and to adjust the exposure settings before you place the film in the patient's mouth. Remove the film or receptor as soon as it has been exposed. You can even tell the patient to remove it as soon as the audible signal stops. Having intraoral images taken is not a comfortable procedure for many patients, even in the hands of an experienced operator. Making the time they have the film or receptor in their mouths as short as possible increases their cooperation.

Increasing Success

One of the most common problems that students have with patients is establishing credibility as authority figures. As soon as patients experience the procedure as unpleasant, they begin to question whether it is really necessary or whether you are competent to do it. They may believe, rightly or not, that their discomfort is your fault. For ways to prevent any unpleasant or argumentative experiences, refer to Box 1-1.

Box **1-1** **INCREASING SUCCESS**

- Begin with the easiest images, probably the maxillary anterior periapicals. When these have been exposed successfully, the patient will be more likely to accept that any difficulty with other films is not the fault of an inept operator.
- Be as quick and gentle as possible but speak with authority. Do not be intimidated. Be sure of what you are doing. If you prepare yourself in advance by learning as much as you can and pay close attention to what you are doing, you have every reason to be confident.

INFECTION CONTROL

No patient should be treated or imaged without first having a complete medical history taken. The medical history has become even more important with the increasing incidence of various infectious diseases such as human immunodeficiency virus (HIV), hepatitis, and tuberculosis. The history should include routine medical questions, a radiation history, and a social history. Certain information elicited from a medical history may alert the radiographer to patients who are at a greater risk of medical complications from dental procedures because of certain disease states or medications. Regardless of what the medical history reveals, appropriate infection control procedures are needed for *every* patient so that exposure to infectious agents for the operator or cross-contamination to other patients is avoided.

During a radiographic examination, you will be working directly in the patient's mouth. Immediately after you place the film or receptor in the mouth, you make adjustments of the tubehead and press the exposure button with hands that are now contaminated with the patient's saliva. If the x-ray equipment is not properly disinfected or wrapped with barrier material, it is a potential source of cross-contamination.

Sound infection control procedures must be followed at all times.

1. Disinfect any flat surface on which films or the image receptor is placed and cover it with a barrier. Place an appropriate barrier on all parts of the x-ray unit that will come in contact with the operator's hands during the procedure, such as the control panel, the exposure button, the beam-indicating device (cylinder), the buttons on the patient's chair, any door handles, and light switches. The barrier technique is recommended for any equipment or surface that has small grooves or hard to clean areas. Plastic bags or plastic wrap works well. Tape may be used to hold the barriers in place.
2. Digital image receptors are used more than once and must be appropriately protected from being contaminated by the patient's oral fluids. Securing a small plastic bag around the receptor often works best.

3. Instruments used in the patient's mouth should be sterilized after use with each patient and kept in a closed container for future use. Disposable film or receptor holders should be appropriately discarded.

4. Exposed films should be placed in a disposable container, such as a cup, *not in the operator's pocket.*

5. The operator should wear gloves, a mask, protective eyewear, and an appropriate gown or cover for clothing during the procedure.

6. Although there are no vaccinations against tuberculosis, HIV, or herpes, there is an acceptable vaccination against hepatitis B and D. Dental professionals should give serious thought to the potential consequences of not being vaccinated because of expense, inconvenience, or fear. Some instructional programs require appropriate vaccination against hepatitis for their students.

7. Infection control procedures for the darkroom are described in Chapter 2.

SUMMARY

Remember that radiography is a skill. You will not be competent immediately; competency takes practice. If this were not true, there would be little need to devote so much time to learning and practice. While practicing, you will have access to experts (your instructors) who are available specifically to help you acquire the skills you need. Take advantage of their expertise. Do not be afraid to ask for guidance and feedback; that is how you learn.

Making mistakes is an important part of the learning process. If you make mistakes during the time you are practicing, someone will be there to give you feedback. If you have the opportunity to practice on manikins, "DEXTERS" (DXTTR),* or skulls before making films of patients, take advantage of that practice time.

STUDY QUESTIONS

1. Which radiographic technique records the most accurate image of tooth crowns, roots, and supporting structures in a selected area?
   A. Bitewing
   B. Occlusal
   C. Extraoral
   D. Periapical

2. When the parallel technique is used, the central ray makes a right angle (90°) with which structure(s)?
   A. The film or image receptor only
   B. The long axis of the tooth only
   C. The film or receptor and the long axis of the tooth
   D. The portion of the bite block that the patient closes down on

3. The *primary* diagnostic use of interproximal (bitewing) radiographs is to
   A. Register the appearance of supporting structures such as alveolar bone
   B. Detect caries between the teeth and evaluate crestal bone levels
   C. Check for developing and unerupted teeth
   D. Check for changes at the apices of teeth needing root canal treatment

---

*DXTTR (Dental X-Ray Teaching and Training Replica), Dentsply Rinn Corporation, Elgin, Ill.

4. The standard film size used for adult bitewings and posterior periapical images is no.
   A. 1
   B. 2
   C. 3
   D. 4

5. A no. 1 size film would most likely be used to image which of the following areas on an adult patient?
   A. Incisors and canines
   B. Maxillary premolars
   C. Mandibular molars
   D. Any area if the palate or floor of the mouth is shallow

6. The premolar bitewing film or receptor should be placed to include which of the following anatomic structures at the anterior edge of the image?
   A. The contact between the first and second molar
   B. The mesial half of the maxillary canine
   C. The distal half of the mandibular canine
   D. The distal half of the mandibular first premolar

7. Which of the following anatomic structures must be captured in a maxillary premolar periapical image?
   A. All premolars and the canine, with the premolars centered on the image
   B. All premolars plus the first and second molars; contacts between the premolars must be open
   C. The distal half or one third of the canine and the premolars
   D. All premolars and the first molar; contacts between the second premolar and first molar must be open

8. One of the most common problems associated with correct positioning of mandibular periapicals or bitewings is
   A. Not having the patient bite hard enough
   B. Using the wrong size film or receptor
   C. Catching your glove between the bite block and teeth as the patient bites
   D. Positioning the film or receptor too close to the lingual surface of the teeth

9. When using x-ray film, film-bending in the apical area is a common problem to try to avoid in each of the following views except one. Which one is the exception?
   A. Maxillary molars
   B. Maxillary premolars
   C. Mandibular premolars
   D. Bitewings

10. Incorrect horizontal angulation causes
    A. A long, stretched-out image
    B. Overlapped images because the lingual aspect of one tooth is superimposed on the facial aspect of the adjacent tooth
    C. Short, blunted images because the x-ray beam is not perpendicular to the long axis of the teeth
    D. Overlapped images because the x-ray beam is not perpendicular to the film or receptor

2

Image Processing and Quality Assurance

Obtaining an image with digital radiography will be covered in Chapter 7. This chapter will concentrate on processing film-based images. The reader is referred elsewhere for a discussion of image processing related to digital images. One place to find such information is on the website: http://www.learndigital.net.

FILM COMPOSITION

Radiographic film is similar to photographic film in many respects. The final image on the film is produced when energy (light or radiation) interacts with the emulsion (chemicals) in the film. To understand film processing, it is necessary to understand some basic concepts about the film itself and the chemicals used in processing.

Inside the plastic or paper cover of a film packet, black paper wrapping surrounds the semiflexible plastic film (Fig. 2-1). If you have the opportunity, open a film packet and look at the contents when you read this section.

The plastic film has a green coating of gelatin and chemicals. The film is a series of layers, beginning with a base of thin polyester plastic (Fig. 2-2). The plastic base is transparent but has a blue tint to modulate the bright light transmitted through the film from the view box.

The Emulsion

A coating called the **film emulsion** is attached to both sides of the base. The emulsion is a homogeneous mixture of gelatin and grains of silver halide crystals. Silver bromide (AgBr) and silver iodide (AgI) are two types of silver halide used in the emulsion; halides are chemical compounds that change when exposed to light or radiation. These grains of silver halide are suspended in the gelatin similar to the way fruit is suspended in the gelatin you eat. When the silver halide grains are exposed to light or x rays, they store energy from the radiation.

The gelatin is transparent so that it can transmit light and porous so that the processing chemicals can reach the crystals. The gelatin holds the crystals in place until some of the crystals are removed in the fixing process.

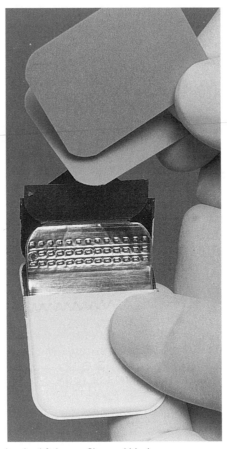

Figure 2-1 Contents of film packet: lead foil, x-ray film, and black paper.

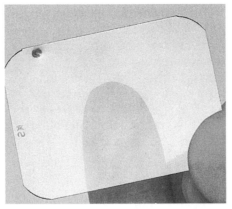

Figure 2-2 Semitransparent polyester plastic film base. This film has *not* been exposed to light or radiation. When it was processed, all of the emulsion and chemicals were removed to leave the transparent base only.

FILM SPEED

How efficiently film responds to radiation determines how much radiation is needed to produce an image, and this is referred to as **film speed.** Very efficient film, known as fast or high-speed film, requires less radiation because the film responds more quickly. Currently, the highest speed radiographic film that is on the market is American National Standards Institute (ANSI) speed group F; an example of that film type is InSight.* The use of the fastest speed film available is recommended so that patients' exposure to radiation is reduced. However, some dental practices continue to use ANSI speed group D film; an example is Ultra-speed.† The film speed, the film size, the number of films in each film packet (one-film packets or two-film packets), and the expiration date are printed on the outside of the film box.

The F speed film is more sensitive (higher speed) and reduces the radiation required for an image by as much as 60% compared with D speed film. The higher speed is accomplished with a different grain configuration and a different base, which is thinner.

LATENT IMAGE FORMATION

Various areas on the film receive more or less radiation, depending on the attenuation differences of the objects irradiated. Another discussion of attenuation may be found in Chapter 6. In this section, attenuation means the way that different tissues stop different numbers of x rays. Thus, exposed films have areas in which silver halide crystals contain various levels of stored energy. The stored energy cannot be seen, but the pattern formed by the energized and nonenergized crystals creates an image within the emulsion. This unseen pattern or image is called the **latent image.**

Pretend you are a white-skinned person wearing a shirt made of lace and you are exposed to the summer sun for 2 hours without sunblock. The areas where the lace was thick and dense will stop the sun's rays. The thinner, cut out areas in the lace will allow the sun to reach your skin. After 2 hours, any sunburn probably won't be visible yet, but the image of the lace will be present in the layers of your skin. This unseen image of the lace is the latent image. After about 6 hours, you will probably see the pattern of the lace on your skin. Skin areas where the lace was cut out might be red, areas where the lace was thin might be pink (where a medium amount of light reached the skin), and areas where the lace was thick enough to block most of the sun might still be white. This ability of the lace to absorb different amounts of radiation based on different thicknesses or densities is called *attenuation*. A similar situation occurs with the oral tissues where teeth, bone, and soft tissues all absorb radiation differently.

The exposed film with its latent image is ready for processing. If the film is never processed, the stored energy will eventually dissipate, and the image will fade. Film should be processed as soon after exposure as possible to avoid any fading. If the film cannot be processed immediately, storage in a refrigerator is recommended until processing can be completed.

CONCEPTS OF FILM PROCESSING

Developing

The chemical reactions of film processing begin with the developer. When the film is placed in the developer, the gelatin softens and swells, and the developer permeates the gelatin to reach *all* of the silver halide crystals. The energized crystals (those that the x rays struck) are easily excited and readily react with the developer chemicals. In simplified terms, the reaction causes the silver halide to separate into bromide

---

InSight, Eastman Kodak, Rochester, N.Y.
†Ultra-speed, Eastman Kodak, Rochester, N.Y.

(or iodide) and metallic silver, which is black. The black metallic silver precipitates into the gelatin and is deposited on the film. If the x rays have been attenuated (stopped) by a dense object such as an amalgam restoration, dental enamel, or bone, then the silver halide crystals are not energized, do not react with the developer, and are washed away. The corresponding area on the film will be white (clear); that is, no reaction will take place in that area of the film.

Recall the analogy of the fruit in the gelatin. Let's imagine that the emulsion is made up of gelatin and fruit: the pieces of fruit represent the silver halide crystals. All fruit struck by radiation is cooked; all other fruit is not cooked. When the gelatin is exposed to developer, the developer softens the gelatin enough to allow the cooked (energized) pieces of fruit to sink to the bottom of the gelatin (like the black metallic silver, which then adheres to the plastic portion of the film). The uncooked fruit remains suspended in the gelatin until the fixing process, when it is removed, or washed away.

Fixation

In the **fixation** step of the film processing, fixer permeates the gelatin, coming in contact with all crystals. The energized crystals that are now "developed" have completed a chemical reaction and are not available for further reaction. The *nonenergized* and *undeveloped* crystals are removed from the emulsion and expelled with the fixer chemicals. The energized and developed crystals are fixed and preserved on the film.

In the edible gelatin model, the fixer spreads through the gelatin, removes all the uncooked fruit, and hardens and shrinks the gelatin so that the cooked fruit is trapped in place. The uncooked fruit (undeveloped silver halide) floats in the fixer tank and continues to accumulate each time this procedure is followed.

To review, the **developer** precipitates black metallic silver from *exposed and energized silver halide crystals* into the emulsion, making the dark areas on the film. The **fixer** removes *unexposed, nonenergized, and undeveloped crystals* from the film, creating the white or clear areas. Therefore, if a film is overexposed or overdeveloped, it will be dark. If a film is underexposed, underdeveloped, or overfixed, it will be light. More information on film and image characteristics appears in Chapter 6.

TECHNICAL ASPECTS OF FILM PROCESSING

The darkroom has tanks of chemicals and water for processing by hand, an automatic processor, or both. Both methods use the same principles and almost identical chemicals. We discuss manual processing first and then describe differences related to automatic processing.

Manual Processing

Film processing refers to the entire sequence of (1) converting the latent (invisible) image to a visible one and (2) preserving the visible image so that it does not disappear later. Because the reactions are chemical, the best results are obtained under optimal conditions.

Developing

Conditions that are of particular importance in developing films are the *temperature of the developer* and the *amount of time* the reaction is allowed to continue. The speed of the developing process depends on the temperature. The higher the temperature,

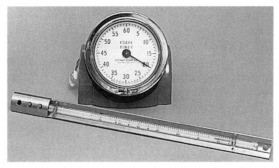

Figure 2-3 Manual timer *(top)* and nonmercury thermometer. The thermometer should measure the developer temperature in the developing tank, either with manual or automatic processing techniques.

the quicker the development, that is, the shorter the developing time should be. *Optimum developing time and temperature for manual processing is 4½ to 5 minutes at 68° F (20° C).* To ensure proper time and temperature, an accurate thermometer and time are mandatory (Fig. 2-3).

Consider what would happen if you changed the time but not the temperature. The longer the films were developed, the more silver halide crystals would precipitate, energized or not. This would cause all areas on the film to become darker and less visible. The same thing would happen if you increased the temperature alone. Films developed for 5 minutes at 75° F (24° C) instead of 68° F would be darker. At 68° F, films developed for only 3 minutes would be too light. This may seem like a minor point, but many patients are needlessly overexposed to radiation because of underdevelopment of films. Radiographers may be tempted to increase exposure times when the finished radiograph is too light rather than checking that the developing time and temperature are correct. Using optimum time and temperature development techniques may significantly reduce the exposure of patients to x rays.

Rinsing

After being developed, the films should be rinsed in clean, circulating water for 30 seconds. Without thorough rinsing of films after development, the fixer will be quickly contaminated with developer, which will cause problems that are discussed in the next section.

Fixing

The fixing time for manual processing should be at least 10 minutes, that is, twice as long as the usual developing time. Fixing for less than 10 minutes or using weak or contaminated fixer will not stop the chemical reaction sufficiently to maintain proper color and clarity for permanent storage; the gray color on the film will eventually turn brown or brownish-yellow, and the transparency of the films will decrease. If films lose their transparency (become opaque), they will not transmit light, which makes them difficult to interpret or "undiagnostic." Fixer that is not washed off may also cause brown discoloration with age.

If the film has to be viewed right away, it may be read outside the darkroom after being developed for 5 minutes and fixed for 3 minutes (i.e., a "wet reading"). The film must then be returned to the fixing solution for 7 minutes more. A word of caution about wet readings is necessary: the films are still covered with a coating of fixer, even if they have been rinsed briefly in water. Drops from these wet films contain a residue of fixer and will stain clothing and other films. The stain may not be visible immediately; as the fixer oxidizes with air, the brown color appears.

Washing and Drying

After the films have been fully fixed, they must be washed and dried. The object of washing is to remove residual processing chemicals and metallic silver from the radiographs. If these chemicals are not removed, the radiograph will discolor with age, which will impair its value as a permanent record. Films should be washed in a separate compartment in clean, running water. Wash time should be no less than 20 minutes, and the circulating water should run at a rate sufficient to replace itself every 6 minutes.

After a complete wash the films are dried. In some offices, films are dried by merely hanging them on a rack in the darkroom above a drip tray. Other offices use an ordinary fan to dry the films. The fan, however, should not blow directly on the films because lint or dust may become permanently embedded in the emulsion. Commercial dryers equipped with a fan and a heating element are also available.

Chemicals are available to speed up the drying process. Wetting agents reduce the surface tension of water, allowing the films to dry faster. Manufacturers' instructions should be followed if wetting agents are used.

Manual Processing Checklist

In most darkrooms, the developer is in the left tank, the water bath is in the center tank, and the fixer is in the right tank. *Always* check where everything is before processing. The fixer can be identified, even under a safelight, by its odor and feel. Its acidic properties give it a strong smell similar to vinegar (acetic acid), and it feels slippery (Procedure Box 2-1).

CHEMICAL COMPOSITION OF SOLUTIONS

Both the developer and the fixer are made up of specific chemicals that serve particular functions. Tables 2-1 and 2-2 are charts of the chemicals and their functions.

CARE OF SOLUTIONS

Daily Care/Quality Assurance

If digital imaging is not available and film-based imaging is the only imaging system used, the most recent recommendations for a quality assurance program are outlined in the National Council on Radiation Protection and Measurements Report No. 145. Dentists and dental educators are encouraged to obtain a copy of this report and adopt the most recent guidelines.

Each day before any patient films are processed, the chemicals should be checked for quality (Box 2-1). This will reduce needless patient exposure to radiation because of processing problems. The check can be done using two "check films" and a stepwedge. A **stepwedge** is a device with small, graduated increases in the thickness of its material (usually aluminum, if it is a commercial product). When placed over an x-ray film and exposed, the stepwedge produces a gradient of gray tones on the film, from very dark (where the material is thin) to very light (where the material is thick). The thin portion allows many more x rays to pass through it; thus, more film emulsion is exposed. This area of the film will be black. The thick portion attenuates, or stops, x rays; thus, this area of the film will appear lighter. A simple homemade stepwedge using lead foil can be constructed as described later.

PROCEDURE *Box* **2-1**

Steps in Manual Processing

The steps in manual processing are summarized as follows:

1. **Stir the solutions.** Stirring will equalize the temperature and evenly mix the chemicals. Use different paddles to stir each chemical so that the chemical will not become contaminated.
2. **Check the solution levels.** If the developer or fixer is low, add the appropriate replenisher. *Do not add water to raise the level.* Solutions that are too low may not completely cover the films attached to the top portion of the film holder, creating artifacts on the films.
3. **Check the temperature of the solutions.** It should be between 65° F (18° C) and 75° F (24° C); 68° F to 70° F (20° C to 21° C) is optimal. If the temperature is outside the 65° F to 75° F range, regulate the temperature of the running water appropriately and wait for the chemical temperatures to adjust.
4. **Label the film hanger** or rack with the *patient's name* and the *date of the exposure*. The plastic wrapper from one of the films can be labeled with a pen or marker and clipped to the film hanger for identification. If more than one film hanger is used, make a separate label for each one.
5. **Turn off the white lights and turn on the safelights.** Until now, overhead lighting was needed. Check for proper safelighting before opening the film packets. The procedure for checking safelighting is discussed later.
6. **Remove the exposed film from the packet or cassette.** Clip the film onto the hanger. *Check to see that the film is clipped tightly* by running your finger along the edge. Residual emulsion on the clips may cause films to become detached and lost in the chemicals. If any of the films are loose, reclip them or put them on another hanger, and check later to see how the problem can be corrected.
7. **Set the timer** according to the temperature of the developer and the manufacturer's recommendations. *Optimum time/temperature processing is 68° F (20° C) for 4½ to 5 minutes.* If rapid-processing chemicals are used, consult the manufacturer's recommendations for the time. A chart should be posted next to the tanks with correct developing temperatures and appropriate developing times.
8. **Immerse the films in the developer and start the timer.** Agitate the film hanger to break up residual air bubbles and to allow the developer to completely engulf the films.
9. **When the timer goes off, remove the films and rinse them** in running water in the rinse tank by agitating the film hanger up and down for approximately 15 to 30 seconds.
10. **Immerse the film hanger in the fixer** tank and agitate for approximately 5 seconds. *Set the timer for 10 minutes.* If the films need to be viewed quickly, they can be removed from the fixer after 3 minutes. However, they must be returned to the fixer for an additional 7 minutes after the wet reading.
11. **Wash the films in circulating water for 20 to 30 minutes.** Although the timing of the wash is not as critical as that for developing and fixing, the minimum wash time is 20 minutes. The water must be circulating such that the water in the tank changes every 6 minutes. There is no maximum wash time, but the longer the film is in the water, the softer the emulsion will get. Eventually, the emulsion could be washed off completely. Films left in the water overnight could be blank the next day.
12. **Remove the films from the wash, and place them in a dryer or hang them over a drip pan in a place where they will remain undisturbed until thoroughly dry.**
13. **When the films are dry, place them in an appropriately labeled mount.** The mount should have the patient's name, the date the films were exposed, and the radiographer's name.

How to Construct a Stepwedge

To make the stepwedge, tape six pieces of lead foil from inside the film packets to the end of a tongue blade. The first two pieces should be approximately 1 inch long, the second two approximately ¾ inch long, and the third two approximately ½ inch long. Tape these foil pieces in three steps, with one step having six layers, the second

Table **2-1** | **Developer Composition**

Function	Chemical	Chemical Activity
Activator	Sodium carbonate	Swells and softens the emulsions so that the reducing agents may work more effectively.
Reducing agents	Metol	Builds up gray tones quickly.
	Hydroquinone	Builds up black tones more slowly than Metol, giving better contrast to the blacks and whites.
Restrainer	Potassium bromide	Keeps the reducing agents from developing unexposed, nonenergized silver halide.
Preservative	Sodium sulfite	Prevents rapid oxidation of the other chemicals.
Solvent	Water	Dissolves chemicals.

Table **2-2** | **Fixer Composition**

Function	Chemical	Chemical Activity
Acidifier	Acetic or sulfuric acid	Stops development by neutralizing developer; provides required acidity.
Fixing agent	Ammonium thiosulfate	Clears away the unexposed silver halide crystals.
Hardener	Aluminum chloride or sulfide	Shrinks and hardens the emulsion.
Preservative	Sodium sulfite	Maintains chemical balance of the fixer chemicals.
Solvent	Water	Dissolves chemicals.

Box **2-1** Simple Daily Quality Assurance

1. Process an unexposed film. This film should be clear. If not, the cause of the problem should be identified and corrected before proceeding. Problems are usually caused by light leaks in the darkroom or by chemical fog owing to outdated or improperly stored film.
2. Expose a check film using a stepwedge and your usual exposure factors. Process the film. This daily check film should be compared with a control film. If there is no visible difference, the patient's films can be processed. The control film is made using the same stepwedge, the same exposure factors, and fresh chemicals (see following).

having four layers, and the third having two layers of lead. Cut the excess foil from the sides and tape the foil layers to the tongue blade (Fig. 2-4).

How to Make a Control Film

A control film must be made in fresh solutions. Place a film on a flat surface, such as the arm of the dental chair, with the embossed dot facing up. Place the stepwedge on top of the film, and set the cylinder over the film (Fig. 2-5). Expose the film using the setting for a molar bitewing. Process the film in fresh solutions as usual. The control film should be dated and taped to a view box for reference until the solutions are changed again and a new control film is made. Check films made on a daily basis should be compared with this control film.

Check Film

A check film should be exposed at the beginning of every day and compared with the control film. If there is a visible difference, patient films should not be processed until the source of the problem is identified and corrected. Poor quality check films

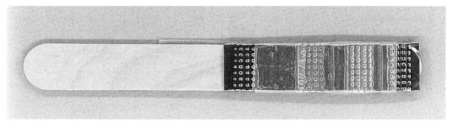

Figure 2-4 Tongue depressor or blade, with foil adapted and taped.

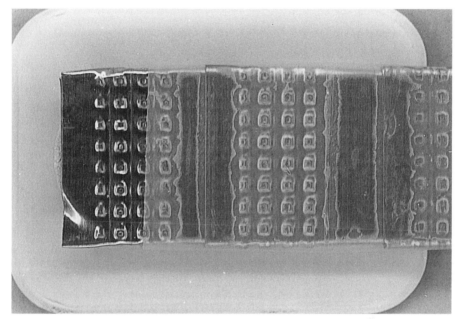

Figure 2-5 Stepwedge placed over x-ray film.

may indicate contaminated solutions, weak solutions, or mechanical problems with the x-ray equipment (Fig. 2-6).

Preparation and Mixing

Developer and fixer solutions can be prepared from powders or concentrated liquids that are mixed with water, or they may come premixed. Regardless of the type used, the manufacturer's instructions should be followed. Each set of chemicals has instructions enclosed in the package or printed on the bottles. If the same chemicals are used consistently, it is wise to post a copy of the mixing instructions near the tanks or processor for reference.

Replenishing Chemicals

As the chemicals are used, they lose their effectiveness. They weaken with use, exposure to air, or contamination with water or another processing chemical. Poor quality films may result from inadequate care of the chemicals. To guarantee the highest quality films, the chemicals should be replenished as they are used.

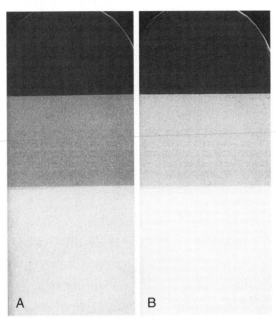

Figure 2-6 **A,** Image of stepwedge properly exposed in fresh solutions. **B,** Weak or depleted developer solution has produced this lighter stepwedge image.

Developer

It is recommended that 6 ounces of developer be added to a 1-gallon tank each morning, regardless of whether the tank has been used. If the tank solution is at its maximum volume, 6 ounces of developer should be removed before adding the replenisher. After the replenisher is added, the developer must be stirred to avoid uneven developing. Developer replenisher may be normally prepared developer solution or a special mixture, as specified by the manufacturer. Manufacturer's instructions on preparing replenisher should be followed.

Fixer

Replenishment of the fixer is not as critical as replenishment of the developer. However, even though it may not be necessary to replenish the fixer daily, it may be beneficial to maintain the same schedule for both solutions to ensure that replenishment of the fixer is not forgotten. If the tank solution is at the maximum volume, 3 ounces of fixer should be removed before replenishing with 3 ounces of replenisher. The fixer should also be stirred on replenishing. Manufacturer's instructions on preparing replenisher should be followed. Keeping the fixer at proper strength will ensure adequate clearing and hardening of the emulsion. Replenishment of the chemicals should be incorporated into the daily maintenance routine.

Changing Chemical Solutions

Even though replenishment will prolong the life of the chemicals, this procedure should not be repeated indefinitely. *Changing the chemicals completely and on a regular basis is necessary.*

Some people change the processing chemicals according to a time schedule. This is acceptable if the time period does not go beyond the life of the chemicals, which is affected by the number of films processed, the amount of exposure to air, the replenishment schedule, and dilution with water or other chemicals. Because these factors can vary from office to office, some chemicals may be thrown away before necessary and others may be used after they are exhausted. The greatest hazard lies in the temptation to increase the exposure time when films are consistently light without checking the quality of the processing solutions. As a result, patients receive unnecessary radiation.

An alternative to changing the solutions according to a time schedule is to rely on the appearance of the check films. This method was described earlier under the section discussing daily care. If there is a visible difference in the density on the check film, the solutions should be changed. If it seems that the solutions are changed quite frequently with this process, they may have been replenished inadequately, that is, either too infrequently or in insufficient amounts. The temperature of the solutions may have damaged the chemicals, or the chemicals may have been exposed to air. These problems are usually easily identified and corrected.

THE DARKROOM

Standard Requirements

The darkroom should be clean, efficient, and well-equipped (Box 2-2). Spots, streaks, film fog, and other artifacts on the processed radiograph can often be traced to poor darkroom conditions and unseemliness. Although it is a tempting place to store film, the darkroom is not recommended for this purpose because of potential reactions between chemical fumes and the film emulsion, which may result in chemical film fog (an overall graying of the film).

There should be adequate space for working, particularly at the counter where films are unwrapped and loaded onto a film rack. The temperature of the room should never exceed 90° F (32° C); temperatures higher than this would be harmful to both the chemicals and the film. A temperature of 70° F to 80° F (21° C to 27° C) at 70% humidity is recommended. Inadequate humidity can cause film artifacts, as will be discussed later.

An automatic processor and film duplicator are recommended as standard equipment. If they are not available, space for their future placement should be allowed.

Box **2-2** A**dequate** D**arkroom** E**quipment**

- A "light-tight" room with a revolving or locking door or maze and with no cracks around doors, corners, or cabinets that would allow light leaks.
- Hot and cold running water, with mixing valves to adjust the temperature.
- Processing tanks and film hangers or racks.
- A source of white light and *proper* safelights at the appropriate distance from the work surface (at least 4 feet).
- A timer that is accurate *in minutes and seconds.*
- An accurate *nonmercury* thermometer that is easy to read and is kept submerged in the developer. The mercury in a thermometer will permanently damage the metal lining of the tanks if it comes into contact with them. Additionally, mercury is a toxic environmental hazard to be avoided.
- Adequate storage space for chemicals, film hangers, and cassettes.
- A film-drying rack and a film dryer.

Lighting

The darkroom should be totally dark when all the lights are off. White light may leak into the room through any opening such as the door, joints in walls, partitions, keyholes, and air vents. Damaged safelights may also be a source of light leaks. If the darkroom door is not a revolving type, it should have a lock to eliminate accidental opening. Some darkroom entryways use a maze of walls rather than a door. These are usually "lightproof."

Some types of fluorescent lights have a short afterglow that could fog the first few films opened after the room lights have been turned off. These should be replaced. Although extraneous light should be eliminated, the room should contain a source of white light (regular room lighting) and a safelight, each with its own switch. It is also desirable to have an illuminator (view box) in the darkroom.

Safelights are devices that provide enough illumination in the darkroom to work by and to process films without danger of fogging the film. X-ray film is sensitive to both radiation and visible light (white light); it is most sensitive to blue and green light and least sensitive to yellow and red light. Consequently, safelights usually contain regular light bulbs with red, yellow, or brown filters covering the bulb. These filter or remove the kinds of light to which the film is most sensitive: the light in the blue–green range.

Commercially available darkroom filters include the Kodak ML-2,* which is a light orange filter, closer to green than to red in the visible light spectrum; it transmits the most light of all the safelight filters. As a result, it is easier to work using this filter because of greater visibility. However, this type of filter *cannot be used with extraoral films* because they are sensitive to light nearer the green part of the light spectrum and would be fogged.

The Kodak GBX* is a deep red filter that, unlike the ML-2, can be used in darkrooms in which both intraoral and extraoral films are processed. The GBX filter removes light nearer the green–blue spectrum, thus protecting sensitive extraoral films. All film is somewhat sensitive to any light. If light fogging is to be avoided, bulb wattage and distance to the work surface must also be controlled. If the safelighting is *direct* (shining down onto the work surface), the bulb should be no brighter than 15 W (the usual wattage in a refrigerator light). If the safelighting is *indirect* (shining up toward the ceiling, then reflected down), the bulb should be no brighter than 25 W. The distance from the light to the work surface should be at least 4 feet, regardless of whether direct or indirect illumination is used.

Quality assurance in checking the darkroom for light leaks and proper safelights is simple. To check for light leaks around doors, lights, walls, and vents, simply go into the darkroom and turn off *all* the lights. Wait 2 or 3 minutes for your eyes to adjust to the darkness. Then look around the room carefully. If you see light coming in from anywhere, you have a light leak that must be corrected.

Coin Test

The "coin test" can be used to check the safelights. With the safelights on and the white light off, unwrap a piece of film. Lay it on the counter and place a coin in the center. Wait between 3 and 5 minutes (approximately the time it would take you to unwrap a complete series, load it onto a rack, and place it in the developer). Process the film as usual. If the image of the coin is visible on the processed film, light is coming in from somewhere and will fog (expose) the film. Safelight bulbs should be

---

Eastman Kodak, Rochester, N.Y.

checked for correct wattage, the distance of the safelights to the work surface should be checked, and the safelight filters should be checked for cracks.

AUTOMATIC FILM PROCESSING

Manual processing for intraoral films is being replaced by automatic processing for a number of reasons:

- An automatic processor can shorten the processing time to as little as 4 to 5 minutes.
- The automatic processing cycle produces consistently good end results *if* the equipment and chemicals are properly maintained. In addition, less opportunity exists for operator error.
- Automatic processors usually require less space than manual equipment, and some have a **daylight loading system** that does not require a darkroom.

An automatic processor is usually constructed of a series of rollers that transport the films through various compartments (developer, fixer, rinse water) and a blower to dry the films (Fig. 2-7).

The processor contains a heating element that maintains a constant temperature in the developer. The rollers are set to rotate at a speed according to the temperature of the developer so that optimal images are produced. Although this mechanism can be thought of as time/temperature developing, the temperatures of the developer in automatic processors range from 85° F to 105° F (29° C to 40° C), which significantly reduces the developing time and the overall processing procedure. Automatic processor developer is manufactured to withstand these higher temperatures.

While moving the film through the processor, the rollers provide a massaging action that contributes to the speed and uniformity of processing. In addition to these transport rollers, special squeegee rollers remove processing solutions from the film surfaces, reducing the amount of solution carryover from one tank to the next. This process prolongs the life of the fixer and removes most of the wash water from the film emulsion before the film enters the drying section. Warm, dry air is blown onto the film before it exits the processor.

Because the total time is reduced in automatic processing, the chemical concentration and temperature of the solutions must be increased. The automatic processor commonly used in dentistry maintains temperatures of approximately 83° F to 85° F (28° C to 29° C) for a 4½ - to 5-minute cycle. For larger, 90-second processing machines commonly used for extraoral films only, the developing temperature is about 95° F to 101° F (35° C to 38° C).

To prevent the emulsion from softening and sticking to the rollers, a special hardening chemical, glutaraldehyde, is added to the developer. Sulfate compounds are also added to the developer to minimize the swelling of the emulsion. If the emulsion has absorbed too much developer, the films will get stuck in the rollers.

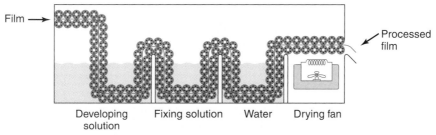

Figure 2-7 Schematic drawing of typical automatic film processor.

Maintenance of Automatic Processors

A rigid schedule for replenishment is far more critical with automatic processors. For example, weak fixer will not shrink the emulsion enough to keep the films moving through the rollers. Films may stick in the fixer or dryer rack, impeding the path of the following films. The smaller amounts of developer or fixer solution in an automatic processor tank demand regular replenishment.

Automatic processors also demand routine preventive maintenance. Experience has shown that the two greatest causes of automatic processor breakdown are (1) failure to keep the rollers clean and (2) inadequate replenishing. A schedule should be established for daily cleaner films and replenishment, as well as for monthly cleaning and solution changes. Guidelines appropriate for maintenance of all automatic processors follow.

Replenishment

Solutions should be replenished at the beginning of each day, regardless of the amount of time of use, and on a regular basis according to the number of films processed. After approximately four complete series or four panoramic films, 4 to 6 ounces of processing chemicals should be added. Failure to add this amount will result in exhausted developer and fixer and, consequently, undiagnostic images.

Cleaning the Rollers

The rollers should be cleaned with warm running water weekly. The rollers should be soaked for approximately 10 to 15 minutes before being placed back in the processor. Two extraoral-sized "cleaning" films should be run through the processor before patient films are processed. Commercially available clear acetate cleaning sheets can be bought for just such a purpose.

Changing the Solutions

The solutions should be changed every *2 to 6 weeks*, depending on the rate of use and the frequency of replenishment. It is wise to empty only one compartment at a time, beginning with the fixer. Cleaning solutions recommended by the manufacturer should be used. If there are no recommendations or if those solutions are not available, the following cleaning solutions can be used: (1) special developer cleaner for the developing rack and compartment, (2) warm running water for the fixer rollers and compartment, and (3) household bleach solutions for the wash compartment. All racks should be rinsed thoroughly with warm running water before they are put back in the processor. The stopper or plug should be removed from one compartment at a time. Each compartment should be totally cleaned and rinsed and the *stopper should be replaced* before proceeding. This will prevent backflow of chemicals into the wrong compartment. After a thorough cleaning has been performed, each compartment should be filled with clear water and the processor should be run for approximately 5 to 10 minutes. After the water is drained, the fixer should be replaced first, followed by the developer. If the developer accidentally splashes into the fixer, the contamination is not as damaging as when the reverse occurs.

Monthly Cleaning

Monthly cleaning includes cleaning the rollers, as described in the section on changing solutions. This is also the time to check the unit (particularly the dryer) for dust and to lubricate moving parts.

Helpful Hints

The most important factor in maintaining the processor is regular preventive maintenance. Suggestions to help prevent problems commonly associated with automatic processors are listed in Box 2-3.

Box **2-3** **Preventing Problems in Automatic Processors**

- Keep the cover open slightly, particularly over the motor, when the processor is *not in use*. Accumulated fumes will fog films if not vented, and the moisture around the motor will cause premature rusting and breakdown. Be sure to replace the cover tightly before processing films.
- Lubricate the moving parts as indicated in the owner's manual.
- Check the temperature of the solutions regularly. A few degrees' difference in the developer temperature will change the density of the films.
- Check each day to see that the rollers are locked in proper position to prevent loss of films.
- *Replenish the chemicals* as described previously.
- Feed the films slowly into the machine and keep them straight. If they turn sideways even slightly, they may merge and stick together.
- Count 10 to 15 seconds after feeding each film into the processor before inserting another film.
- Alternate slots or sides when possible.
- Check to be sure that the black paper has been completely removed and that double-pack films have been separated; place only the films into the processor.
- Do *not* put wet films into the processor because they will contaminate the rollers.

TROUBLESHOOTING: DIAGNOSING PROCESSING ERRORS

Processed films may not have the expected quality. Table 2-3 lists different problems, possible causes, and appropriate corrections. Most of these conditions pertain to both manual and automatic processing. Exposure errors and radiographic examples of errors that may cause similar appearances are discussed in Chapter 9.

MOUNTING FILMS

Detailed instructions on film mounting will be discussed in Chapter 3, but characteristics of the film mount are discussed here.

Preparing the Mount

Processed films are normally placed in a film holder, either cardboard or plastic, that arranges the films in an anatomically oriented pattern and protects them from scratches and careless handling. Mounting films routinely and correctly reduces the potential for incorrect interpretation, such as confusing the right side with the left.

Looking at a set of films is also more efficient than viewing one at a time. Although each film is viewed individually, an overview of the complete survey gives the operator the opportunity to look for symmetry and to compare sides for such characteristics as bone pattern, eruption sequence, and the size and shape of the teeth (Fig. 2-8).

Table **2-3** | **Troubleshooting for Processing Errors**

Condition	Possible Causes	What to Do
1. Light films (low density or contrast)	A. Underdevelopment 1. Temperature too low 2. Time too short 3. Inaccurate thermometer or timer B. Exhausted developer C. Diluted developer	 1. Check temperature. 2. Check time (if possible). 3. Check timer and thermometer. B. Do check film.* C. Do check film.
2. Dark films (high density)	A. Overdevelopment 1. Temperature too high 2. Time too long 3. Inaccurate thermometer or timer B. Light leak in darkroom or processor C. Exposure of films to white light	 1. Check temperature. 2. Check time. 3. Check thermometer and timer. B. Check inside darkroom.* Do coin test. C. Turn overhead lights off.
3. Grayish films (film fog)	A. Light leaks B. Improper or defective safelights C. Exposure of films to white light before complete fixing D. Exposure of films to unwanted radiation E. Chemical fog overdevelopment (time) F. Outdated film	A. Check inside darkroom for leaks.* Do coin test. B-C. Check safelights* for correct wattage or light leaks due to cracks. D. Check storage area of films and check for films left in x-ray cubical while exposing. E. Check temperature (it may have increased and changed development time). F. Discard old film.
4. Yellow or brown films	A. Exhausted developer B. Exhausted fixer C. Incomplete fixing D. Insufficient washing	A. Do check film.* B. Do check film.* C. Check fixing time. D. Rewash.
5. Streaks	A. Careless rinsing before fixing B. Exhausted chemicals C. Contaminated developer or wash water D. Contaminated rollers	A. Rinse thoroughly. B. Do check film.* C. Do check film. D. Run cleaning film through processor; clean rollers if necessary.
6. Greenish films	A. Contaminated or exhausted fixer B. Insufficient washing C. Films stuck together (uneven developing)	A. Replenish or change fixer. B. Rewash. C. Replace in fixer and continue processing.
7. Black or white lines	A. Film bending B. Rough film handling	A. Curve but do not crease film if possible. B. Be gentle when inserting film into holders.
8. Lightening or treelike marks (static electricity)	A. Excessively dry air (most commonly seen on extraoral films)	A. Humidify darkroom. Use Static Guard on clothing/hair.
9. Spots	A. Water droplets on film B. Premature contact with developer (black spots) C. Premature contact with fixer (white spots)	A. Check counter for cleanliness. B. Check counter for cleanliness. C. Check counter for cleanliness.

*See section on quality assurance for specific checks and tests.

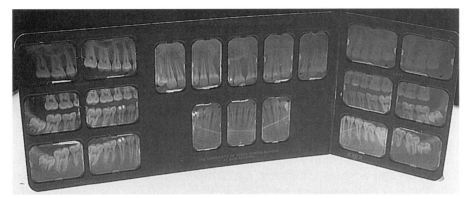

Figure 2-8 Complete set of periapical and bitewing radiographs. Note that the anterior windows are for no. 1 size film. No. 2 size film would not fit properly in these windows.

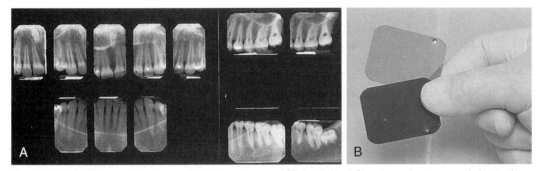

Figure 2-9 **A,** Opaque x-ray mount, with appropriate areas filled with black films to mask extraneous light. **B,** The film blank, which appears black in this figure, is used for this purpose. Exposing a film to light and then processing it will result in a black film.

The mount should be opaque to eliminate extraneous light from around the films. Eliminating extraneous light enables the eye to detect the subtle differences in density that may indicate the presence or absence of pathologic conditions. The film mount (Fig. 2-9, A) should contain the right number and size frames to hold the prepared films. Empty frames should be blocked out with opaque material such as film blanks (Fig. 2-9, B).

The **film mount** should be labeled before use. If films become separated from the patient's chart, they cannot be identified if they are not labeled. The information on the mount should include three things:

1. *The patient's full name*, not just the last name and initial.
2. *The date the films were exposed.* Even if the films are processed on a different date, the exposure date should be the one recorded on the mount. This is a radiographic record of the patient's intraoral condition on the date of the exposure, not on the processing date.
3. *The name of the radiographer.* This is the person who may be able to furnish information should future questions arise. Recording the name also gives a quality of ownership for a skill performed and a means of quality assurance for technique. Radiographers may be a little more particular with technique if their names are attached for others to see. If the operator is consistently making the same error, remediation may be in order. Thus, the error can be identified, and the operator can be given instructions for correction.

DUPLICATING FILMS

For many reasons, a practitioner may desire a copy or duplicate set of radiographs. Preauthorization for treatment, population mobility, and protection from liability may dictate the need for more than one copy of a radiographic survey.

Intraoral film is available in *double-film packets;* that is, two pieces of film are in one packet. They are exposed in the normal manner, and the films are separated before processing. This way, two identical sets of films are obtained, and the patient is not exposed to extra radiation.

An alternative method is to copy the radiographs using duplicating film and a film duplicator as shown in Figure 2-10. Duplicating film has emulsion on one side only and is sensitive to light, particularly ultraviolet light. The reaction of the emulsion is the opposite of that of radiographic film. When exposed to radiation or light, x-ray film becomes dark. Duplicating film, on the other hand, becomes lighter with increasing exposure to light.

Duplication is performed in the darkroom under safelights. Radiographs are placed on a duplicator, and the duplicating film is placed carefully on top with the emulsion side (which is normally gray or lavender in color) against the radiographs. If available, film organizers, which look similar to film mounts but are especially designed for duplicating, should be used to organize the films (Fig. 2-11). The organizers are helpful because they blacken the areas around each film, eliminating extraneous light transmission.

A source of light (usually ultraviolet) is present in the duplicator. The light passes through the original radiograph and strikes the duplicating film. Light areas of the radiographs allow increased light transmission to the duplicating film. The longer the duplicating film is exposed to light, the lighter the duplicating film will become. This is the opposite of x-ray films, which become darker when exposed to light.

This process is also helpful in producing acceptable radiographic copies (Fig. 2-12) of films that are overexposed and too dark to interpret. However, it is not always successful in making darker duplicates of overly light radiographs.

The duplicating film is then processed normally. If the duplicates are not as good as the original films, the process can be repeated without additional radiation exposure to the patient until the desired outcome is achieved.

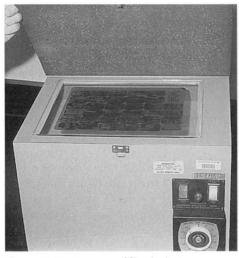
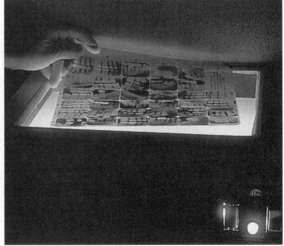

Figure 2-10 Two types of film duplicators.

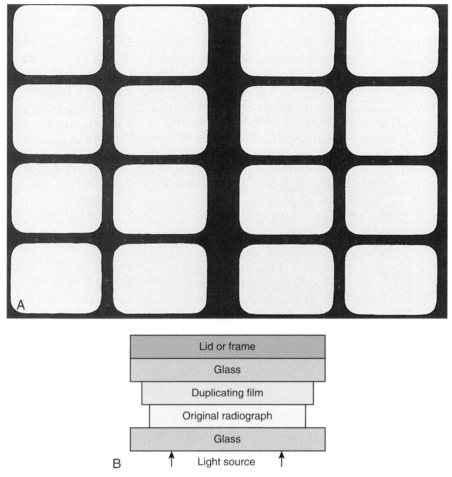

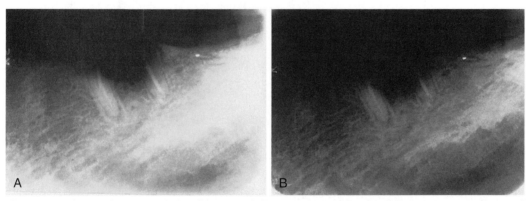

Figure 2-11 A, X-ray film organizer on which to place films for duplication. Films to be duplicated are centered in the clear area, and an edge of the film is taped lightly to hold them in place when the duplication film is placed over them. **B,** The basic arrangement for using duplicating film. Note that the direction of the light source is from below, as would occur when using a duplicating machine. *(B: From Miles DA, Van Dis ML, Razmus TF:* Basic principles of oral and maxillofacial radiology, *ed 1, Philadelphia, 1992, Saunders.)*

Figure 2-12 A, This film was duplicated from the dark film seen in *B*. **B,** More detail is seen in *A*, especially around the root tips. Exposing the dark film *B* and the duplicating film to the ultraviolet light longer than usual results in the lighter film *A*.

Helpful Hint

It is very important to obtain good contact between the duplicating film and the radiographs to prevent blurring and fuzziness of the image. Regular film mounts should not be used as organizers because they hold the radiograph away from the duplicating film slightly, which prevents good contact. They also "cut off" the edges of the films, leaving an incomplete view on the duplicates. The radiographs should be placed on the duplicator with the dot downward so that good contact with the duplicating film is made. Care should be taken to ensure that the original radiographs are arranged in the correct position before duplicating them. No raised dot exists on the duplicating film to help identify film orientation in terms of left and right sides. The duplicate film should be labeled immediately with the patient's name, the date the originals were made, and which side is right or left.

INFECTION CONTROL FOR PROCESSING FILMS OR PHOSPHOR PLATES

In the Darkroom

Films that have been in the patient's mouth are contaminated with saliva. They must be transported safely into the darkroom and processed without contaminating the darkroom door, processors, or any darkroom surfaces. To do this, with gloves on,

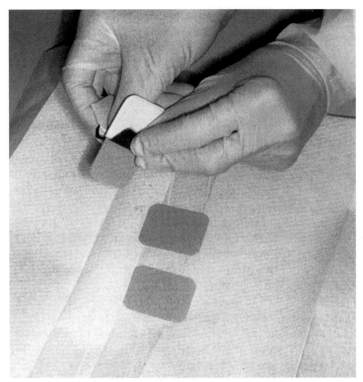

Figure 2-13 The film drop-out technique is the recommended method for handling saliva-contaminated films in the darkroom. The operator should open the film packet, pull the black paper–film combination out of the wrapper, and then allow the film to fall out onto a paper towel on the countertop without actually touching the film. The wrapper is then disposed of properly. *(From Miles DA, Van Dis ML, Razmus TF:* Basic principles of oral and maxillofacial radiology, *ed 1, Philadelphia, 1992, Saunders.)*

the operator should place the exposed films into a disposable receptacle such as a paper cup *without touching the exterior surface of the cup.* The contaminated gloves are removed, and the operator should wash his or her hands. *Touching only the outside of the cup,* the operator may then transport the films into the darkroom.

Once in the darkroom, the operator should put on fresh gloves and proceed to unwrap every film packet with gloves on. The operator should allow the film to drop out of the wrapper onto a paper towel without touching the film itself (Fig. 2-13). Once *all* of the films have been unwrapped and dropped out of the packets, the operator should dispose of all the film wrappings. After this is done, the operator may then remove the gloves and wash his or her hands. The films themselves may be handled with clean, dry, ungloved hands and placed onto film processing racks or into the automatic processor (Fig. 2-14).

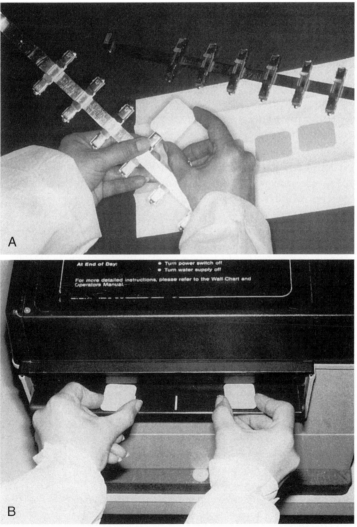

Figure 2-14 The operator should remove the gloves and wash the hands after all films have been dropped out and the wrapping properly discarded. Note that the operator handles the films by the edges for both processing techniques. For manual processing, **A** shows individual films being attached to film rack. **B** shows films being inserted into an automatic processor intake tray. *(From Razmus TF, Williamson GF: Current oral and maxillofacial imaging, ed 1, Philadelphia, 1996, Saunders.)*

Similar handling of reusable phosphor plates is necessary to avoid plate contamination. All phosphor plates, regardless of the system used, must be wrapped individually in a barrier and unwrapped with clean gloves before being placed into the plate reading system. Further discussion of photostimulable phosphor plate systems can be found in Chapter 7.

Daylight Loaders

Daylight loading system is designed with cloth openings or sleeves that allow an operator to insert the hands and films into the unit and work in the daylight. The films are protected from white light with a filter, but the operator can see through the filter into the unit. Getting exposed films into a daylight loader without contaminating the unit with saliva is a real challenge and requires close attention to detail.

Contaminated films can be placed in a disposable receptacle as already described. It is important to make sure the film packet surfaces are dry; they must be blotted with a paper towel if they are still damp with saliva. With clean, ungloved hands, the operator can open the daylight loader filter window. Clean paper toweling on a plastic liner should be inserted into the bottom of the loader (Fig. 2-15). Next, the film receptacle and powderless gloves should be placed into the daylight loader. The lid is then closed, and the hands are inserted into the cloth openings. Once the hands are inside the unit, the gloves should be put on, and the films should be unwrapped in a manner similar to that described for the darkroom. Once the films are unwrapped, the operator should remove the gloves and leave them inside the loader but away from the films. The films can then be inserted into the processor with ungloved hands. When all the films have entered the processor, operators may withdraw their hands, open the filter window, and put on clean gloves to properly dispose of all the contaminated items that are inside the loader.

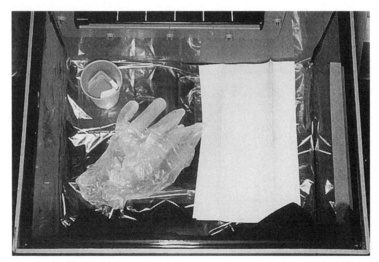

Figure 2-15 The daylight loader should be prepared for processing by covering the bottom with plastic wrap. The film receptacle, gloves, and a paper towel should be placed onto the plastic surface through the lid before the hands are inserted through the sleeves. *(From Razmus TF, Williamson GF:* Current oral and maxillofacial imaging, *ed 1, Philadelphia, 1996, Saunders.)*

STUDY QUESTIONS

1. The latent image on a radiograph is
   A. An unseen image produced by silver halide crystals that have been exposed to radiation and that contain various levels of stored energy, making a pattern
   B. The image seen on the film after removal of the unexposed silver halide crystals in the developing solution
   C. The image seen on the film after removal of the exposed silver halide crystals in the developing solution
   D. The image seen on the film after the film has been in the fixer at least 3 minutes

2. During the chemical processing procedure, the fixer
   A. Removes the metallic silver deposited during the developing process
   B. Removes the unexposed silver halide crystals, leaving a white (clear) area where those crystals used to be
   C. Precipitates the exposed crystals onto the base of the film, creating black (dark) areas
   D. Softens the emulsion to "set" energized crystals and remove nonenergized crystals

3. A stepwedge may be used to
   A. Check the darkroom for light leaks
   B. Determine film speed
   C. Determine processing times when chemical temperatures vary
   D. Check the quality of processing chemicals

4. The emulsion is softened, and exposed silver halide crystals precipitate from within the gelatin onto the film base during the
   A. Latent period
   B. Developing cycle
   C. Fixing cycle
   D. Washing cycle

5. After processing, you find a check film to be too light. The temperature was appropriate for the developing time. No log shows how long the chemicals have been used. Which of the following is an appropriate step to take?
   A. Increase exposure time to darken the films
   B. Increase the developing time
   C. Change the chemicals
   D. Increase the fixing time

6. After doing a coin test, you see a slight but noticeable well-defined white circle on the processed film. This indicates
   A. Chemical film fog from improper film storage
   B. Weak or exhausted chemicals
   C. Inadequate exposure time before processing
   D. A light leak or unsafe safelighting

7. The primary reason that automatic processors are much faster than manual processing is that automatic processors
   A. Have rollers that act as squeegees
   B. Skip the wash cycle
   C. Have higher developing temperatures
   D. Have lower fixing temperatures

8. Given that exposure errors are not the problem, processed films that are too dark may be the result of
   A. Developing time that is too long or developer that is too warm
   B. Weak or exhausted developing solution
   C. Underfixation or weak fixing solution
   D. Fixing time that is too long or fixer that is too warm

9. The reducing agent in the developer responsible for building the black and gray tones is
   A. Potassium bromide
   B. Metol or hydroquinone
   C. Ammonium thiosulfate
   D. Sodium carbonate

10. The fixing agent that clears the unexposed crystals is
    A. Acetic or sulfuric acid
    B. Sodium sulfite
    C. Ammonium thiosulfate
    D. Aluminum chloride or sulfide

11. You retrieve films from a patient's chart and find them to be brownish, opaque, and difficult to interpret. This could be caused by any of the following reasons except one. Which one is the exception?
    A. Inadequate washing time
    B. Inadequate fixing time
    C. Exhausted fixer
    D. Overdevelopment

3

Film Mounting and Normal Radiographic Anatomy

The knowledge of normal anatomic landmarks is indispensable to the members of the dental team because it is this knowledge that facilitates the mounting of radiographs in their proper location and sequence. An error in image mounting could result in improper treatment of the dental patient. This chapter assumes that the student has already received instruction in basic anatomy, including the bony anatomy of the maxilla and mandible. The student must be able to identify normal anatomic landmarks in the maxilla and mandible on radiographs to be able to detect abnormal findings. Normal structures encountered on dental images can sometimes resemble pathologic conditions. This chapter identifies the common radiographic anatomic landmarks seen on intraoral images. Not all of the structures identified appear each time on each image. The landmarks on dental images vary widely because of differences in technique and patient anatomy. Chapter 12 compares normal anatomy with certain pathologic conditions that may have similar radiographic appearances.

Many of the illustrations in this chapter repeat landmarks. This is to reinforce your learning. The structures vary in appearance depending on the angulation of the x-ray beam or how the image receptor was placed. Some of the illustrations in this chapter also have questions for you to answer; a figure reference to remind you of the answer often follows the questions.

Characteristics of film mounts and how to label them were described in the previous chapter. What follows are helpful hints to assist you with mounting films.

MOUNTING DENTAL RADIOGRAPHS

For the new student of dental radiography, the mounting of radiographs can be frustrating (Procedure Box 3-1). Some clinicians or institutions like to have the raised (embossed) dot on the films facing upward (like a pimple), and some like it downward (like a dimple). The American Dental Association recommends that radiographs be mounted and viewed from the facial aspect, that is, from the outside inward, as if you are looking at the patient's face. A catchy phrase to help you remember is *"You want a pimple, not a dimple."* A pimple sticks out; a dimple is a depression.

PROCEDURE *Box* **3-1**

Suggested Mounting Procedure

Step 1. Collect the dry films and sit at a view box in a quiet atmosphere with a prepared mount. Some viewing areas are large, almost tablelike; other view boxes are smaller, about the size of the mount. If you are at a tablelike viewing area, all your films will fit onto the viewing area for sorting. If you have a small view box, place your films on a paper towel or piece of paper. Placing them directly on a countertop puts them at greater risk of being scratched if you drag them across the surface top.

Step 2. Turn all the films so that the embossed dot is *raised toward you*. The American Dental Association recommends that radiographs be mounted and viewed from the facial aspect, that is, from the outside inward, as if you are looking at the patient's face. If you hold a mounted set of films in front of the patient, the structures in the images will match the structures in the patient's jaws. The films that match the *patient's right side* structures will be on *your left side,* and the *patient's left side* structures will be on *your right side*. Think of looking at the images as if you were standing in front of the patient, looking at him or her.

Step 3. Group all of the maxillary anterior periapical films together, all of the mandibular anterior periapical films together, all of the maxillary posterior periapical films together, all of the mandibular posterior periapical films together, and all of the bitewing films together (use Box 3-1). Set the bitewings aside temporarily.

Step 4. Turn the periapical films so that all of the occlusal or incisal surfaces of the maxillary films point downward and the roots point upward, and turn the occlusal or incisal surfaces of the mandibular films upward with the roots pointing down.

Step 5. Identify the maxillary central incisors (two identical-looking teeth) and the mandibular incisors (four similar-looking teeth). Then find the remaining anterior images and identify them as maxillary or mandibular; arrange them according to how the teeth appear in a patient's mouth (incisors at the midline, canines to the distal of the incisors).

Step 6. Find the posterior periapical images and identify them as maxillary or mandibular; arrange them according to the natural arrangement of teeth and anatomic structures.

Step 7. Orient the bitewings according to left and right; use the periapical films to help you. For example, if the mandibular right first molar has a crown on it in the periapical view, you will know that the right molar bitewing should also contain an image of the mandibular first molar with a crown on it.

Step 8. Slip the films into the mount, making sure that the embossed dot is still facing up as you look at the mounted films.

Step 9. *Final check*: Make sure all the dots are raised as you look at the front of the mount. The patient's name and date of exposure should be clearly seen on the front of the mount. The overall curve of the occlusal plane (occlusal, incisal edges) should turn slightly upward as if the patient were smiling at you.

If you hold a mounted set of films that have the embossed dot up toward the observer, and you stand in front of the patient, the structures in the images will match the structures in the patient's jaws. The films that match the *patient's right side* structures will be on *your left side,* and the *patient's left side* structures will be on *your right side*. Think of looking at the images as if you were standing in front of the patient, looking at him or her. If the raised dot is up, facing the observer, the patient's right side is seen on the left portion of the x-ray mount.

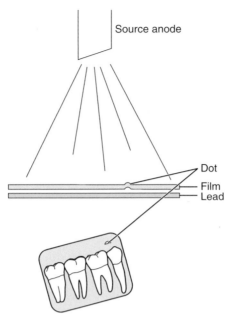

Figure 3-1 Orienting the films so that the embossed dot is raised makes it easier to determine which parts of the film are anterior and which parts are posterior. Remember, the raised dot should feel like a pimple, not a dimple.

If you happen to be in an office or institution that prefers to look at mounted films with the embossed dot downward (like a dimple), it is as if you are sitting on the patient's tongue, looking outward. In this case, the patient's right side structures are also on your right side. This is quite a rare occurrence in today's dental practices, but you may encounter it.

However, because the raised dot is always oriented toward the tubehead during exposure (so that the sensitive side of the film packet faces the x-ray source), it is reasonable to maintain this orientation when viewing the processed images. Fig. 3-1 demonstrates the orientation of the dot and the x-ray source. Thus, "right is left, and left is right" when the embossed dot faces upward. This is the same orientation as your patient's face: the patient's right side is on your left side, and the patient's left side is on your right. The midline structures will be in the middle of the mount, and the most posterior structures will be on the left and right edges. It is customary to place all the maxillary periapicals along the top portion of the mount, and the mandibular structures are placed along the lower side of the mount. Bitewings films are often sandwiched between the maxillary and mandibular posterior views (see again Fig. 2-8 in Chapter 2).

Many instructors teach their students to "put the dot in the slot" when placing an x-ray film packet in a film-holding device. By always orienting the dot toward the occlusal surface ("in the slot" of the holder), you make sure that the dot will never be superimposed over the apical areas on periapical films. Additionally, you will be able to identify the occlusal/incisal aspects of the films. Please note that this technique does *not* apply to bitewing films because all occlusal edges are in the middle of the bitewing film, not on the image edges. Your instructor may favor placing the dot in the mandible on a bitewing film or in the maxilla, or your instructor may have no preference for the dot orientation for bitewings.

Figure 3-2 illustrates both the correct orientation of the dot in a periapical view (A) and a possible position on a bitewing film (B).

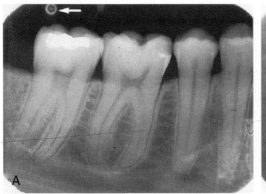 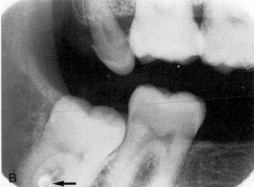

Figure 3-2 An illustration of the correct **(A)** and incorrect **(B)** orientation of the raised dot in a periapical view.

Let us now look at the anatomic landmarks you might find in each type of image (Box 3-1). Once you are able to identify these landmarks, mounting your films will be easier.

Box **3-1** Helpful Hints for Anatomic Landmark Identification in Intraoral Images

1. The teeth are oriented with the longer side of the film vertical for anterior teeth and horizontal for posterior teeth.
2. Mandibular anterior teeth have smaller crowns and shorter roots than maxillary anterior teeth.
3. The four mandibular incisors usually fit on one image, whereas the four maxillary incisors are larger and may not all fit on one image.
4. The maxillary central incisor image shows the median palatal suture, which is seen as a distinct radiolucent (dark) line between the maxillary incisors. This structure is not present between the mandibular central incisors.
5. Mandibular molars usually have only two roots, the image of which is very distinct. Maxillary molars have three roots, and it may be difficult to distinguish all three of them easily.
6. If tooth roots curve, they usually (although not always) curve distally (posteriorly).
7. Maxillary images have large radiolucent (dark) areas representing anatomic cavities: the nasal fossa in the anterior area and the maxillary sinus in the posterior region near the apices. These anatomic cavities are not present in the mandible.
8. The posterior border of the maxilla has an area called the tuberosity that looks like a rounded corner (see Fig. 3-31). The mandible does not have this structure.
9. Some teeth may have restorations that will help you match periapicals and bitewings on a given side of the patient.
10. The overall appearance of a complete mouth survey or even a bitewing survey presents the occlusal plane in an upward curve that looks like a smile.

Digital images are often displayed in an electronic array in the software program that accompanies the image receptor. The arrays often resemble film mounts. Because it is commonplace to display the image that was just acquired and the operator knows what image was just exposed, it is easy to then place that image in the appropriate place in the electronic array.

TEETH AND ADJACENT STRUCTURES

The Tooth

Enamel, dentin, cementum, and pulp tissue are the components of a tooth. Of the four tissues, enamel is the hardest. Next are the dentin and cementum. The pulp is soft tissue and thus is not visible on the image but is represented by a dark space

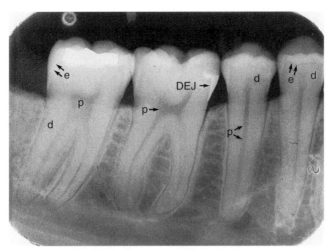

Figure 3-3 Mandibular periapical image: dentin *(d)*, enamel *(e)*, pulp space *(p)*, and dentinoenamel junction *(DEJ)*.

within the tooth (Fig. 3-3). In contrast, the enamel appears white on the film. It is very dense and attenuates (stops) more x rays than the other dental tissues; therefore, it can be easily distinguished from the dentin. A distinct and often abrupt interface between enamel and dentin in the crown, or coronal, portion of the tooth is called the dentinoenamel junction (DEJ). The DEJ is apparent in Figure 3-3.

Dentin is less dense than enamel but has a density similar to both cementum and bone. The cementum is a thin layer of tooth structure that covers the entire root surface. The interface between the dentin and the cementum in the root portion of the tooth is not visible radiographically. The radiographic density of dentin and cementum is between that of the white enamel and the darker pulp space and, therefore, appears gray.

Bone, Periodontal Ligament Space, and Lamina Dura

Bone, like dentin, is usually less dense than enamel and, therefore, usually appears gray on radiographs. Bone supporting the teeth (the *alveolar bone*) appears as irregularly shaped lines in random patterns called *trabeculae* that surround the marrow spaces. The trabecular pattern of bone is extremely variable; even normal variations can look very different from one another. This type of bone is also called *cancellous* bone.

Cortical bone is bone without marrow spaces and thus is usually denser and more distinct than cancellous bone. Examples of cortical bone are the crests of the alveolar process and the lamina dura and the outer layer of the jaws, such as the inferior border of the mandible. The alveolar process itself consists of the cortical crests, the cancellous bone, and the lamina dura. The *lamina dura* (literally, *hard layer*) is the bone that lines the sockets where teeth are present. On occasion, the bone referred to as the lamina dura can be relatively dense, or white, similar to enamel (Fig. 3-4).

The periodontal ligament (periodontal membrane) or PDL, like the pulp tissue, is not visible on the radiograph. However, the space it occupies is apparent as a thin dark line. Therefore, it is termed the *periodontal ligament space* or *periodontal membrane space*. It appears on a radiograph as a continuous dark line around the root of the tooth from one interproximal area to the next (see Fig. 3-4). Not all PDL spaces can be seen on each tooth in a set of intraoral images. Angulation of the x-ray beam

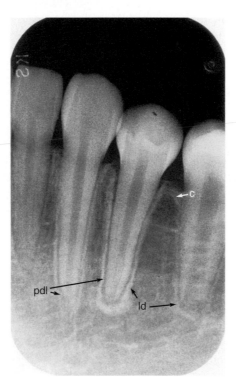

Figure 3-4 Periodontal ligament *(pdl)*, the thin radiolucent line adjacent to the root surface; lamina dura *(ld)*, the white radiopaque line between the pdl and the cancellous bone; and cortical bone *(c)*, which, in this example, is the alveolar crest.

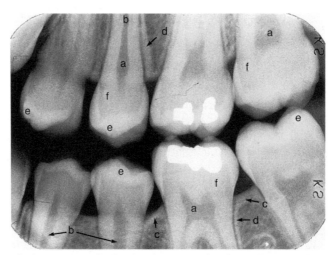

Figure 3-5 Left premolar bitewing. *a*, Pulp chamber. *b*, Root canal (pulp canal). *c*, The alveolar crest is continuous with which structure? *Answer:* The lamina dura. *d*, Lamina dura (surrounds entire root). *e*, Enamel. *f*, Dentin.

and tooth anatomy influence how well the PDL space is seen. It is most obvious when the x rays enter at a 90° angle to the teeth and the image receptor.

When healthy, both the periodontal ligament space and the lamina dura are continuous around the root. The lamina dura is also continuous with the alveolar ridge crest (crestal cortex). Figures 3-3 through 3-5 demonstrate this.

MAXILLARY AND MANDIBULAR ANATOMIC LANDMARKS

Figs. 3-6 through 3-16 identify various maxillary anatomic landmarks and, in some instances, invite the reader to identify them (Box 3-2). Mandibular anatomic landmarks are displayed in Figs. 3-17 through 3-28 (Box 3-3).

Box **3-2** Identifying Maxillary Anatomic Landmarks

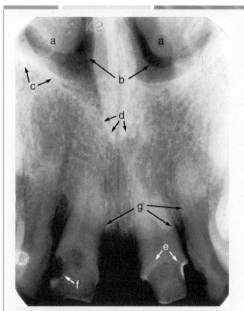

a. Inferior turbinate bone.
b. Inferior nasal meatus.
c. Lateral wall of the nasal fossa (cavity).
d. Anterior nasal spine.
e. Crown preparation.
f. Carious lesion or nonradiopaque restoration.
g. Soft tissue outline of the nose.

Figure 3-6 Maxillary central incisor view.

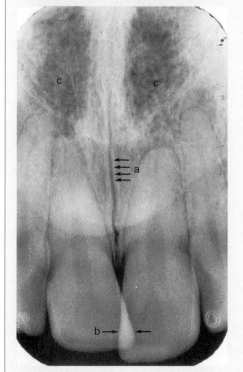

a. Intermaxillary suture (median palatine suture).
b. Overlapped enamel (crowded teeth).
c. Nasal fossa. Can you identify the anterior nasal spine? Can you identify the soft tissue of the nose? Can you identify the intermaxillary suture in Fig. 3-6?

Figure 3-7 Maxillary central incisor view.

Continued

Box **3-2** Identifying Maxillary Anatomic Landmarks—cont'd

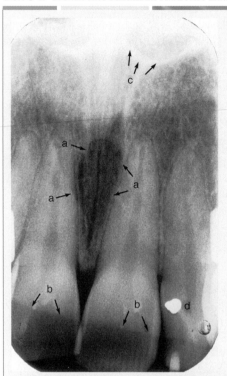

a. Incisive (nasopalatine) foramen.
b. Soft tissue outline of the upper lip.
c. Wall of the nasal fossa.
d. Small amalgam filling in lingual pit of left lateral incisor.

Figure 3-8 Maxillary central incisor view.

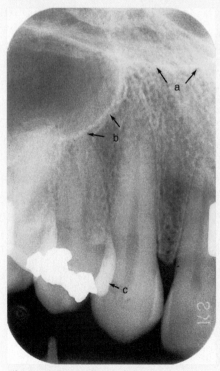

a. Lateral wall of the nasal fossa.
b. Maxillary sinus (anterior wall). The lateral wall of the nasal fossa and the anterior wall of the maxillary sinus form an inverted Y, called the *Y line of Ennis*. The arms of the Y are the sinus wall and nasal fossa wall, and the tail is the continuation of the nasal fossa wall.
c. What does *c* represent? *Answer:* The lingual cusp of the maxillary right first premolar, usually superimposed on the distal aspect of the canine in this view.

Figure 3-9 Maxillary right canine view.

Box **3-2** IDENTIFYING MAXILLARY ANATOMIC LANDMARKS—cont'd

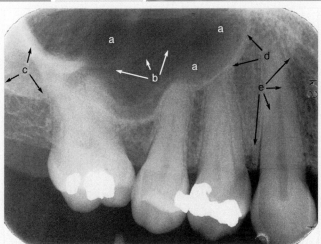

Figure 3-10 Maxillary right premolar view.

a. Right maxillary sinus.
b. Vascular channel (blood vessel).
c. Zygoma (cheek bone).
d. Anterior wall of the maxillary sinus (remember, it comes as far forward as the canine as seen in Fig. 3-9).
e. Nasolabial fold (a soft tissue shadow that runs from the corner of the nose to the corner of the lip).

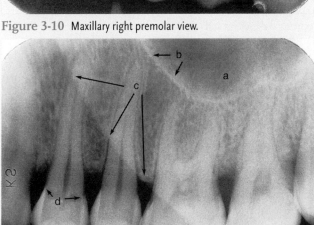

Figure 3-11 Maxillary left premolar view.

a. Left maxillary sinus.
b. What is this? (See Fig. 3-10, *d.*) *Answer:* The anterior wall of the maxillary sinus. It extends superiorly upward in the anterior (front) region.
c. What is this? (See Fig. 3-10, *e.*) *Answer:* The nasolabial fold.
d. What is this? *Answer:* The cementoenamel junction (CEJ), the point where the enamel meets cementum.

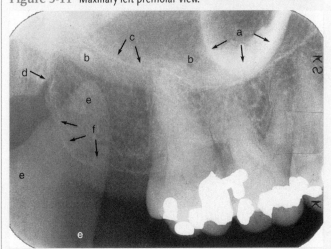

Figure 3-12 Maxillary right molar view.

a. Zygomatic process (U-shaped "strut" of the cheekbone).
b. Body of the zygomatic bone.
c. Floor of the maxillary sinus (fine white line is zygoma superimposed over it).
d. Hamular notch (indentation between the tuberosity and the hamular process of the sphenoid bone).
e. Coronoid process of the mandible (it swings down and forward when the patient opens wide).
f. Maxillary tuberosity.

Continued

Box **3-2** IDENTIFYING MAXILLARY ANATOMIC LANDMARKS—cont'd

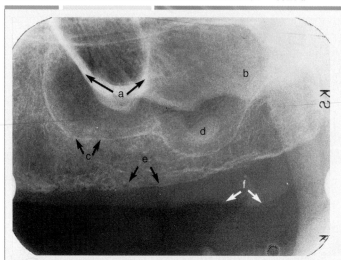

a. Zygomatic process.
b. Body of the zygomatic bone.
c. Floor of the maxillary sinus.
d. Root tip left over from an extraction.
e. Edentulous alveolar crest.
f. Soft tissue outline of the gingival (edentulous) ridge.

Figure 3-13 Maxillary left molar view. (The coronoid process and tuberosity are the most posterior structures.)

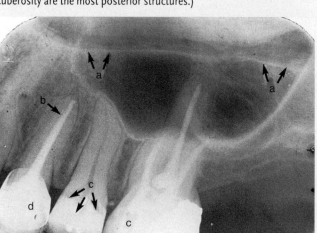

a. Floor of the nasal cavity.
b. Gutta percha (rubbery root canal filling material).
c. Radiopaque (light) tooth-colored filling material.
d. Temporary stainless steel crown.
e. Amalgam (silver) fillings.

Figure 3-14 Maxillary left molar view.

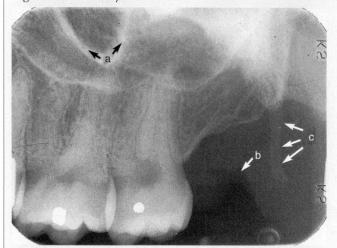

a. Zygomatic process.
b. Soft tissue outline.
c. Hamulus (hamular process); bony projection from the medial pterygoid plate of the sphenoid bone.

Figure 3-15 Maxillary left molar view.

BOX 3-2 IDENTIFYING MAXILLARY ANATOMIC LANDMARKS—cont'd

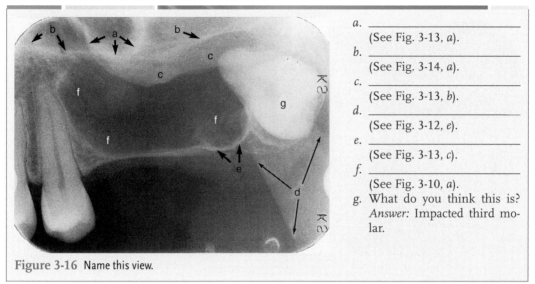

a. _____
   (See Fig. 3-13, *a*).
b. _____
   (See Fig. 3-14, *a*).
c. _____
   (See Fig. 3-13, *b*).
d. _____
   (See Fig. 3-12, *e*).
e. _____
   (See Fig. 3-13, *c*).
f. _____
   (See Fig. 3-10, *a*).
g. What do you think this is?
   Answer: Impacted third molar.

Figure 3-16 Name this view.

BOX 3-3 IDENTIFYING MANDIBULAR ANATOMIC LANDMARKS

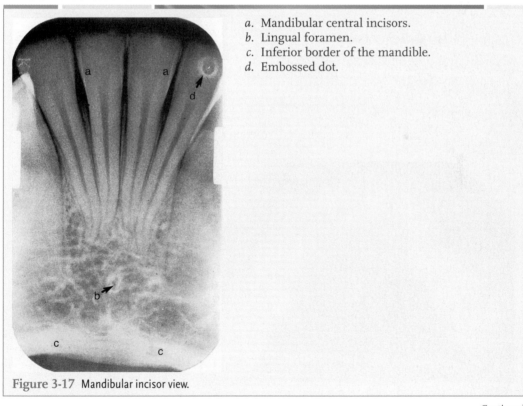

a. Mandibular central incisors.
b. Lingual foramen.
c. Inferior border of the mandible.
d. Embossed dot.

Figure 3-17 Mandibular incisor view.

Continued

Box **3-3** Identifying Mandibular Anatomic Landmarks—cont'd

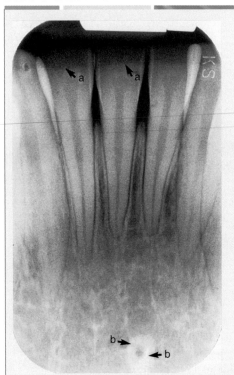

a. Soft tissue outline of lower lip.
b. Genial tubercles (opaque "doughnut") surrounding the lingual foramen (*dark dot;* see Fig. 3-17).

Figure 3-18 Mandibular incisor view.

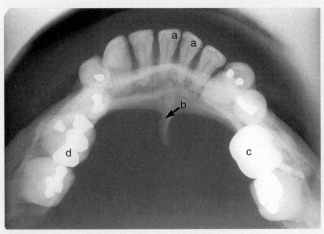

a. Mandibular central incisors.
b. Genial tubercles.
c. Gold crown.
d. Amalgam filling.

Figure 3-19 Mandibular occlusal radiograph.

Box 3-3 IDENTIFYING MANDIBULAR ANATOMIC LANDMARKS—cont'd

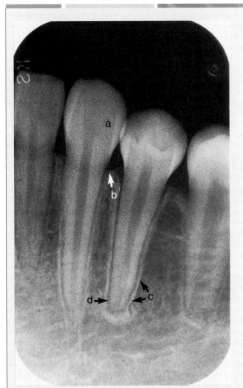

a. Mandibular left canine.
b. Alveolar crestal bone.
c. What is this? (See Fig. 3-4.)
d. What is this? (See Fig. 3-4.)

Figure 3-20 Mandibular left canine view.

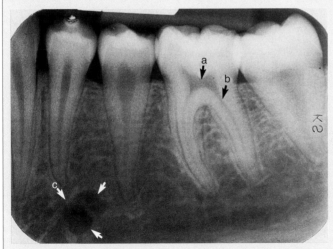

a. Pulp chamber.
b. Root canal (pulp canal).
c. Mental foramen (exit for contents of mandibular canal; almost always lies near the apices of the premolars).

Figure 3-21 Mandibular left premolar view.

Continued

Box **3-3** Identifying Mandibular Anatomic Landmarks—cont'd

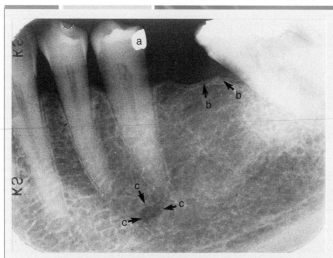

a. Small amalgam (silver) filling.
b. Alveolar crest.
c. What is this? *Hint:* It is the radiolucent (dark) area near the apices of the mandibular premolar teeth (see Fig. 3-21).

Figure 3-22 Mandibular left premolar view.

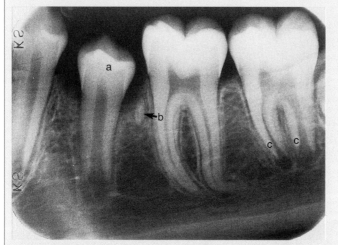

a. Erupting second premolar.
b. Retained root tip of second primary molar.
c. Developing apices of second molar. *Note:* The mental foramen, so prominent in Fig. 3-21, is *not* seen in this image.

Figure 3-23 Mandibular left premolar view.

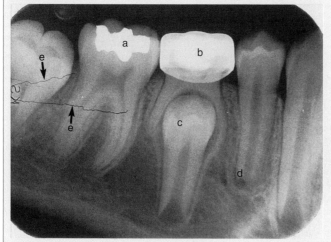

a. Amalgam filling.
b. Stainless steel crown on second primary molar.
c. Developing second premolar.
d. Developing apex of first premolar, which erupts around age 9 and finishes root formation about 2 to 3 years later. Therefore, this patient's age is _____ years. *Hint:* The second molar, or "12-year molar," erupts around age 12.
e. Artifact, possibly dust, thread, or static.

Figure 3-24 Mandibular right premolar view.

Box 3-3 IDENTIFYING MANDIBULAR ANATOMIC LANDMARKS—cont'd

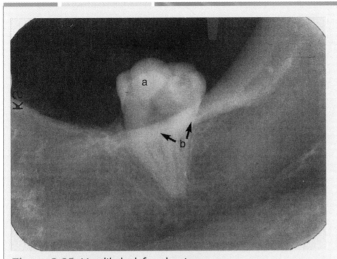

Figure 3-25   Mandibular left molar view.

a. Mandibular third molar (wisdom tooth).
b. External oblique ridge.

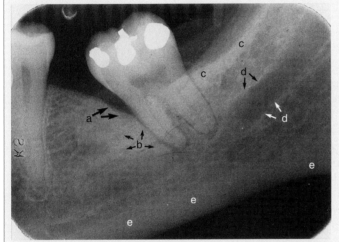

Figure 3-26   Mandibular left molar view.

a. Vertical bone defect.
b. Alveolar bone.
c. External oblique ridge.
d. Mandibular canal (inferior alveolar canal).
e. Inferior border of mandible (lower cortical border).

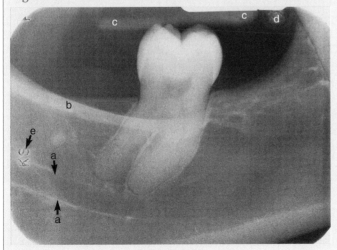

Figure 3-27   Mandibular right molar view.

a. Mandibular canal.
b. External oblique ridge.
c. Plastic bite block of film holder.
d. Embossed dot.
e. Manufacturer's film code.

Continued

Box 3-3 IDENTIFYING MANDIBULAR ANATOMIC LANDMARKS—cont'd

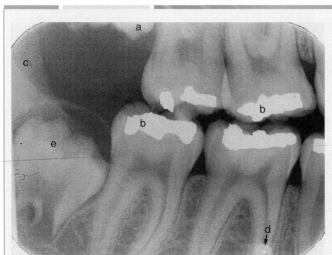

a. Developing unerupted maxillary third molar.
b. Amalgam fillings.
c. Ascending ramus.
d. Embossed dot.
e. Developing mandibular third molar.

Figure 3-28 Mandibular right molar bitewing.

Maxillary Images

The tooth that is centered in Figure 3-29 is a maxillary lateral incisor. Is it in the left or right side of the maxillary dental arch? First, you must determine which side of the image is anterior (toward the midline, or mesial) and which is posterior (or distal).

Which tooth is the central incisor? It is the one to the right of the lateral incisor. Therefore, the midline, or the front (anterior) part of the mouth, is to the right side of the image, if one assumes that the embossed dot is facing up. The maxillary canine (canines have big, long roots) is to the left of the lateral incisor and is distal to it. Recall that the lingual cusp of the first premolar, in Figure 3-29, is usually overlapped on the distal part of the canine. Therefore, we are looking at the *patient's right side*. If you look at patients from the front, their central incisors are to the right (mesial, toward the midline) of their right lateral incisors, and their canines will be to the left of (distal to, posterior to) the lateral incisors.

How does the knowledge of normal anatomy confirm this conclusion? Look at the structure labeled *a* in Figure 3-29. It is the maxillary sinus. It begins near the maxillary canine region. Therefore, *d* must be the maxillary canine. It has the correct shape, and its root length is appropriately longer than that of the lateral incisor. What is *b* then? It is the nasal cavity or fossa (see Figs. 3-6 through 3-9).

The arrows pointing to structure *c* in Figure 3-29 then demonstrate the right ala (side, or "wing") of the nose.

In Figure 3-30, structure *a* is the maxillary canine. What is *b*? It is the nasolabial fold, or the crease in the skin between the corner of the nose and the corner of the lip. This fold always runs obliquely downward in an anterior (front)-to-posterior (back) direction. Therefore, this must be a maxillary left premolar view. How can we confirm this?

Look at the structure labeled *c*. This is the maxillary sinus. Notice that it rises in the region of the premolar. The section rising is the anterior wall of the maxillary sinus (see Fig. 3-9, *b*); it is higher in the anterior region. With the correct identification of both the maxillary sinus and the shadow of the nasolabial fold, you can properly mount intraoral images of partially edentulous or even completely edentulous regions.

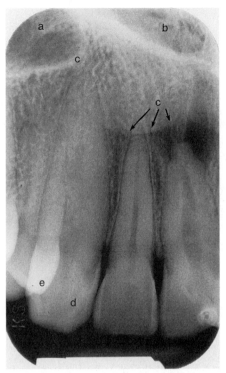

Figure 3-29 Maxillary right lateral incisor view.

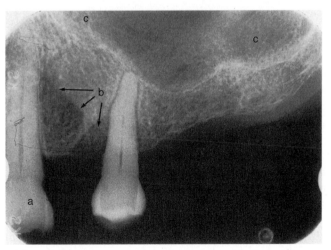

Figure 3-30 Maxillary left premolar view.

In Figure 3-31, what is the structure labeled *a*? It is the coronoid process. Is it anterior or posterior in the mouth? It is posterior. What is the structure labeled *b*? It is the tuberosity. It, too, is a posterior structure. Therefore, the left side of the image is the posterior and the right side is the anterior. Thus this must be a maxillary *right* molar view because as you look at a patient's right side, the more posterior structures will be on your left-hand side.

In Figure 3-32, what is the structure labeled *a*? What is the structure labeled *b*? What is this view? Identification of this view is a bit tricky.

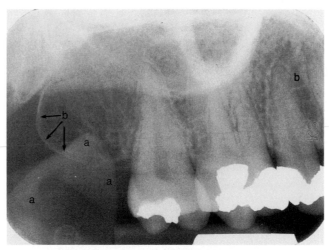

Figure 3-31 Maxillary right molar view.

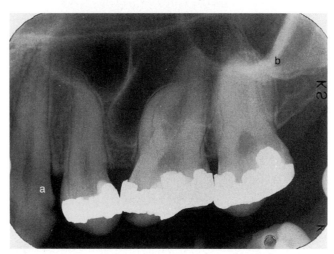

Figure 3-32 Maxillary left molar view.

The maxillary first premolar has been extracted. The operator decided to use one image to record all the teeth from the canine to the second molar. Therefore, this is a premolar view that records all the posterior teeth. This view was possible only because the operator knew that both the first premolar *and* the third molar had been previously extracted. The structure *a* is the canine; *b* is the zygomatic process. Can you identify the floor of the nasal cavity?

Mandibular Images

The mandibular central incisor view (Fig. 3-33) should not be difficult to identify because no other image will contain four mandibular incisors. As long as the embossed dot *(arrow)* is raised, you can identify *a* as the mandibular *right* central incisor, *b* as the mandibular *right* lateral incisor, and *c* as the mandibular *left* central incisor.

Is Figure 3-34 a maxillary or a mandibular canine view? What anatomic space, or lucency, is seen in a *maxillary* canine view? The maxillary sinus and/or the nasal

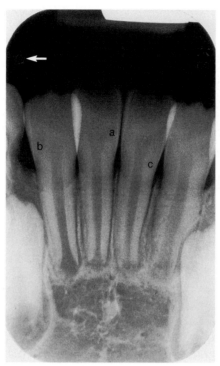

Figure 3-33 Mandibular incisor view.

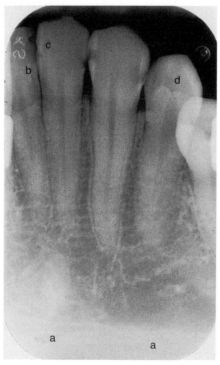

Figure 3-34 Mandibular left canine view.

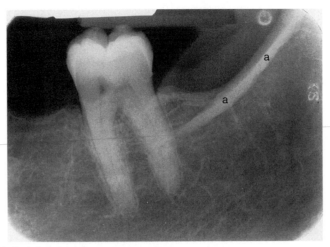

Figure 3-35 Mandibular left molar view.

cavity. Is it seen here? No. What is the structure labeled *a* (see Fig. 3-17)? It is mandibular cortical bone and the inferior border of the mandible. Therefore, because the image shows no sinus or nasal cavity, but it does show a view of the mandibular cortex, this must be a mandibular view, in which *b* is the mandibular left central incisor, *c* is the mandibular left lateral incisor, and *d* is the mandibular left first premolar. We can conclude that this is the *left* mandibular canine view.

Figure 3-35 is a molar view. Can you identify the structure labeled *a*? It is the external oblique ridge (see Figs. 3-25 to 3-27) and is in the posterior part of the mandible. Therefore, this is a mandibular left molar view. The anterior part of the mouth is to your left. The external oblique ridge always runs obliquely downward from posterior to anterior. This is not a maxillary view because there is no sinus seen.

SUMMARY

These illustrations demonstrate that you must always rely on your knowledge of normal anatomy to arrange and mount images that you expose. Remember that the embossed dot on film should always be raised. It will be the only time in your life that you want a pimple instead of a dimple! You can feel the bump of the dot with your fingers. An incorrectly mounted radiograph could result in misidentification of teeth and the wrong dental procedure being performed on a patient.

Review this chapter until you feel confident that you can identify the normal anatomic landmarks accurately. Refer to this chapter if you have any doubts about the correct orientation of images as you mount them.

STUDY QUESTIONS

1. Which of the following structures is considered to be radiolucent (dark)?
   A. Zygomatic process
   B. Lamina dura
   C. Dental enamel
   D. Mental foramen

2. Which of the following structures is considered to be radiopaque (light)?
    A. Periodontal ligament space
    B. Maxillary sinus
    C. Pulp chamber
    D. Genial tubercles

3. When you view mounted images with the raised dot facing you, which of the following statements is true?
    A. The patient's left side is on your left
    B. The patient's left side is on your right
    C. You are looking at the patient's teeth as if you were sitting on the patient's tongue looking outward
    D. You cannot tell left from right unless the films are labeled

4. Which of the following is a helpful hint for mounting radiographs?
    A. Maxillary central incisors have shorter roots and smaller crowns than mandibular incisors
    B. The longer side of the film is oriented vertically for posterior teeth
    C. The overall appearance of the survey will have an upward curve like a smile
    D. Mandibular molars have three roots, whereas maxillary molars have only two

5. Which of the following structures would you expect to see on a mandibular premolar periapical image?
    A. Mental foramen
    B. Maxillary sinus
    C. Nasal cavity
    D. Intermaxillary suture

6. You would expect to see all of the following structures on a maxillary molar periapical view except one. Which one is the exception?
    A. Maxillary sinus
    B. Maxillary tuberosity
    C. Inferior alveolar canal
    D. Zygomatic process

7. Have you answered the questions for Figure 3-16?

4

X-Ray Properties and the Generation of X Rays

THE DISCOVERY OF X RAYS

The first three chapters taught basic techniques of radiographic imaging. But how did the "magic" happen? How were the x rays produced? What properties do they possess that allow them to record the patient's image on film or an image receptor? We'll begin with the discovery of x rays.

Wilhelm Conrad Roentgen (pronounced "rent-gen") was a Bavarian physicist who lived from 1845-1925. He discovered x rays while experimenting with Hittorf-Crookes tubes. These sealed glass tubes were partially evacuated; only small amounts of air were inside. Each tube contained a cathode and an anode. When Roentgen applied high-voltage currents to one of these tubes, he noticed that a fluorescent screen near the tube glowed. Roentgen placed various materials, including his own hand, between the tube and the screen to determine whether the "rays" coming from the tube could be obstructed. The resulting image of his hand bones on the fluorescent screen changed medical history. Roentgen had discovered x rays on November 8, 1895.

PROPERTIES OF X RAYS

X rays themselves are not unique. They are part of a spectrum of electromagnetic radiation, some rays of which are visible and some invisible (Fig. 4-1). However, x rays have properties that make them especially useful in medicine and dentistry. X rays can

1. Penetrate matter
2. Produce a **latent image** on film or an image receptor
3. Produce **fluorescence** in certain materials
4. Produce **ionization** of matter

The remainder of this chapter discusses the properties of x-ray *penetration* and *ionization*. The production of a latent image and the production of screen fluorescence are discussed in other chapters.

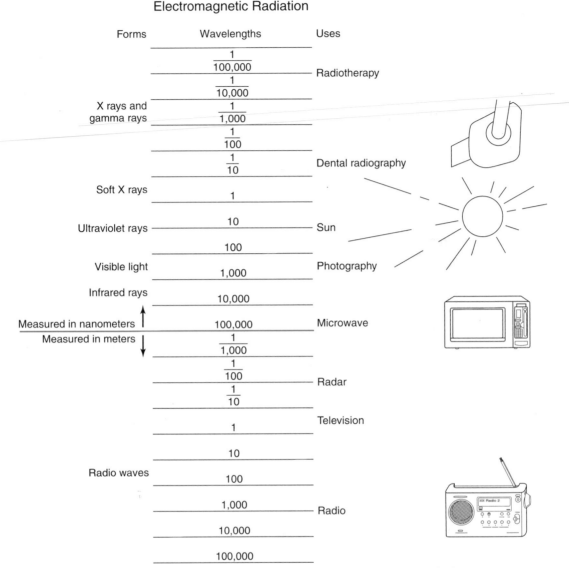

Figure 4-1 Electronic spectrum showing the various wavelengths of commonly used types of radiation.

Particulate Radiation

X rays are "packets" of energy that travel, with properties of *both* waves and particles. An x ray as a particle or bundle of energy is termed an x-ray **photon.** The x-ray photon has no mass or charge and moves in straight lines at the speed of light (186,000 miles per second). These x-ray photons interact with electrons in the x-ray tube, in the patient, and on the image receptor.

Interactions of x rays with the electrons within the tubehead or the patient are called ionizations. Ionization is the process whereby electrons are removed from atoms through collisions with x-ray photons. The atoms that lose electrons become positively charged ions. Both the positive ions (ionized atoms) and the negatively charged ions (electrons) are unstable structures. The electrons ejected from the atom can speed off to interact with other atoms, tissues, and chemicals. The positive ions can also interact but usually return to a stable state. The importance of

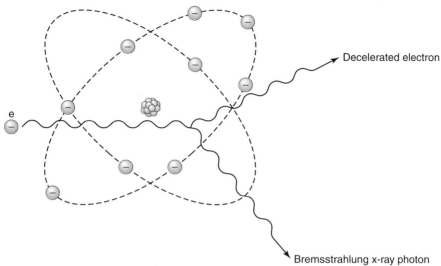

Figure 4-2 Bremsstrahlung radiation. This radiation occurs in the target anode material. The incoming electron (from the cathode) slows as it is drawn to the nucleus of the atom. Some of the energy lost in the deceleration is emitted as an x-ray photon with energy equal to that lost by the electron.

the process of ionization in biologic tissues is discussed in Chapter 5. This chapter explains how x rays are produced by collisions of high-speed electrons with a metal "target" in the dental x-ray tube. The physics of such interactions is termed *quantum physics* or *quantum theory*, the discussion of which is beyond the scope of this book. However, some basic interactions that produce the types of radiation called bremsstrahlung radiation and characteristic radiation are described here.

Bremsstrahlung Radiation

Bremsstrahlung radiation is produced when an electron passes near the nucleus of an atom. The negatively charged (–) electron is deflected by the positively charged (+) nucleus. The energy lost by the deceleration of the electron is emitted in the form of a photon of radiation called *bremsstrahlung* (from the German word for *braking*) radiation. This process is diagrammed in Figure 4-2. Braking radiation is the primary kind of radiation produced in the dental x-ray tubehead.

Characteristic Radiation

Characteristic radiation results when an electron within an atom is ejected from the inner orbit of the atom by an incoming high-speed electron. With the loss of the electron from the inner orbit, the atom becomes very unstable (and positively charged, or ionized). The vacancy left by the ejected electron is soon filled by an electron from an outer orbit. As this new electron "drops down" into the inner orbit, some of its energy is emitted as a specific kind of x radiation called characteristic radiation. This radiation is specific to, or characteristic of, the particular atom in which the interaction occurs. Each element emits a particular characteristic energy when its atoms are bombarded. This process is diagrammed in Figure 4-3.

Characteristic radiation makes up only a small portion of the x rays produced in a dental x-ray unit. However, a process similar to the production of characteristic radiation occurs when x-ray photons interact with the patient's tissues. The incoming x-ray photon ejects an electron from its orbit in the patient's molecule, another

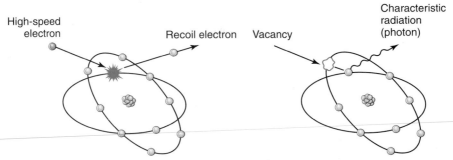

Figure 4-3 The incoming high-speed electron ejects an *inner* electron from the atom; this vacant position is then filled by an *outer* electron. Energy left over by the difference between these two electrons is given off as characteristic radiation with an energy specific to the atom being bombarded.

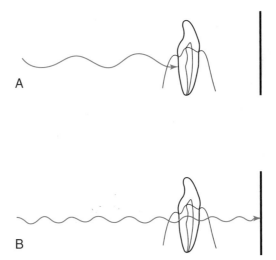

Figure 4-4 X ray **A** has a long wavelength; that is, the distance between its peaks is greater than for x ray **B**. It is therefore less energetic and less penetrating and will usually be stopped within the object it enters. Its energy will be deposited in that object. X ray **B** has a shorter wavelength and is therefore more energetic and more penetrating; it proceeds through the material to strike the image receptor and registers a portion of the image of that object.

electron fills the vacancy, and radiation is emitted from the patient. The interaction of patient tissues and radiation from x rays is presented in more detail in Chapter 5.

Electromagnetic Radiation

Examples of electromagnetic waves or radiation are radiowaves, microwaves, cosmic rays, and visible light (see Fig. 4-1). Visible light is a spectrum of colored rays with different wavelengths. The visible rays are those seen in the colors of a rainbow; the invisible rays are *ultraviolet* (above our eyes' range) and *infrared* (below our eyes' range). X rays, too, are an invisible spectrum that has its own range of wavelengths, which determines the frequency of the waves. The shorter the wavelength, that is, the more waves that pass a particular point in a given time, the higher the wave frequency. High-frequency, short-wavelength x rays are more penetrating; low-frequency, long-wavelength x rays are less penetrating. Figure 4-4 shows two x rays with different wavelengths and frequencies. The shorter wavelength radiation (*B*) is more penetrating than the longer (*A*). An x ray is made more or less penetrating in a dental tubehead by the selection of a high or low kilovoltage.

Kilovoltage

A **volt (V)** is a unit of electrical potential that can be considered a measure of work capacity. In an electrical system, the potential difference between a negatively and a positively charged pole creates an electrical "pressure." The greater the electrical potential, the more pressure or potential energy in the system. Higher voltages mean greater energies. Normal household voltage is 120 V; some extraoral x-ray units may require 220 V.

The x-ray machine converts 120 V to the several thousand volts needed to generate x rays by means of a step-up transformer. A transformer is an electromagnetic device that changes current from low to high voltage or vice versa. A step-up transformer raises the voltage, whereas a step-down transformer lowers it (Fig. 4-5). The electrical potential between the **cathode** (negative side) and **anode** (positive side) in an x-ray unit is increased to such a high level that it is measured in **kilovolts (kV)** rather than V. One kV equals 1000 V. Some dental x-ray machines allow the operator to select a **kilovoltage peak (kVp)**, or maximum, setting in the range of 50 to 100 kV. Other units have predetermined kVp settings: 70 kVp is a common setting, although it may be as low as 60 kVp or as high as 90 kVp.

A higher kVp setting will produce x rays that are more energetic, have greater penetrating power, and have a greater capacity to pass through matter. Low-energy x rays tend to be absorbed by the matter through which they pass, including body tissues. If the x rays are absorbed by the patient, they will not reach the image receptor to make an image. Therefore, kilovoltages lower than 60 kVp are rarely used in dentistry. The amount of energy in an x-ray beam is sometimes referred to as the *quality* of the beam. The kVp setting on the x-ray machine influences the *quality*, or energy level, of the x rays produced.

As mentioned, the kVp settings for dental x-ray machines are usually in the range of 70 kVp. However, for every 15% increase in kilovoltage, the density (or darkness) on the resulting image will double. Although 15 kV is a little more than 15% of 70 kV, a 15-kV rule works well as a baseline. Going from 70 kV to 85 kV essentially doubles the density of the image. Stated another way, *increasing the kilovoltage* by 15 would require *decreasing an exposure* time by one half to keep the image density (darkness) the same. Conversely, decreasing the kilovoltage by 15 requires doubling the exposure time to keep the image density the same.

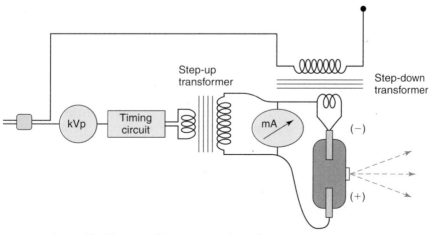

Figure 4-5 Extremely simplified diagram of the circuitry and transformers involved in x-ray production.

Milliamperage

An **ampere (A)** is the unit of electrical current, or the number of electrons flowing, in an electrical circuit. The amount of current needed in an x-ray machine is very low, and the amperage is measured in **milliamperes (mA)**, or $\frac{1}{1000}$ A. Some dental x-ray units offer a choice of milliamperage settings, usually 10 and 15 mA. Other dental x-ray units may have a predetermined single milliamperage setting, perhaps as low as 6 or 7 mA.

The current in the filament circuit in an x-ray machine is used to heat a very thin wire (a **filament**) made of tungsten, similar to the filament in a light bulb. Heating the filament agitates the tungsten atoms; some of the electrons in these atoms escape from their orbits. This action, called **thermionic emission**, can be thought of as a "boiling off" of tungsten electrons. Although the process is different, think of the concept as similar to water molecules escaping as steam from boiling water. The tungsten electrons that have been boiled off form a cloud around the filament, and it is these "free" electrons that are ultimately responsible for generating x rays.

As a greater amount of current is applied to the filament, more heat is generated and more electrons are boiled off. The milliamperage setting in the x-ray unit influences the current flowing through the filament and therefore the number, or *quantity*, of x rays that will be produced in the x-ray tube. The other factor that influences the number (quantity) of x rays produced is the *length of the exposure time*. In some dental x-ray units, the time of exposure is the only factor within the operator's control (Fig. 4-6).

COMPONENTS OF A DENTAL X-RAY TUBE

Cathode

The cathode is the negatively charged end of an x-ray tube. In a dental x-ray tube, the cathode consists of the tungsten filament and a focusing cup (Fig. 4-7).

Focusing Cup

The **focusing cup** has a negative electrostatic charge and is usually made of molybdenum. The shape of the cup and its negative charge repel the electrons (also negatively charged) coming from the filament and keep them suspended in a "cloud" around the filament. When the high-voltage circuit is activated, the focusing cup's charge and shape help direct the electrons toward the anode and prevent them from spreading out and missing the target.

Anode

The anode, the positive end of the x-ray tube, is made of tungsten and copper. A small block of tungsten is embedded in a larger copper stem or sleeve to act as the target for the electrons. Tungsten is used because it has a high atomic number and thus can produce many x rays. In addition, tungsten has a high melting point (remember the heat produced) and a low vapor pressure. It will not melt, or vaporize, unless extremely long exposures are made or unless many exposures are made in a short period of time. Copper is used around the tungsten target to conduct heat rapidly away from the target, thus reducing the wear by heat on the target.

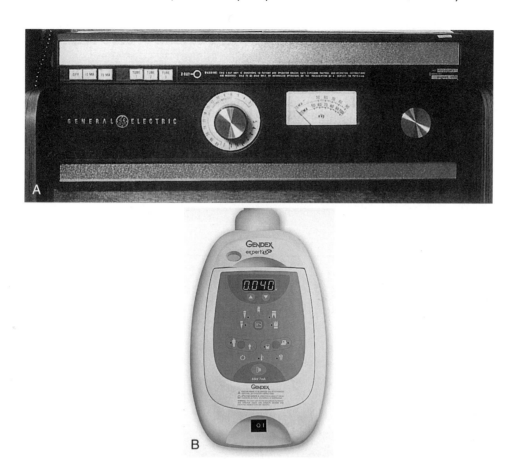

Figure 4-6 **A,** Example of control panel with milliamperage selector, kilovoltage peak selector, and exposure time selector. The panel is capable of controlling as many as three different tubeheads. **B,** Example of a control panel that uses tooth icons for selecting exposure times. Exposure time is the only setting that can be changed. *(A: From Razmus TF, Williamson GF:* Current oral and maxillofacial imaging, *ed 1, Philadelphia, 1996, Saunders. B: Courtesy of Gendex Dental Systems, Lake Zurich, Ill.)*

Filter

In most dental x-ray tubes, an aluminum **filter** in the form of a disk is placed at the port, or opening, of the open-ended cylinder (Fig. 4-8). The small fraction of x rays that is allowed to escape (1%) must pass through this filter. Many of the lower-energy x rays, those with long wavelengths, are prevented from reaching the patient or the image receptor by this added filter. By law, dental x-ray machines operating below 70 kV must have 1.5 mm of added aluminum filtration. Those with a kVp of 70 or above must have 2.5 mm of aluminum filtration. The additional filtration required for the higher kilovolt machines is necessary because of the higher average energy (mean energy) of the x rays produced in these machines. The filtration is necessary to remove low-energy x rays, which add to the absorbed dose in the patient's skin but do not contribute to image formation.

Tubehead Housing

All the structures discussed so far are surrounded by a glass envelope in a vacuum environment. The glass envelope, in turn, is housed by metal (usually lead). The metal insulates the **tubehead** components and reduces the amount of radiation that can leak from the tubehead housing.

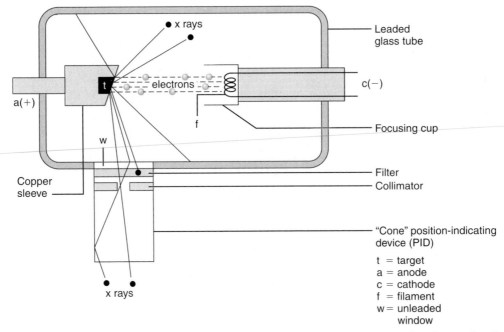

Figure 4-7 Schematic drawing of a conventional dental x-ray tube. The x rays are represented as photons (bundles or packets of energy). The leaded glass does not permit many x rays to exit the tube. In fact, most of the x rays are absorbed by the leaded glass. The photons that are used for diagnosis escape the tube through the unleaded window.

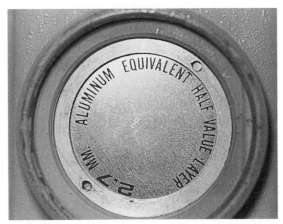

Figure 4-8 This demonstrates the added filtration in an x-ray unit: an aluminum disk placed near the exit on part of the tubehead. The cylinder has been removed so that the disk is visible.

Oil

Within the tubehead, the glass tube is immersed in oil to help absorb the heat created by x-ray production (Fig. 4-9). X-ray production is very inefficient: 99% of the energy used to generate x rays is lost as heat.

Collimator

The **collimator** is a disk of metal, usually lead, that has a small aperture that restricts the size or shape of the x-ray beam as it exits the tubehead (Fig. 4-10). Thus, collimation is the restriction of the x-ray beam size by a lead diaphragm. According to

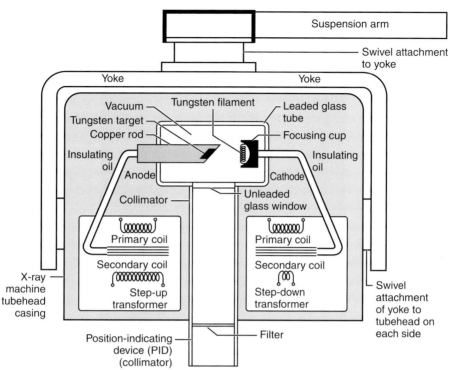

Figure 4-9 Schematic drawing of a conventional x-ray tubehead and its major components. The leaded glass x-ray tube is surrounded by oil to help dissipate the heat produced during the generation of x rays. The tubehead also contains two transformers (a step-up transformer and a step-down transformer). The step-up transformer creates the thousands of volts in the high-voltage circuit, and the step-down transformer helps create the low-milliamperage current. *(Redrawn from Razmus TF, Williamson GF:* Current oral and maxillofacial imaging, *ed 1, Philadelphia, 1996, Saunders.)*

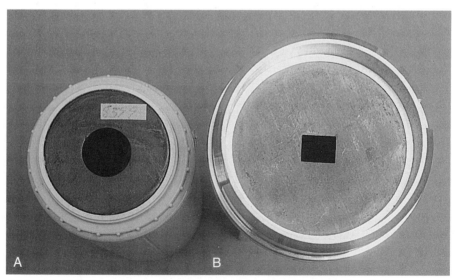

Figure 4-10 A, Lead diaphragm for round cylinder. **B,** Lead diaphragm for rectangular cylinder.

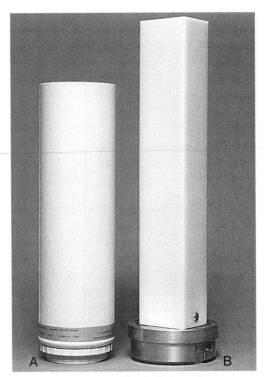

Figure 4-11 Round and rectangular open-ended, lead-lined cylinders. These screw into the x-ray tubehead housing, providing secondary collimation and allowing the operator to aim the x-ray beam.

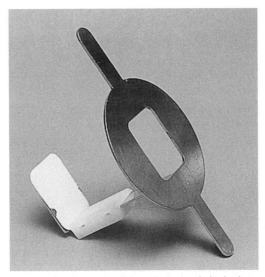

Figure 4-12 Film-holding device that may be used with round open-ended cylinders to further collimate the x-ray beam to a rectangular shape.

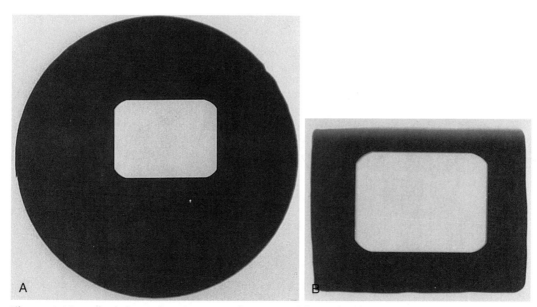

Figure 4-13 A, The dark, round area represents the amount of skin surface that would be exposed using a round open-ended cylinder. The white area is a size no. 2 film. **B,** The dark rectangle is the skin surface area exposed using a rectangular cylinder. The white area is a size no. 2 film. The patient is exposed to less radiation when rectangular collimation is used.

federal regulations, the diameter of the restricted beam must not exceed 2¾ inches (7 cm) at the patient's skin surface.

Lead-lined cones or cylinders effect a second collimation of the x-ray beam. Figure 4-11, A shows an example of a standard open-ended cylinder. This cylinder further directs the x-ray beam to the area of interest. Some manufacturers have introduced rectangular collimating devices (Figs. 4-11, B and 4-12) that reduce the beam size even more and consequently reduce the skin surface area exposed to x rays. The description of the technique in Chapter 1 using the paralleling instruments included examples of rectangular collimators. Figure 4-13 illustrates the dramatic reduction in skin surface area exposed to the beam when a rectangular "cone" is used.

PRODUCTION OF X RAYS

Following is a step-by-step explanation in Box 4-1 of the way x rays are produced in an x-ray tube. Although it seems like a long and complicated process, it occurs instantaneously when the exposure button is pressed. You may want to refer to Figure 4-7 for a review of the dental x-ray tube components.

Box **4-1 Production of X Rays**

1. The operator turns on the x-ray machine.
2. The operator selects the kilovoltage peak and milliamperage settings, if appropriate. Many machines do not allow for such adjustments.
3. The operator selects the exposure time. The exposure time is the length of time the x rays are actually produced. In dental units, this time is usually less than 1 second.
4. The operator pushes the exposure button.

Continued

BOX 4-1 PRODUCTION OF X RAYS—cont'd

5. Electrical current passing through the filament boils off electrons through thermionic emission.
6. The potential difference between the cathode (negatively charged side) and the anode (positively charged side) of the tube is activated. The electrons, which have a negative charge, are attracted to the positive anode at extremely high speeds. Nothing impedes their progress because the x-ray tube is a vacuum tube; there are no air molecules inside it.
7. The electrons from the filament collide with the target at the anode end of the tube. The collision of the high-speed electrons against the target produces energy in the form of x rays.
8. X rays are generated in all directions (360°) from the target. The x rays travel at the speed of light.
9. Most of the x rays produced are absorbed by the leaded glass x-ray tube and the metal housing surrounding the x-ray tube.
10. A small portion of the x rays generated escape the x-ray tube through an unleaded area in the glass (the *window*).
11. These escaped x rays then pass through a filter, which absorbs the less useful, lower-energy x rays in the beam.
12. The x-ray beam then passes through a lead collimator, which restricts the spread of the beam. The x rays that pass through the opening in the collimator (the *port*) travel through the x-ray cone to reach the patient and the image receptor.

STUDY QUESTIONS

1. Which of the following is not a characteristic of an x ray?
   A. It travels with a wavelike motion
   B. It travels at 186,000 miles per second in a vacuum
   C. It causes ionization in matter
   D. It has a mass equal to its density

2. Which of the following statements is false?
   A. X-ray photons with the highest energy have the shortest wavelengths
   B. The kilovoltage determines the energy or quality of the x rays
   C. Changing the milliamperage alters the wavelengths of the x rays
   D. The number of electrons released in the "boiling off" process affects the number of x-ray photons produced

3. A beam that is properly collimated should
   A. Pass through a 1.5-mm aluminum disk at the exit or portal
   B. Pass through a 2.5-mm aluminum disk at the exit or portal
   C. Be restricted to a diameter of 2 inches at the skin surface
   D. Be restricted to a diameter of 2¾ inches at the skin surface

4. X rays are actually produced in the tube by
   A. Radioactive decay of particulate matter
   B. Electrical current passing through a mixture of oil and gases, creating minute explosions
   C. High-speed electrons colliding with electrons in the target, giving off radiation
   D. High-speed photons colliding with electrons in the oil mixture and target

5. What percentage of the energy generated by the collision between electrons from the cathode and the anode is actually converted to x rays?
    A. 1%
    B. 15%
    C. 70%
    D. 99%

6. The term *thermionic emission* refers to
    A. The heating of the tungsten filament to such a degree that electrons "boil off" and form a cloud around the filament
    B. The excessive production of heat that occurs during x-ray production
    C. The ability of the x rays emitted from the x-ray tube to produce reddening of the skin when overexposure occurs
    D. The radioactive contamination that is produced but contained within the x-ray tube during x-ray generation

7. The greater the difference between the negative side and the positive side of the x-ray tube (the greater the electrical "pressure"), the greater the speed of the electrons flying from one side of the tube to the other. The greater the speed is, the greater the impact on collision. This description refers to the effect of changing the
    A. Milliamperage
    B. Kilovoltage
    C. Exposure time
    D. Filtration

8. Filtration is used to
    A. Remove excessive amounts of electrons
    B. Narrow the beam to a specified diameter
    C. Absorb excessive heat during x-ray production
    D. Remove long-wavelength x-ray photons

9. The anode contains the
    A. Positively charged target and is where primary x-ray production takes place
    B. Positively charged filament and is where electrons are released during thermionic emission
    C. Negatively charged target and is where primary x-ray production takes place
    D. Negatively charged filament and is where primary x-ray production takes place

10. Most of the energy during x-ray generation is transferred from kinetic energy (the energy of motion from the high-speed electrons) to energy in the form of
    A. X-ray photons
    B. Heat
    C. Light
    D. Radioactive decay

5

Radiation Biology and Protection

You will frequently hear from your patients, "I've heard x rays are bad for me; they cause cancer. Do you really need to take them?" Aside from educating your patients about the diagnostic importance of dental radiographs, you will have to address their fears of radiation. What will you tell them? What do you, as a person working with radiation, need to know about it to keep your exposure and your patient's exposure to a minimum?

The science of the effects of radiation on living organisms is called *radiation biology*. This chapter discusses these effects as they apply to the biologic molecules and cells of the body. It also discusses how much radiation is involved in dental radiographic procedures, the risks that are involved with these exposures, and how to protect yourself and your patient from unnecessary or excessive exposure to x radiation.

EFFECTS OF RADIATION ON MOLECULES

As a beam of x radiation passes through matter, it gradually loses its energy, weakens, and eventually disappears. The energy of the beam is transferred to the material through which it passes. This transfer of energy is called **absorption.**

Direct Effects

Diagnostic x radiation interacts with matter at the atomic level in body tissues in three main ways. These interactions are called *classic scattering*, the **photoelectric effect**, and the *Compton effect* (Fig. 5-1). The latter two interactions result in **ionization** of atoms; that is, an atom either gains or loses an electron and acquires a positive or negative charge.

Classic Scattering (Coherent Scattering or Thomson Scattering)

When a low-energy x-ray photon approaches an outer orbital electron of an atom, it may not have enough energy to eject the electron from its orbit. Instead, the photon may interact with the electron and cause it to be excited, or to vibrate. The photon transfers all of its energy to the excited electron, and the photon ceases to exist.

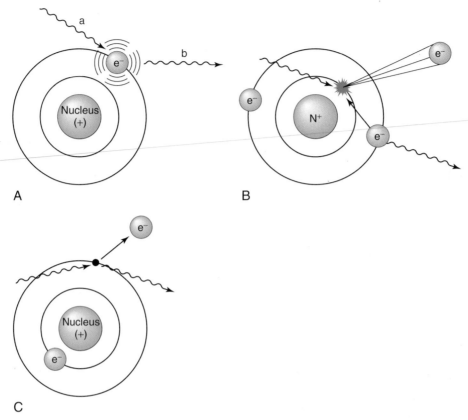

Figure 5-1 Schematic representations of possible interactions between incoming x-ray photons and matter. **A,** Classic scattering. **B,** Photoelectric effect. **C,** Compton effect.

The vibrating electron then radiates its newly acquired energy in the form of another x-ray photon with the same energy level as the first photon. The new photon exits the atom, usually in a different direction (see Fig. 5-1, A), and the atom goes back to its original energy state and is unchanged. The radiation, then, has "scattered," and no ionization has occurred. In diagnostic radiology, little of this classic scattering occurs.

Photoelectric Effect

The photoelectric interaction occurs when an x-ray photon of sufficient energy collides with an inner orbiting electron in an atom. All of the energy from the photon is used to eject the electron from its orbit, and the photon ceases to exist. The atom absorbs the radiation with no scatter. The ejected electron speeds away from the atom as a recoil electron.

When the atom loses one of its inner orbiting electrons, one of the electrons in an outer orbit drops down to fill the vacancy left by the recoil electron. When the other electron moves to another level in the atom, energy is given off in the form of an x-ray photon. Each orbit of every type of atom has a specific energy level, and the photon that is generated in this process will have that specific energy (see Fig. 5-1, B).

The atom is still missing one electron (now one of the outer electrons) and thus has a net positive charge. An atom with a charge is called an *ion,* and it can interact with other atoms and molecules. The photoelectric effect occurs frequently in diagnostic radiography.

Compton Effect

The Compton effect occurs when a photon with sufficient energy collides with an outer orbital electron in an atom, ejecting it from its orbit. In this instance, however, the incoming photon does not transfer all of its energy to the recoil electron but continues in a different direction as a photon with lower energy. The energy of the photon equals the energy of the incident (incoming) photon minus the energy used to eject the electron. Therefore, the Compton effect results in energy absorption by the atom, ionization of the atom, and the release of a newly formed x-ray photon in a different direction (scatter radiation) (see Fig. 5-1, C). The Compton effect and the photoelectric effect occur in nearly equal proportions in dental radiography.

The ionized atoms and the recoil electrons of the photoelectric effect and the Compton effect may cause further molecular interactions in the patient's tissues. These direct effects of radiation may result in

1. Breaking molecules into smaller pieces
2. Disrupting molecular bonds
3. Forming new bonds within molecules
4. Forming new bonds between molecules

These disruptions and new bonds often render a biologic molecule nonfunctional.

Indirect Effects

Molecules not directly affected by x rays can be altered indirectly in tissues that are irradiated. Living organisms consist mostly of water, and usually plenty of oxygen is present in biologic tissues. If an x-ray photon interacts with water and oxygen, compounds called **free radicals** are formed through a process called *radiolysis*. A free radical is uncharged, but highly reactive, and readily interacts with other biologic molecules. Radicals may remove electrons or hydrogen atoms from organic molecules, add new bonds, or initiate intermolecular bonding; any of these interactions may essentially destroy the organic molecule's ability to function normally in tissues.

Examples of radicals created by the radiolysis of water include

$$x\text{-ray photon} + H_2O \rightarrow H^{\cdot} + OH^{\cdot} \text{ (hydrogen radical + hydroxyl radical)} \text{ (initiation)}$$

$$H^{\cdot} + O_2 \rightarrow HO_2^{\cdot} \text{ (hydroxyl radical + oxygen yields a peroxyl radical)}$$

In addition, two hydroxyl radicals ($OH^{\cdot}$) can combine to form hydrogen peroxide (H_2O_2), a chemical toxic to most cells. The reaction would appears as

$$OH^{\cdot} + OH^{\cdot} \rightarrow H_2O_2 \text{ (termination)}$$

An organic molecule, designated as RH, could be altered by either a hydrogen radical or a hydroxyl radical as follows:

$$RH + H^{\cdot} \rightarrow R^{\cdot} + H_2 \text{ (propagation)}$$

$$RH + OH^{\cdot} \rightarrow R^{\cdot} + H_2O$$

The altered organic molecule can then react with other organic molecules, and this reaction chain could continue indefinitely. The effects caused by the radical are not directly the result of an organic molecule being "hit" by radiation. Because the damage is mediated by a free radical, it is referred to as an indirect effect of radiation. The indirect actions of x rays can damage biologic molecules as easily as can the direct actions of a hit. In fact, indirect effects have a higher probability of causing biologic damage than do direct effects. Any changes in an organic molecule, no matter how the molecule is damaged, may result in altered cell function. In summary, indirect effects of radiation include (1) the production of free radicals, which in turn causes (2) the alteration of other molecules. There are causes of free radical formation in the body other than from x radiation. These include chemicals in food, exposure to the sun, and toxins in the air.

EFFECTS OF RADIATION ON CELLS

A cell has two basic components: the nucleus and the cytoplasm. Ionizing radiation may affect either area or both. Damage in the nucleus often affects the chromosomes, which contain deoxyribonucleic acid (DNA). The DNA in each organism is composed of a particular series of bases. The specific order of the DNA bases is the foundation of the genetic code, making each organism unique. Radiation may alter the base sequence of the DNA molecule and make it defective (Fig. 5-2).

Defective DNA may lead to the disruption of the mechanisms for cell division (mitosis). Cell division may be delayed, or the reproductive capacity of the cells may be lost. Errors that are permanently incorporated into the DNA are passed on to future generations of the affected cells as **mutations.** If the defective DNA is contained in a reproductive cell (sperm or ovum), then the defect may be passed along to future generations of organisms. This, then, would be a **genetic effect** of radiation.

Radiation can also affect cellular cytoplasm. Cells may develop the following problems if the cytoplasm is damaged:

1. Increased permeability or rupture of membranes
2. Nonfunctional organelles such as lysosomes, endoplasmic reticulum, or mitochondria
3. Inactivation of enzymes
4. Coagulation of the cytoplasmic fluid

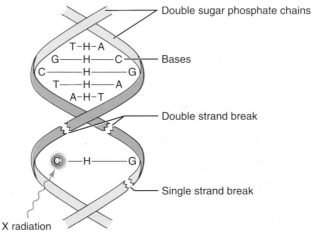

Figure 5-2 X-ray interaction occurs as a "hit" on the target deoxyribonucleic acid (DNA) molecule. The hit damages a portion of the molecule and thus alters the genetic code. The damaged base sequence may be improperly repaired or replaced by a different base sequence, which may make the DNA faulty or nonfunctional. *(Adapted from Kasle MJ, Langlais RP: Basic principles of oral radiography, vol 4, Philadelphia, 1981, WB Saunders.)*

Any one of these changes could result in the disruption of cell function or even cell death.

All body tissues except the reproductive cells are called *somatic* tissues. The **somatic effects** of radiation may occur in the cell cytoplasm or nucleus. If the damage to the cells is severe enough, the organism may become ill or even die. However, somatic effects of radiation are not passed along to future generations of organisms the way genetic effects are. Genetic effects occur only in the reproductive cells.

Cellular Sensitivity to Radiation

Some cells are more sensitive to radiation than others. A cell will be more sensitive to radiation if it has any of the following characteristics:

1.   A high mitotic rate (it undergoes frequent cell division)
2.   A long mitotic history (it undergoes many divisions over time)
3.   A primitive or immature nature (it must undergo further growth or development)
4.   An undifferentiated nature (it is not highly specialized in function)

An exception is the lymphocyte, which is a highly specialized cell that is part of the immune system. It will not divide once it is mature. The small lymphocyte is probably the cell most sensitive to radiation. Table 5-1 lists various groups of cells and their relative radiation sensitivity.

Short- and Long-Term Effects of Radiation

Harmful effects of radiation do not show up immediately. A time lag exists between exposure to radiation and the signs and symptoms of biologic damage. This period, called the **latent period**, may be as short as a few hours or as long as 20 years or more. The length of the latent period depends on the total dose of radiation received and the amount of time it took to receive that dose. The higher the dose and the shorter the dose rate, the shorter the latent period is.

Table 5-1 | **Relative Radiation Sensitivity of Cells and Tissues**

Sensitivity to Radiation	*Cell Type or Tissue*
High	Small lymphocyte
	Bone marrow
	Reproductive cells
	Intestinal mucosa
Fairly high	Skin
	Lens of the eye
	Oral mucosa
Medium	Connective tissue
	Small blood vessels
	Growing bone and cartilage
Fairly low	Mature bone and cartilage
	Salivary gland
	Thyroid gland
	Kidney
	Liver
Low	Muscle
	Nerve

Short-term, or acute, effects of radiation usually result from high doses to the entire body. Symptoms may include nausea, vomiting, diarrhea, fever, loss of hair, hemorrhaging, and even total body collapse. Long-term, or chronic, effects of radiation are usually the result of doses of radiation received over a long period. The effects may not be seen for several months or even years.

Repeated radiation exposure produces **cumulative effects.** Tissues have the capacity to repair radiation damage to a certain degree; however, some damage cannot be repaired, and the damage remains in the tissues. In other words, *radiation itself does not accumulate in tissues, but some of the unrepaired damage might.* Thus one acute exposure of 1 gray (Gy; see explanation of units later in the chapter) would be more biologically damaging than 10 exposures of 0.1 Gy spread over 10 years, even though the total dose for each exposure is 1 Gy. Unrepaired damage can lead to future health problems such as the development of cancer, cataracts, birth defects, or premature aging. Table 5-2 lists critical tissues and organs that might be affected by dental x radiation. More information about these critical organs is discussed later in the chapter.

At one time it was believed that very low doses of radiation were not harmful to patients. It was thought that a certain threshold existed below which no biologic damage occurred (Fig. 5-3). It now appears that no level of radiation is safe. The low doses received by the patient from dental radiography produce very little damage, but damage does occur. The number of cells in the body that are affected by dental radiography is low, and the probability of cell death is even lower. Nevertheless, it is necessary to keep exposure to x radiation to a minimum. Remember, every photon does some biologic damage, every single time.

Table 5-2 | **Cumulative Effect of Repeated Exposure (Organ and Disorder)**

Critical Organ	*Resulting Disorder*
Lens of eye	Cataracts
Bone marrow	Leukemia
Salivary gland	Cancer
Thyroid gland	Cancer
Skin	Cancer
Gonads	Genetic abnormalities

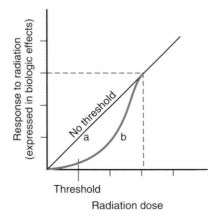

Figure 5-3 The diagonal straight line *a* represents the extrapolation of damage caused by low doses of x radiation in a nonthreshold manner; that is, any amount of radiation will cause some damage. Curve *b* represents a nonlinear threshold approach in which a certain radiation dose must be received before damage can be observed.

UNITS OF RADIATION MEASUREMENT

Before the amounts of radiation associated with dental radiography can be discussed, the way radiation is measured must be defined. To complicate matters, two sets of terminology exist to measure radiation. In 1985 an international system (SI) of measurement was adopted worldwide. However, traditional terminology is sometimes still used, and you may encounter it in older textbooks and journals. Both systems are presented here.

The amount of radiation a person is *exposed to* (not necessarily the amount *absorbed*) is measured in SI units as coulombs per kilogram. This is a measure of electric charge in a certain mass of air. Many people find it more convenient to use the old term, the **roentgen (R).** The roentgen is the unit of radiation exposure that produces one electrostatic charge per cubic centimeter of air.

The amount of radiation actually absorbed by the tissues is the absorbed dose. The SI unit of absorbed dose is called a **gray (Gy).** It is defined as the transfer of 10 joules (a unit of energy and work) per kilogram of tissue. The traditional system uses the term **rad (radiation absorbed dose)** as the unit of measurement. One rad is equivalent to the transfer of 100 ergs (another unit of energy and work) per gram of tissue; 1 Gy equals 100 rads.

Different forms of ionizing radiation have different energies. Some forms of radiation pack a bigger punch than others. For example, x radiation has a different energy level than does α-particle radiation. Therefore, to bring all forms of radiation dosage to the same level, **dose equivalence** is used. Traditionally, the **rem (roentgen-equivalent-man)** is the unit of dose equivalence. It is defined as the absorbed dose of any form of radiation that produces the same biologic effect in a human as does 1.0 rad of x radiation. Therefore, 1 rem of x radiation will produce the same amount of biologic damage as 1 rem of α-particle radiation, even though the energy transferred into the tissue might be different for each type of radiation. The SI unit of dose equivalence is the **sievert (Sv);** 1 sievert equals 100 rems.

Although differences between the units of radiation measurement exist, in dental radiography the differences are extremely small, and the units are virtually interchangeable.

$$1 R = 1 rad = 1 rem$$

and

$$1 Gy = 1 Sv$$

The amounts of radiation involved in dental radiography are much smaller than 1 Gy or 1 Sv and even smaller than 1 rad. Just as a meter can be divided into centimeters or millimeters, the units of radiation measurement can be similarly divided. For example, a centigray (cGy) is one hundredth of a gray, a millirad (mrad) is one thousandth of a rad, and a microsievert (μSv) is one millionth of a sievert. Table 5-3 gives a summary of radiation measurements.

Table 5-3 | **Units of Radiation Measurement**

Quantity	SI Units	Traditional Units	Conversion
Exposure	Coulombs per kilograms (C/kg)	Roentgen (R)	1 C/kg = 3380 R
Dose	Gray (Gy)	Rad	1 Gy = 100 rad
Dose equivalence	Sievert (Sv)	Rem	1 Sv = 100 rem

AMOUNTS OF RADIATION USED IN DENTAL RADIOGRAPHY

The exact amount of radiation produced when taking dental images varies, depending on factors such as the image-receptor sensitivity, the technique used, kilovoltage used, and whether any additional collimation is used. For example, F speed film requires only about 50% as much radiation for a diagnostic image as does D speed film. Digital imaging receptors require even less radiation than dental film to produce a diagnostic image. Rectangular collimation further reduces the amount of tissue exposed to the x-ray beam by as much as 60% to 70% compared with a circular beam.

Extraoral film-based techniques that employ intensifying screens require less radiation than the direct-exposure film in an intraoral film packet. The intensifying screens do just as their name implies: the actions of the x rays are intensified by the screens; therefore, less radiation is needed for a diagnostic image. Digital extraoral imaging receptors are extremely sensitive to radiation and require even less radiation than film-intensifying screen combinations. Cone beam volumetric imaging exposes a patient to higher levels of radiation than standard intraoral or extraoral imaging. Doses from cone beam imaging may range anywhere from approximately 4 to 40 times higher than panoramic imaging. However, doses are less with cone beam imaging than with conventional computed tomography.

It is very difficult to determine the exact doses associated with dental radiography. Keep in mind that **exposure** to radiation is not the same as the dose that is *absorbed*. Measuring absorbed doses is a very complicated procedure. Additionally, it is often difficult to compare one tissue with another because they have different densities, thicknesses, and sensitivities to radiation. In general, the skin receives a higher dose than does the bone marrow. The parotid glands receive more radiation when a round cylinder is used than when a rectangular collimator is used. The thyroid gland receives a measurable dose with intraoral and extraoral imaging.

Scientists have found that one of the best ways, albeit one of the more complex ways, to compare doses is with the *effective dose equivalent* (abbreviated as EDE or sometimes simply E). The effective dose equivalent is calculated to define a risk to the whole body from an estimate of a dose administered to a smaller portion of the body. It essentially puts dose comparisons on common ground. Table 5-4 compares some effective doses associated with dental imaging.

Table 5-4 | **Comparison of Effective Dose Equivalents in Dental Imaging**

Image	14-Image CMRS (Film)	14 CMRS (Digital)	Pano (Film)	Pano (Digital)
EDE (µSv)	78	41	54	45

CMRS, Complete mouth radiographic survey; *EDE*, effective dose equivalent.

RISK VERSUS BENEFIT OF DENTAL RADIOGRAPHIC IMAGES

We are exposed to radiation every day of our lives. Background radiation comes from radioactive materials that naturally occur in the ground and air, and cosmic radiation reaches us from space. The average background radiation dose for the U.S. population is approximately 3.0 mSv per year, although it varies with geographic location. Some areas contain more radioactive materials in the ground than others, and areas of higher elevation, such as Denver, Colorado, receive more cosmic radiation than cities at sea level. The majority of this naturally occurring radiation is in the form of radon in the air. Radiation also comes from man-made sources such as radioactive waste and nuclear fallout. The background dose does not include any radiation received from medical or dental sources or from consumer goods and activities. These man-made sources, including medical and dental imaging, account for another 0.6 mSv of radiation exposure per year for a total of approximately 3.6 mSv annually.

It is often tempting to make comparisons about naturally occurring exposures to radiation and those in dental imaging, particularly when trying to explain the risks to patients. However, it is not a simple comparison to make. Sophisticated calculations are used to make whole-body risk estimates from limited dental exposures. Table 5-5 gives some general examples of background radiation equivalents.

Table **5-5** | **Equivalent Background Exposure from Film-Based Dental Radiography**

Survey Type	Film Speed/Collimation	Background Equivalent
Full mouth survey	D Speed/Round	19 days
Full mouth survey	E Speed/Rectangular	4 days
Panoramic image	Rare-earth screens	3 days

Critical Organs

Although the radiation doses from dental imaging are small, there is a potential for biologic damage every time tissues are exposed to radiation. Some tissues or organs are exposed to more radiation than others when dental images are taken. If these tissues are damaged, the quality of an individual's life declines. These tissues or organs are the **critical organs.**

The skin is the first tissue exposed to radiation from sources outside the body. One of its responses to radiation exposure is a reddening or erythema. This is the same reaction seen in sunburn. (Remember that sunlight is also a form of electromagnetic radiation.) Exposure to radiation increases the risk of skin cancer, yet an increased risk of skin cancer has not been shown for doses of x radiation less than 250 mGy. The dose to the skin of the face is about 10 mGy when the operator uses an open-ended cylinder and D speed film. Therefore, a patient would have to receive at least 25 complete mouth radiographic surveys (CMRSs) in a very short time to significantly increase the risk of skin cancer. Remember that the dose to the skin is substantially reduced with F speed film and rectangular collimation.

Radiation to the lens of the eye may produce cataracts (a cloudiness of the lens). The x-ray dose associated with this problem appears to be about 2 Gy (2000 mGy). The dose to the eye from a CMRS used with an open-ended cylinder and D speed film is about 0.6 mGy; the dose is even lower with faster film or digital imaging. Therefore, scientists no longer consider the eye lens to be a critical organ in terms of dental radiation exposure.

The thyroid gland is fairly resistant to radiation in the adult. However, it is more susceptible to radiation in children. Thyroid cancer has been found in people who were exposed to a dose as low as 50 mGy when they were children. The dose to the thyroid from a CMRS (open-ended cylinder, E speed film) is less than 300 μGy (0.003 mGy). This dose to the thyroid can be further reduced by approximately half with the use of a protective thyroid collar. Leaded thyroid collars should always be used when intraoral images are taken.

Malignant changes in bone marrow may result in leukemia. Development of leukemia may be associated with an x-ray dose of approximately 50 mGy. Active (blood cell–producing) marrow is found in the jaws, skull, and cervical spine. About 13% of the total bone marrow lies in the head and neck areas. The dose to the bone marrow in a CMRS (open-ended rectangle, E speed film) is about 2500 µGy (0.025 mGy). Even though mature bone is fairly resistant to radiation, the risk of bone cancer with exposure to radiation still exists.

The salivary glands in an adult are only moderately sensitive to radiation. However, an association has been shown between tumors in the salivary glands and people who received full-mouth radiographic examinations before the age of 20 years. The doses associated with the parotid salivary glands can be nearly 300 mGy in a CMRS taken with D speed film and a round cylinder. Doses are substantially lower with faster speed film and rectangular collimation. Effective doses to the parotid gland are quite low in panoramic imaging, but they are nearly four times higher in cone beam imaging than in panoramic imaging.

As we have learned, the genetic effects of radiation can have far-reaching results. However, the dose to the reproductive cells from dental imaging is very small: only about 50 µGy (0.0005 mGy) or less for males and 30 µGy (0.0003 mGy) for females. The dose to female patients is lower because the reproductive cells are in a more protected body location. If the patient wears a lead apron, exposure to the reproductive cells is virtually zero (1.0 to 3.0 µGy).

Developing Fetus

The exact amount of x radiation that may produce damage to a developing human embryo or fetus is unknown. It is thought that doses less than 0.01 mGy produce very little risk. Therefore, radiographs may be prescribed for pregnant patients provided that standard radiation protection practices are followed. However, to preserve the woman's peace of mind, some practitioners prefer to postpone nonemergency images until after the delivery.

In summary, some risk of cellular injury is always present when ionizing radiation is used on biologic tissues. Table 5-6 lists some estimates of the probabilities of finding excess fatal cancers associated with dental radiography in a large population. Still, the levels of radiation involved in dental imaging are only about $^1/_{25}$ to $^1/_{1000}$ of the levels associated with biologic damage. Therefore, the benefit of detecting disease in a patient—disease that might not be detected by any other means—far outweighs the risks of receiving small doses of radiation. However, the images must be prescribed, exposed, and processed in an appropriate manner to minimize the patient's exposure to radiation. Although it is difficult to compare the risks of radiation exposure with the risks involved in other daily activities, Table 5-7 provides some comparisons of equivalent risks ("one in a million") that might provide helpful information when you discuss radiation risks with your patients.

Table 5-6 | **Risk of Fatal Cancers per Million Film-Based Dental Radiographic Examinations**

	Bone Marrow	*Thyroid*	*Bone Surface*	*Overall*
Full mouth survey D speed film Round collimation	0.7	0.8	0.5	2.5
Panoramic image Rare-earth screens	0.06	0.06	0.03	0.21

Table 5-7 | **Situations in Which a Person Has Roughly a One-in-a-Million Risk of Dying**

Risk Situation	Cause of Fatality
Being a man, age 60, for 20 minutes	Cardiovascular disease, cancer
Living in New York for 2 days	Air pollution
Living in Denver for 2 months	Cosmic radiation
Living in a stone building for 2 months	Natural radioactivity
Drinking water in Miami for 1 year	Carcinogens
Riding in a canoe for 6 minutes	Accident
Riding a bicycle for 10 miles	Accident
Riding in a car for 300 miles	Accident
Traveling by airplane for 1000 miles	Accident
Traveling by airplane for 6000 miles	Cosmic radiation
Working in a coal mine for 1 hour	Black lung
Working in a typical factory for 10 days	Accident
Smoking cigarettes, 1.4	Cardiovascular disease, cancer
Drinking wine, 500 mL	Cirrhosis
Drinking diet soda, 30 cans	Carcinogens

Modified from Council on Dental Materials, Instruments and Equipment: Biological effects of radiation from dental radiography, *J Am Dent Assoc*, 105:8, 275-281, 1982. Copyright 1982 American Dental Association. All rights reserved. Adapted with permission. Data from Pochin EE. *Why be quantitative about radiation risk estimates?* LS Taylor Lecture Series, no 2. Washington, DC, NCRP Publications, 1978 and Wilson R. Risks caused by low levels of pollution. *Yale J Biol Med* 51:37-51, 1978.

RADIATION PROTECTION FOR THE PATIENT

Despite the low risks to the patient from dental radiography, it is best to keep exposure to ionizing radiation to a minimum. Therefore, the **ALARA** concept (as low as reasonably achievable) should be kept in mind when exposing dental images. Remember, the operator controls the amount of radiation the patient receives; all exposure should be kept as low as possible. In the following paragraphs, ways to adhere to the ALARA principle are discussed.

Receptor Speed

If film is used, the fastest possible speed should be used for periapicals and bite-wings. E speed film (which is no longer manufactured) reduced patient exposure by at least 40% compared with D speed, and F speed film reduces exposure by approximately 20% compared with E, for a reduction of approximately 60% compared with D speed film. Digital imaging receptors are even more sensitive to radiation than film and require less exposure than even F speed film. An intraoral **charge-coupled device (CCD)** image receptor requires only about one tenth of the radiation of D speed film to make a diagnostic image.

Selection Criteria

Using selection criteria to determine the number and type of images for each patient will minimize radiation exposure. Using sound professional judgment in prescribing images for specific reasons based on the patient's history and clinical examination rather than prescribing images routinely or according to arbitrary time-tables is an effective method of reducing x-radiation doses. This concept is known as using selection criteria for prescribing images. The American Dental Association's Council on Scientific Affairs has determined that, "Diagnostic radiographs should

Table 5-8 | **Examples of Selection Criteria for Prescribing Radiographs**

Type of Patient	Child (Mixed Dentition)	Adult
New patient	Individualized examination consisting of panoramic examination with posterior bitewings *or* posterior bitewings with selected periapical views	Individualized examination consisting of posterior bitewings and selected periapicals; a full mouth survey is appropriate when patient presents with clinical evidence of generalized dental disease or a history of extensive dental treatment
Recall patient with no clinical caries and low risk factors for caries	Posterior bitewing examination at 12- to 24-month intervals	Posterior bitewing examination at 24- to 36-month intervals
Recall patient with clinical caries or high risk factors for caries	Posterior bitewing examination at 6-month intervals until no carious lesions are evident	Posterior bitewing examination at 12- to 18-month intervals

be used only after clinical examination, consideration of the patient's history and consideration of both dental and general health needs of the patient. Routine use of radiographs as part of periodic examination is an inappropriate practice." Clinicians should always specify a reason for the images they order based on subjective patient complaints and the objective signs in the patient's oral cavity. Table 5-8 gives an abbreviated example of recommended guidelines for prescribing radiographs. The complete guidelines can be found on the U.S. Food and Drug Administration web site (www.fda.gov/cdrh/radhlth/adaxray-1.pdf) or the American Dental Association web site (www.ada.org/prof/resources/pubs/jada/reports/report_radiography.pdf).

Kilovoltage

Using an x-ray beam with low **kilovoltage** results in higher patient doses, primarily to the skin. The lower-energy x-ray photons are absorbed by the patient's tissues and do not reach the image receptor and, therefore, do not contribute to the diagnostic image. Most contemporary dental x-ray units do not allow adjustment of kilovoltage; most are fixed at 70 kVp, although some are as low as 60 kVp. However, it is recommended that units should be operated using *at least* 60 kVp.

Filtration

Units operating at 70 kVp or more should have **filtration** equivalent to 2.5 mm of aluminum. Units operating at less than 70 kVp should have the equivalent of 1.5 mm aluminum. Filtration removes the low-energy x rays from the beam. These low-energy x rays are absorbed by the patient's tissues and do not contribute to image formation. Removing these low-energy photons before they reach the patient reduces radiation exposure.

Beam Collimation

The x-ray **beam** should be collimated so that it is no more than 7 cm (2³⁄₄ inches) in diameter at the patient's face. Rectangular collimation further reduces the amount of tissue irradiation because of the reduced area of skin surface exposed and the reduction in the number of overlapping fields. Rectangular collimation can result in a dose reduction of 50% to 90%, depending on the anatomic site being imaged. The 2003 National Council on Radiation Protection and Measurements (NCRP) Report indicates that "rectangular collimation of the beam shall be used routinely for periapical radiography. Each dimension of the beam, measured in the plane of the image receptor, should not exceed the dimension of the image receptor by more than 2 percent of the source-to-image receptor distance. Similar collimation shall be used, when feasible, for interproximal (bitewing) radiography."

Cylinders

Open-ended circular or rectangular lead-lined cylinders are preferred for directing the x-ray beam. A long (12- to 16-inch) cylinder will reduce exposure to the patient more than a short (8-inch) cylinder will because there will be less divergence of the beam. The 2003 NCRP Report indicates that beam indicators "*shall not* be less than...20 cm (8 inches) and *should* not be less than 40 cm (16 inches)." *Pointed plastic cones are NOT recommended and are illegal in some states:* the x rays interact with the plastic cones as they exit the unit housing and substantially increase the amount of scatter radiation produced (Fig. 5-4).

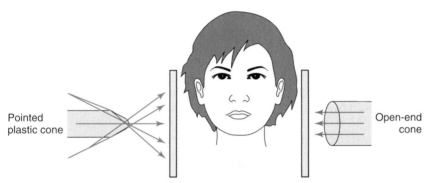

Pointed plastic cone

Open-end cone

Figure 5-4 X-ray interaction with the slopes of the pointed cone scatter more x rays in a wide pattern, resulting in a greater skin surface radiation dose.

Technique

The use of receptor-holding devices is recommended. These devices usually result in a more stable positioning of the receptor. In addition, the patient's hands are not exposed to radiation. If rectangular collimation is being used, receptor holders with a positioning guide are mandatory to avoid "cone cuts."

Retakes should be kept to a minimum. If you are in doubt about the placement of an image receptor or the position of the tubehead, do not press the exposure button. Be sure you are producing the best image that you can. Patients should be observed at all times during exposures. Additionally, all images should be evaluated before retaking any of them. For example, if the apex of a mandibular first premolar is not seen on the premolar image, it might be captured in the canine view, even though the canine view is not intended to show the premolars. Retaking the premolar view to get an ideal image when the information is available in another image is not in the patient's best interest. However, if the information needed is *not* available anywhere in the survey, it must be obtained so that an appropriate diagnosis can be made.

Proper Chemical Processing

If a film-based system is used, a quality assurance program such as the one outlined in Chapter 2 will help ensure that film processing is adequate. The best technique in the world will not produce films of good quality if chemical processing standards are not acceptable.

Protection

Thyroid collars should be used on all patients for intraoral imaging. Recommendations by the 2003 NCRP Report indicate that "thyroid shielding shall be provided for children and should be provided for adults when it does not interfere with the examination." The report also indicates that a leaded apron may not be necessary during dental radiography *if* other avenues for radiation reduction are "rigorously followed." Many patients may prefer to wear one for peace of mind.

RADIATION PROTECTION FOR THE OPERATOR

People who work with radiation are entitled to protection from radiation. Exposure limits have been established for occupationally exposed workers. The **maximum permissible dose (MPD)** is the dose of radiation to the whole body that produces very little chance of somatic or genetic injury. The current MPD for whole-body exposure per year for occupationally exposed personnel is 0.05 Sv (50 mSV).

Occupationally exposed women who are pregnant are allowed an MPD of only 0.005 Sv (5 mSv) per year. Therefore, during their pregnancies, female radiation workers should be protected as much as possible from any potential exposures.

A film badge service is a good way to keep track of occupational exposure. Badges are worn by personnel at all times while at work. The badges are regularly sent to the company providing the exposure measurement service. Written reports of the exposure recorded on the badges are provided. If proper safety precautions are followed, no one in a dental office should receive radiation doses anywhere near the MPD.

It is preferable that the operator stand behind an appropriate barrier while exposing images. The barrier should have a window or other means of monitoring the patient during the exposure. If no barrier is available, the operator should stand at least 6 feet away from the patient and in an area that lies between 90° and 135° to the primary x-ray beam. These are areas of minimum scatter radiation (see Fig. 1-3 to review these areas).

Dental personnel should never hold image receptors for patients. If assistance is necessary, ask a family member or guardian to help. Be sure to protect the helper with a lead apron and, if they are available, leaded gloves. Dental personnel should never hold the tubehead for stability. If the equipment is unstable, it should not be used until it is professionally repaired.

The operatory that contains the x-ray unit should be constructed so that it protects the people in surrounding areas from radiation. Most dental offices have a fairly low radiation workload. This means that low milliamperage and exposure times are used, and images are not constantly being exposed. Shielding or barrier requirements are based on radiation workloads, kilovoltage used, distances involved, and occupancy factor (who is in the area and how often). Regular construction materials such as plaster, cinderblock, or at least $2^{1}/_{2}$ inches of drywall will provide adequate protection from the radiation produced by dental units. Wood paneling alone does not provide adequate protection, but wood paneling over drywall would be acceptable. Guidelines for barrier construction to provide a safe working environment for everyone can be found in the NCRP Report no. 35.

RISK MANAGEMENT AND DENTAL IMAGING

Liability (legal accountability) has become a major concern in all service industries. Proceeding with ignorance; carelessness; lack of professional skills; or disregard for established rules, regulations, or principles constitutes malpractice. The following discussion addresses these issues as they relate to dental imaging.

Prescribing Images

The decision to obtain dental images for patients and the number or types of images to be obtained are to be determined by licensed dentists as part of their contractual duty to their patients. The decision to prescribe images must be based on the concept that the benefit derived from the diagnostic images outweighs the risk of exposing the patient to radiation. The concept of using selection criteria has been adopted by most major dental specialty groups in the United States and Canada, as well as by the American and Canadian Dental Associations.

The decision whether to order radiographs cannot be reasonably accomplished without first obtaining a patient history to determine whether any reasons exist not to prescribe them. In addition, the patient should be examined clinically to determine the need for images and the number and types of images to obtain. The patient history and clinical examination together should contribute significantly to the diagnosis, treatment, and prevention of disease. As stated many times in this chapter, taking images based on a predetermined timetable is not accepted as appropriate treatment. Just as taking radiographs that are not necessary is unsound practice, so is providing treatment without images that are needed for proper diagnosis and treatment. Both situations may be considered malpractice. In addition, images that are not diagnostically usable are also a source of malpractice.

Certification

The 1981 Consumer–Patient Radiation Health and Safety Act addresses the legal responsibility for quality and maintenance of equipment, certification of all persons using ionizing radiation equipment, and the accreditation of educational programs to train such personnel. The Act states that equipment must be properly maintained and must be inspected regularly, according to state statutes. It also leaves dentists to assume vicarious liability for the radiographic services provided by their employees. Using operators who are not certified according to state law leaves both the employee and the employer open to legal problems of statute violations and malpractice. All employees exposing patients to ionizing radiation must be verified as competent in technique and protection procedures. Students in training programs must be properly supervised by appropriate personnel as they practice their technical skills.

Informed Consent

Before exposing any patient to ionizing radiation, the operator must obtain and document the receipt of informed consent from the patient. To receive the consent, the operator needs to provide the patient with an explanation of the procedures, why it is necessary, what alternative diagnostic aid is available, what the risks are, and an estimation of the prognosis. This explanation must be in understandable language, and patients must be in full control of their senses (e.g., not under the influence of drugs or alcohol and mentally competent). If the patient is a minor, the parent or guardian must be informed about the procedure and must give consent. A patient's consent may be implied or expressed. When the procedure has risks associated with it, such as from ionizing radiation, receiving expressed consent is strongly recommended. A consent form signed by the patient and dated is the best documentation.

Confidentiality

Images are an integral part of the patient's record. The clinician has the obligation to ensure the privacy of the patient's information under state laws and under the 1996 Health Insurance Portability and Accountability Act (HIPAA). The clinician has primary custodial rights to the patient's records; in other words, they belong to the dentist. However, the patient has property rights, which means the patient has reasonable access to those records. The patient has the right, and must give permission, to have the records forwarded to other professionals such as specialists or a new dentist if the patient moves, to third-party providers, and, possibly, to the courts in litigation procedures. Prudent practice dictates forwarding quality duplicates of the records, including images, while keeping the originals with the patient file. Electronic patient records and electronic (digital) images simplify such transfers.

SELECTED REFERENCES

ADA Council on Scientific Affairs: An update on radiographic practices: information and recommendations, *J Am Dent Assoc* 132:234-238, 2001.

Aroua A, et al: Radiation exposure in dental radiography: a 1998 nationwide survey in Switzerland, *Dentomaxillofac Radiol* 33:211-219, 2004.

Ludlow JB, et al: Dosimetry of 3 CBCT devices for oral and maxillofacial radiology: CB MercuRay, NewTom 3G and i-CAT, *Dentomaxillofac Radiol* 35:219-226, 2006.

Napier ID: Reference doses for dental radiography, *Brit Dent J* 186:392-396, 1999.

Radiation Protection in Dentistry: *National Council on Radiation Protection and Measurements (NCRP) Report No. 145,* 2003.

White SC: 1992 Assessment of radiation risk from dental radiography, *Dentomaxillofac Radiol* 21:118-126, 1992.

STUDY QUESTIONS

1. The units of absorbed dose are expressed in
   A. Rads or grays
   B. Roentgens
   C. Rems or sieverts
   D. RDEs

2. Ionization is associated with each of the following interactions except one. Which one is the exception?
   A. Photoelectric effect
   B. Compton effect
   C. Thomson scattering
   D. They all cause ionization

3. The maximum permissible dose for a radiation worker is
   A. 0.10 Sv/yr
   B. 0.05 Sv/yr
   C. 0.005 Sv/yr
   D. 0.001 Sv/yr

4. X radiation affects the incidence of cancer and other abnormalities by
   A. Producing specific types of cancer or other abnormalities
   B. Storing radiation within tissues, resulting in continual damage
   C. Increasing the incidence of each disease in the patient
   D. Increasing their incidence among the general population

5. Damage to a living organism that is produced by photons striking the organism and producing a molecular change may be caused by
   A. Breaking molecules into smaller pieces
   B. Disrupting molecular bonds
   C. Forming new bonds within molecules
   D. Forming new bonds between molecules
   E. All of the above

6. The damage described in Question #5 is a description of which kind of radiation absorption?
   A. The somatic effect
   B. The genetic effect
   C. The direct effect
   D. The indirect effect
   E. Both the direct and indirect effects

7. Mutations from radiation exposure can occur
   A. Only in reproductive organs as genetic abnormalities
   B. In both somatic and reproductive tissues
   C. Only in the "critical organs"
   D. Only in the cytoplasm

8. Which of the following combinations would produce the least biologic damage from radiation?
   A. A large dose of radiation given over a short period of time
   B. A large dose of radiation given over a long period of time
   C. A small dose of radiation given over a long period of time
   D. A small dose of radiation given over a short period of time

9. Certain cells and tissues are more sensitive to radiation than others. Which of the following has the lowest sensitivity?
   A. Small lymphocytes
   B. Nerve and muscle
   C. Bone marrow
   D. Skin and oral mucosa
   E. Salivary glands

10. Each of the following can reduce radiation exposure to the patient except one. Which one is the exception?
    A. Using the fastest image receptor possible
    B. Using proper darkroom and processing procedures when using film
    C. Using rectangular collimation
    D. Using an 8-inch cylinder on the x-ray machine

6

Image Characteristics

Up to this point you have learned how to position, expose, process, and mount a radiograph. You have discovered some of the properties of x rays and how x rays interact with matter, the patient, and film emulsion. You know how x rays are generated in the x-ray tube. You have produced your first radiographs!

How do you judge the quality of your image? What does a "good" image look like? What are the characteristics that constitute a diagnostically useful image?

In the next few chapters, these questions are answered. Film qualities, patient factors, and technical and processing errors that directly affect the image quality are described. This chapter describes the visual characteristics (film qualities) of the x-ray image that make it diagnostically useful. These image characteristics are outlined in Box 6-1.

Box **6-1** **Image Characteristics**

Visual Characteristics
- Contrast
  - Film
  - Subject
- Density
- Detail

Geometric Characteristics
- Unsharpness/magnification
  - Geometric
  - Motion
- Distortion

VISUAL QUALITIES OF AN X-RAY IMAGE

Contrast

An x ray is basically a black and white picture that also includes multiple shades of gray. The darkest area of the image is black and the lightest is white, as viewed on a lightbox. In radiologic terms, *black* or *dark* is referred to as **radiolucent** and *white*

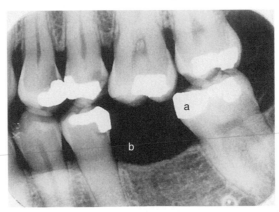

Figure 6-1 Bitewing radiograph. The white area *(a)* is an amalgam, and the dark area *(b)* represents air and soft tissue of the cheek.

or *light* is called **radiopaque.** Figure 6-1 is a bitewing radiograph. The white area marked *a* is an amalgam restoration (a silver filling). The dark area, *b*, represents air and soft tissue of the cheek. Because the x rays pass through the cheek and expose a lot of the image receptor (recall Chapter 2), this area is black. On the other hand, the x rays are stopped completely by the silver filling. No emulsion is exposed; thus no image is recorded. This area is then white. These two regions of the film highly contrast with each other: one is black and one is white.

   Contrast is also defined as the difference between the shades of gray, or optical densities, that can be measured on the image. The overall contrast on a radiograph is the product of both the image contrast and the subject contrast, and the subject contrast includes the patients and their anatomic structures. Except for choosing the type of film or receptor to use, the clinician has little control over image contrast. If you are using a digital receptor, then you may alter the image contrast in software programs after the image is acquired. Furthermore, as presented earlier, attenuation (stopping) of x rays by an object or patient also affects the contrast of an image. Although nothing can be done to change the patient's thickness or tissue differences, the kilovoltage, milliamperage, and/or exposure time may be altered to compensate for different patient characteristics, such as a large person versus a small person.

Film Contrast

   Film contrast depends on three things: (1) the type of film, (2) the processing of the film, and (3) the density of the film. The film type applies primarily to extraoral x-ray films. Each film type has its own inherent contrast; each is evaluated by a method that generates a graph called a *characteristic curve.* The discussion of this curve is beyond the scope of this book, but a detailed description can be found in other dental radiology texts.

   Film processing, as described in Chapter 2, can also influence the contrast of a film. A developing time that is too long will darken the film, and the subtle shades of gray will be lost; the overall image will be uniformly dark (Fig. 6-2). Similarly, under-processing because of insufficient time, low temperatures, or exhausted chemicals will decrease film contrast. The underprocessed film will be uniformly light (Fig. 6-3). Again, the different shades (contrast) are lost or not differentiated by our human visual system.

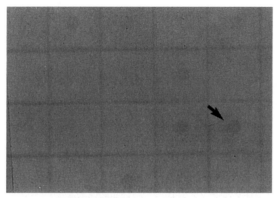

Figure 6-2 Darkened film. Details, seen here as dots, are still visible, but there is little contrast. The *arrow* indicates one of the dots. This image has too much density because the development time was too long. Compare this with Figure 6-3.

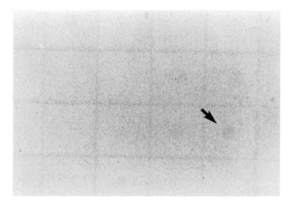

Figure 6-3 This image is uniformly light gray. Contrast is lost in this image. The dot indicated by the *arrow* is barely visible. This image has insufficient density because of insufficient development time or temperature or weak chemicals.

The degree of darkness or lightness of a film is called the film **density**. Some clinicians like dark films, but others prefer them lighter. The correct density of a film should enable the observer to view the grays of soft tissue and bone and the blacks and whites of airways and metallic restorations (Fig. 6-4). Density is further discussed later in this chapter.

Subject Contrast

Obviously, all patients are not alike; each one has a different height, weight, and bone structure. Even if the same exposure factors are used, a radiograph taken of a child will be very different from that of a 200-lb adult. The **subject contrast** depends on (1) the thickness of the subject, (2) the density of the subject, (3) the atomic number of the tissue(s) of the subject, and (4) the kilovoltage used. On many x-ray units, the operator can adjust only the time of exposure. Changing the time will change only the number, or quantity, of x rays produced. Changing the kilovoltage, if the unit allows that adjustment, will alter the penetrating power, or quality, of the x rays. Higher kilovoltages will better enable the x rays to pass through the patient's tissues. Therefore, kilovoltage is the only exposure factor over which the operator has control that directly affects subject contrast. Exposure time coupled with milliamperage

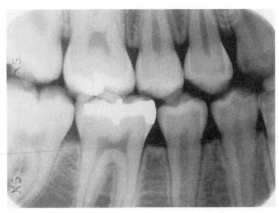

Figure 6-4 Black areas between teeth represent soft tissue such as the cheek or gingiva. Bright white areas are restorations. Note the distinct density (darkness) differences between the enamel, dentin, and pulpal tissues.

controls only the number of x rays produced and thus has the most impact on the density (overall darkness) rather than on the contrast (different shades of gray) of the image.

Density

As you can see from the previous discussion, contrast and density cannot be readily separated. Contrast is really the difference between densities. Radiographic density refers to the degree of darkness of a radiograph. This density depends on several things, including (1) the amount of radiation reaching the film, either the quantity (milliamperage and exposure time) or the quality (kilovoltage) of the radiation; (2) the distance from the x-ray tube to the patient; (3) the patient (subject) thickness; and (4) the developing conditions.

Amount of Radiation

The amount of radiation reaching the image receptor depends on the quantity of x-ray photons produced and their opportunity to reach the receptor. The more x-ray photons that strike the receptor, the more dense, or dark, is the resulting image. Recall from Chapter 4 that the *milliamperage influences the number of x rays produced* in an x-ray tube, and that longer exposure times allow more x rays to reach the receptor. The product of the milliamperage and the time of exposure measured in seconds is expressed as **milliampere-seconds (mAs).** This product has the greatest effect on the quantity of radiation produced, that is, the number of x rays made.

If two films are to have the same mAs product, they should have the same density. If other factors are constant, an exposure made at 10 mA and 0.3 second will produce the same density as one made at 15 mA and 0.2 second.

$$10\,mA \times 0.3\,s = 3\,mAs$$
$$15\,mA \times 0.2\,s = 3\,mAs$$

The **kilovoltage peak (kVp)** also influences the amount of radiation reaching the receptor. The higher the kilovoltage peak, the more energy the beam will have and the greater will be the penetrating power of the resultant x rays. A greater penetrating power means that more x rays will pass through the patient and reach the receptor rather than be absorbed by the patient's tissues. As a rule of thumb, if you increase the kilovoltage peak by 15 kV, you must decrease the exposure time by half to keep the densities of the images similar. If you decrease the kilovoltage peak by 15 kV, you must double the time of exposure to maintain similar densities.

For example, if you produce one image at 75 kVp and 0.5 second and you want to produce a second image at 90 kVp, you must reduce the exposure time of the second film by half to a new time of 0.25 second so that the two images have similar densities. On the other hand, if you produce one image at 85 kVp and 0.3 second and you want to produce a second image at 70 kVp, you must double the exposure time for the second film to 0.6 second.

Distance the X Rays Travel

The distance the x rays travel is called the source (x-ray tube)-to-film distance or source-to-receptor distance. It is also called the target-to-film distance or target-to-receptor distance. The intensity (its ability to create darkness or density) of the x-ray beam varies inversely as the square of the distance from the source. This means that the intensity of the beam is reduced the farther away the x-ray source is from the object being imaged. This is called the inverse square law and is written as follows:

$$I = \frac{1}{d^2}$$

where I = intensity (density) and d = distance.

A simple formula will help calculate the new exposure times to use if you change the source-to-film distance, for example, if you change from an 8-inch cylinder to a 16-inch cylinder.

$$\frac{I_1}{I_2} = \frac{(d_2)^2}{(d_1)^2}$$

Think of what happens as you move a flashlight farther away from an object. The light becomes dimmer on that object. Light, which is also a form of electromagnetic radiation, also follows the inverse square law.

The farther away one moves the x-ray tube or source, the less intense the x-ray beam becomes. To maintain the same radiographic density on an image, you must increase the exposure time accordingly. Figure 6-5 illustrates this concept. For example, one exposure is made at 8 inches and 0.4 second and has an intensity (I_1) of 1. When the tubehead is moved 16 inches away, the new intensity (I_2) will be one fourth as much as I_1 or $\frac{1}{4}$ because we doubled the distance (d) from 8 to 16 inches.

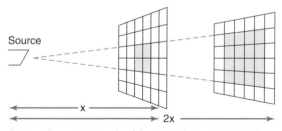

Figure 6-5 With the formula, $I = 1/d^2$, a ratio is made of the original intensity, I_1, to the new intensity, I_2, which can be written where d_2 is the new distance: $I_1/I_2 = (d_2)^2/(d_1)^2$. Notice that the "exposed" squares increase in number from 4 to 16 as the distance is doubled, and the resulting intensity (darkness) of the 16 squares is lighter than the original 4.

$$\text{New I}_2 = \frac{8^2}{16^2}$$

Remember that $8/16$ can be reduced to $1/2$ to make the math easier. Therefore,

$$\text{New I}_2 = \frac{1^2}{2^2} = \frac{1}{4}$$

Consequently, we would have to increase our exposure time by a factor of 4 (4 × 0.4 second) to 1.6 seconds to maintain the same image density. Using our formula, this would be

$$\frac{I_1}{I_2} = \frac{(d_2)^2}{(d_1)^2}$$

or

$$\frac{0.4}{x} = \frac{(16)^2}{(8)^2}$$

Reducing the fraction $16/8$, the formula becomes

$$\frac{0.4}{x} = \frac{(2)^2}{(1)^2}$$

or

$$\frac{0.4}{x} = \frac{4}{1}$$

$$x = 0.4 \times 4$$

$$x = 1.6$$

In more simple terms, whatever change you make to the distance, square it, then apply the square to the time. So, if you double the distance, square it to 4 (2 × 2) and multiply the time by 4. If you halve the distance, square the half ($1/2 \times 1/2 = 1/4$) and multiply the time by $1/4$.

Scale of Contrast

The x-ray film's range of useful densities is called its *scale of contrast.* If a radiographic film is mostly black and white, it has only two useful densities and thus has a *short contrast scale.* If a radiographic film has many shades of gray, including black and white, then it has a *long contrast scale.* In general, high-kilovoltage techniques produce longer scales of contrast, with more shades of gray, or more useful densities on the image. Low-kilovoltage techniques (65 kV or less) have short contrast scales: black, white, and fewer shades of gray. In other words, high kilovoltages produce low-contrast (more shades of gray, **long-scale contrast**) images, whereas low kilovoltages produce high-contrast (fewer shades of gray, mostly black or white, or **short-scale contrast**) images. Figure 6-6 shows a comparison of short- and long-scale contrasts. Some extraoral films are manufactured for high contrast (short contrast scale) and some for less contrast (long contrast scale).

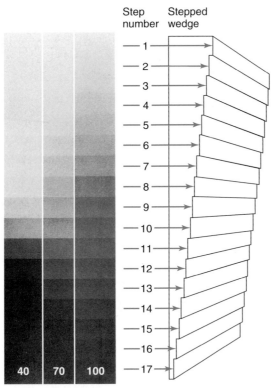

Step number | Stepped wedge

Figure 6-6 Radiographs taken at 40 kV are predominantly black and white; that is, they have high contrast (short-scale contrast). Those taken at 100 kV show many shades of gray (long-scale contrast) and, therefore, low contrast.

Detail

Receptor **detail** is also known as **resolution.** An image has good detail or high resolution if small objects can be easily identified without distortion, overlap, or unsharpness. The detail or sharpness of an image depends on several characteristics, including (1) the focal spot size in the tubehead, (2) the radiographic contrast, and (3) certain geometric characteristics. In general, intraoral film demonstrates greater detail or resolution than extraoral film. Digital image receptors now demonstrate a resolution similar to high-speed intraoral film.

Focal Spot Size

The focal spot size is determined by the size and the angulation of the target anode. The smaller the focal spot size is, the better the resolution, or detail, of the resulting image. Figure 6-7 shows a diagram of a conventional dental x-ray tube focal spot. As you can see, the **effective focal spot** can be made smaller than the **actual focal spot** by angling the tungsten target (anode) approximately 20°. A typical tungsten anode has an effective focal spot size of about 1 mm. This size is inherent to the machine and cannot be altered.

GEOMETRIC CHARACTERISTICS

Geometric Unsharpness

A certain amount of image unsharpness is present in every radiograph. Casting an image of teeth onto a dental radiograph is similar to casting a shadow. If an object is close to a flat surface and a light is shined on it, its shadow's size will be close to

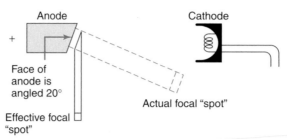

Figure 6-7 The target, when viewed from below (where the x rays would exit), appears smaller than viewed from the cathode because of the angulation of the anode. The technique of angling the target anode 20° reduces the size of the effective focal spot and results in better resolution.

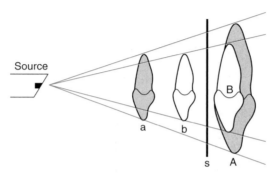

Figure 6-8 Object *a* is farther from the screen(s). Its shadow, *A*, is thus enlarged and is bigger than the shadow *(B)* cast by object *b*. Shadow A is more magnified than shadow B.

the actual size of the object. If the object is moved away from the flat surface (closer to the light source), then its shadow will be magnified. So it is with x-ray imaging; Figure 6-8 helps illustrate these points.

Even an object such as a tooth, which is placed as close as possible to the film, will have both an **umbra** (the shadow or image of the object) and a **penumbra** (area of unsharpness around the shadow) (Fig. 6-9). Placing the object near the image receptor, or *reducing the object-to-receptor distance,* helps reduce geometric distortion or unsharpness by reducing magnification. In addition, *increasing the source-to-receptor distance* reduces magnification.

Motion Unsharpness

Unsharpness caused by patient movement can also be considered a geometric problem. The results of patient movement are seen in Figure 9-26 in Chapter 9. Some clinicians believe that motion unsharpness can be caused by x-ray tubehead movement; but even if the tubehead is moving or rocking, no perceptible unsharpness should occur in the x-ray image. Figures 6-10 and 6-11 show images of two paper clips. Both images were exposed using settings of 70 kV and 15 mA for 0.13 second (8 impulses). An operator, wearing a protective lead apron and lead gloves, physically rocked the tubehead during the exposure. No blurring is seen in either figure. The x-ray photons traveling at the speed of light for 0.13 second are not altered significantly from their straight-line paths to create motion artifacts that would be visible to the human eye.

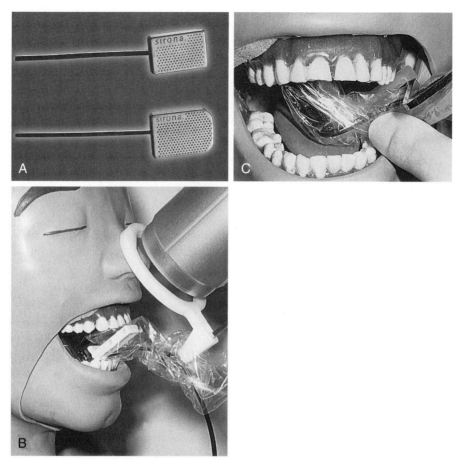

Figure 7-1 A, A rigid cabled intraoral sensor. **B,** Sensor being placed in oral cavity using a film holder. Notice the plastic infection-control barrier. **C,** Final position of sensor with cone aligned with the indicator ring just as with an x-ray film. *(A: Courtesy of Sirona Dental Systems LLC, Charlotte, N.C.).*

A CMOS chip is already in every computer made, and manufacturers have now managed to put an image receptor on the same chip! They work extremely well for video cameras and digital cameras. However, they are less efficient than CCDs at gathering x-ray information. Nonetheless, because the CMOS technology has matured during the lifetime of this textbook, today one cannot distinguish any clinical difference in images produced by these two main types of solid-state detectors. The CMOS chip has a microprocessor on it, as well as the sensor/receptor. This means that less imaging "real estate" is available on the chip than on the CCD. This additional component also produces more system noise, which must be filtered out in image processing software before display on the monitor.

Sensor Arrays

For digital imaging, two main types of sensor arrays (arrangements) exist: linear arrays and area arrays (Figs. 7-2 and 7-3). Linear array detectors can be placed beside each other in any width. Some panoramic imaging systems arrange these linear detectors in a 6- × 12-inch format to approximate the size of a standard panoramic film.

Area array detectors are used with intraoral digital x-ray systems and video cameras. Although once quite small, area array detectors now have the approximate size of dental x-ray films, both size no. 1 and size no. 2 films. These detectors allow

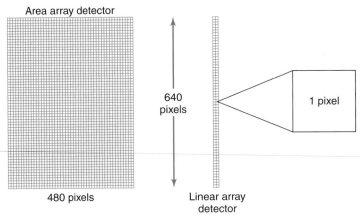

Figure 7-2 Two types of charge-coupled device (CCD) detector arrays. The area array is used in intraoral video cameras and digital x-ray systems. The linear array is used in desktop scanners and fax machines.

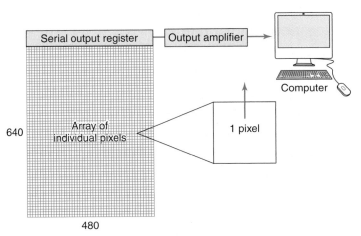

Figure 7-3 Diagram of an area array detector. The electronic image is stored as different numbers of electrons in each pixel. The pixel numbers are read in the serial register as electric signal strengths. Each pixel is assigned a gray level (value). The output amplifier enhances the signal for "sampling" by the analog-to-digital converter (ADC) for display on the monitor.

for the acquisition of images in both the vertical and horizontal orientation. Thus, the operator can display a full-mouth series of images in a manner similar to the arrangement of a film-based complete mouth survey.

Area array CCDs currently fall into two categories: those that use a *scintillator*, or a material that emits light when exposed to x rays (similar to an intensifying screen in extraoral radiography), sandwiched to the CCD, and those that do not. In the systems that use a scintillator, the x rays strike the screen material and cause photoelectrons to be produced. One x-ray photon will produce hundreds of light photons, which are then gathered in the CCD and transmitted by a cable to the computer for processing.

In contrast, the systems that do not use a scintillator are termed *radiation hardened*. These systems gather x rays directly onto the CCD. Although the image is considered to be more detailed (have higher resolution), the life of these radiation-hardened systems may be shortened by the direct bombardment of the sensor by the x rays.

How Images Are Generated

How are the images generated? What actually happens in the CCD when x rays strike it? The x-ray beam passes through the object of interest, in this case a tooth, and the beam is attenuated (stopped) to varying degrees by the different materials in the tooth (see Chapter 6). In digital imaging, the x rays that are not absorbed by the patient's tissues strike the amorphous silicon instead of film emulsion. The energy in the x rays breaks the chemical bonds in the silicon, and electrons are ejected from their orbits and attracted to a *potential well.* This well is positively charged to attract and hold the electrons. The well is "divided" into rectangular sections, corresponding to pixels. Each rectangular area represents a different pixel. Each well will hold different amounts of electrons, depending on how many electrons were ejected from their orbits in the different areas of the silicon (Fig. 7-4).

Circuitry in the sensor called the *polysilicon gate* consists of two layers. The electrons in the wells, which are embedded in the silicon dioxide, remain in these wells for only a few milliseconds before an electronic gate is opened. When the gate is opened, the electronic signal strength of each well is read by a serial register and sent to an output amplifier to enhance the signal (Fig. 7-5). The signal is transferred to the analog-to-digital converter (ADC) for conversion to a visible image. CMOS receptors actually have a small amplifier at each pixel address and thus can detect the number of incident x-ray photons independently at each pixel site.

The ADC converts the electronic information to a digital signal by assigning a number that corresponds to the signal strength from each well. The number corresponds to a gray level (amount of darkness or lightness), and the numbers usually range from 0 to 255. The information is forwarded to a frame grabber, which is an electronic circuit board that allows the computer monitor screen to display the image in pixels created by the various gray-level number assignments. The image is displayed almost instantaneously, and the monitor screen is refreshed constantly and rapidly. A typical screen image has about 307,200 pixels (640 × 480), each of which is assigned a gray level or value. Computer software is used to enhance the image (see the section on image processing later in this chapter). The overall process is diagrammed in Fig. 7-6.

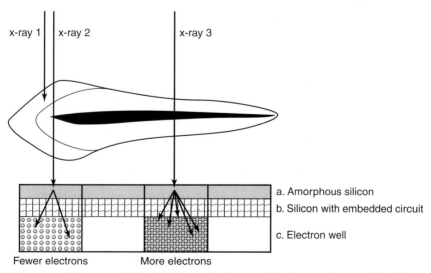

Figure 7-4 Fewer x-ray photons reach the digital sensor in the area of tooth enamel compared with the root area. When the x rays collide with the silicon (layer *a*), electrons are ejected from their orbits and are attracted to the positively charged potential well. Each rectangular area of the well represents a different and separate pixel and contains different numbers of ejected electrons. When the electronic circuit (*b*) is opened, the electronic signal can be read.

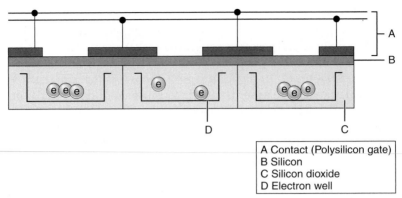

A	Contact (Polysilicon gate)
B	Silicon
C	Silicon dioxide
D	Electron well

Figure 7-5 Three wells, or pixels, are represented here. The circuitry called the polysilicon gate consists of layers *A* and *B*. The electrons *(e)* stored in the wells *(D)*, embedded in silicon dioxide *(C)*, remain in these wells for only a few milliseconds before the electronic gate is opened to transfer the charge in the wells to the analog-to-digital converter (ADC) for conversion to a visible image.

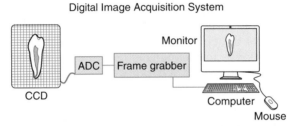

Figure 7-6 Diagram of a typical direct digital system with charge-coupled device (CCD), analog-to-digital converter (ADC), and frame grabber. The ADC device converts the electronic signal to a digital signal by assigning a gray-level value that corresponds to the signal strength. The frame grabber circuitry allows the monitor screen to display the image pixels.

A wireless direct digital sensor has been developed that uses radio frequency transmission to eliminate the need for a cable connected to the computer. The image is instantly transmitted to the computer via radio waves. However, caution must be used if more than one sensor is being used in an area because sometimes cross talk is present; that is, the computer has a hard time telling which sensor is sending information to it, and patient information may potentially be mismatched.

Storage Phosphor Imaging

Storage phosphors are simply reusable materials like those used in intensifying screens that convert x rays to light for detection by a receptor. In storage phosphor imaging systems, a plate coated with the phosphor is the image receptor used to capture the image. This plate is then placed in a device that uses a laser scanner to read the light signal stored on the plate in the phosphor (similar to a latent image on film), and the signal is then displayed on a computer monitor (Figs. 7-7 through 7-9).

Unlike the CCD, which is usually attached to the computer by a cable, the reusable phosphor plates have no cables and thus may be placed in the mouth like x-ray film. The plate is not as thin as film, but it is thinner than the average CCD receptor. The scanning device adds to the cost of the system, and the plate used for an exposure must be "recycled" to remove the image scanned before replacing it in the mouth for the next image. Therefore, this type of imaging is less rapid than CCD image capture and display. In addition, each phosphor plate must be wrapped and

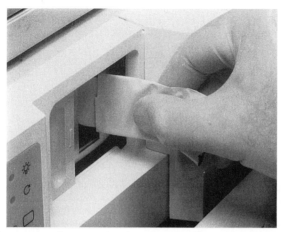

Figure 7-7 A clinician placing a digital storage phosphor plate in an optical scanner to be read by a laser beam. The light information on the storage plate is converted by the laser into a readable gray-scale image on the computer screen. *(Courtesy of Dr. Robert Langlais, San Antonio, Tex.)*

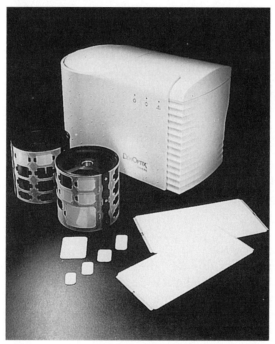

Figure 7-8 An optical scanner that uses a drum to mount the plates. Note that the scanner can accept the equivalent of all intraoral film sizes, including occlusal, and it can also scan a panoramic-size image. *(Courtesy of Gendex Dental Systems, Lake Zurich, Ill.)*

unwrapped in a protective barrier for infection control purposes, which, again, reduces the productivity of image acquisition.

Indirect Digital Imaging

Of course, you can digitize a film-based radiograph or any other document to obtain an image for display on the computer. Digitizing is done all the time in the publishing industry. Desktop scanners capture and digitize the light signal of whatever is placed inside them and are commercially available to anyone. If clinicians wish to

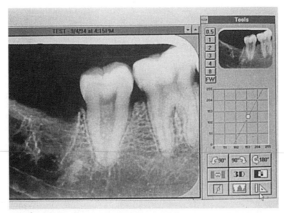

Figure 7-9 Storage phosphor image. *(Courtesy of Dr. Robert Langlais, San Antonio, Tex.)*

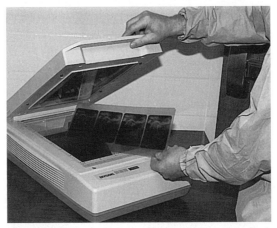

Figure 7-10 A typical desktop scanner that can also be used for digitizing images from paper, slides, or radiographs. This is an indirect method of digital imaging.

record x-ray film images this way, they need only to add a transparency module to the scanner, which allows the light to be transmitted through the x ray to be recorded (Fig. 7-10). This is similar to placing a film on a duplicator lightbox, closing the lid, and having the computer grab the image, digitize it, and display it on the monitor. Figure 7-11 illustrates the difference between direct and indirect image acquisition.

DIGITAL IMAGE PROCESSING

Digital imaging has distinct advantages over film. The signal is displayed on a computer, which eliminates the need for x-ray film, developing solutions, running water, a darkroom, and film mounts. The image is stored in the computer, which eliminates the need for filing films in the patient chart; this is an advantage as more and more clinicians opt to go paperless in their practices. Perhaps one of the primary advantages of digital imaging is that the images may be processed, or enhanced, after they have been acquired. Some of these enhancements include contrast and/or brightness alteration and digital subtraction. Obviously, you cannot do this with traditional film-based radiographs. Digital images can be sent electronically by email

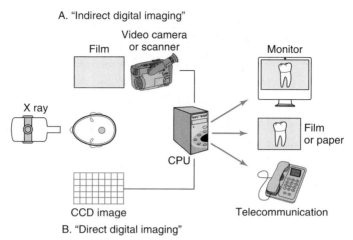

Figure 7-11 Indirect vs. direct digital imaging. On the indirect side (A), a film can be placed in a scanner or imaged by a video camera and digitized. Another electronic device has been added to the imaging chain to capture the image for display on a monitor. Indirect digital imaging is inferior to direct imaging because the additional devices add electronic noise to the image, degrading it. A direct capture with an intraoral charge-coupled device (CCD) as shown on the *B* side is preferable. However, once the image is obtained and in the computer, it can be (1) displayed on the monitor, (2) printed on film or paper, or (3) sent electronically to a third party.

or other electronic means, which is useful for consultation or insurance purposes. This process has been termed *teledentistry* by some authors.

It is the digital system software or image processing that truly affects patient care, and that is the part of the imaging system that may seem daunting to operators who were taught to use x-ray film. The software operations are, for the most part, very similar to most image software programs, such as Adobe Photoshop, Aldus Persuasion, and MacPaint.

Most image processing software programs for performing electronic image processing or image enhancement allow the operator to change the following image variables either together or separately:
- Brightness
- Contrast
- Image size (zoom)
- Image orientation
- Sharpness
- Inversion (white to black and vice versa)
- Pseudocolor alteration

These are all useful tools and are all available in desktop publishing software. Nothing is proprietary about these enhancements. Figure 7-12 illustrates some of these.

DIGITAL IMAGE PROPERTIES

Resolution

In imaging, resolution can be thought of as a detail in an image (see Chapter 6). Resolution should be high enough to allow you to distinguish between small objects that are close to one another. Resolution is usually defined in numbers of line pairs per millimeter (lp/mm). Dental x-ray film has a resolving power between 12 and 20 lp/mm.

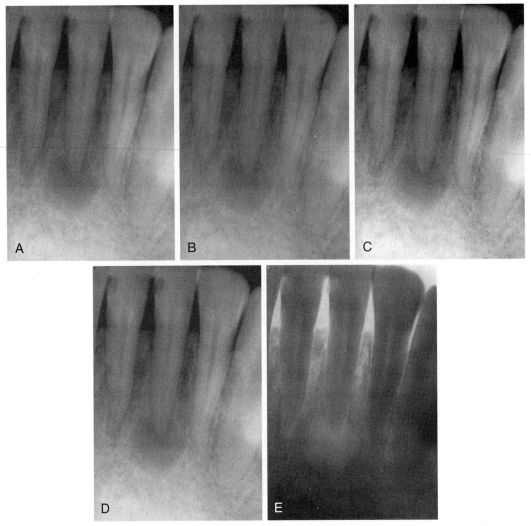

Figure 7-12 Examples of software enhancements of an image. **A** is the original image; **B** has reduced brightness; **C** has enhanced contrast; **D** has been sharpened; and **E** shows inversion (switching of black and white).

A typical CCD system is closer to 10 lp/mm. Because the unaided human eye can resolve only about 8 to 10 lp/mm, the CCD appears to have sufficient resolution for dental tasks and treatment decisions.

X-Ray Sensitivity

The typical digital imaging receptor is much more sensitive to light or x rays than is conventional dental x-ray film. Exposure times for most systems are about 50% less than for E speed x-ray film and about 70% less than for D speed film. Consequently, the absorbed x-ray dose to the patient is substantially reduced with little or no perceptible loss of image detail. An exposure time for a molar view with a digital system can be as low as 0.10 to 0.05 second! Compare this with the typical 0.20 second required for a molar view with the use of E speed film.

Because the sensors are so sensitive to radiation, consideration should be given to the x-ray machine that is being used with digital imaging systems. Ideally, an x-ray generator to be used with a solid-state electronic detector should have the following characteristics:

- Low kilovoltage peak (70 kVp or less)
- Low milliamperage (5 mA or even less)
- An extremely accurate timer capable of producing very short exposure times accurately
- The smallest focal spot (target) feasible
- Direct current (DC) circuit

Wide Dynamic Range

The dynamic range is the digital imaging equivalent to exposure latitude with x-ray film. For a CCD, the dynamic range is a linear one; thus the latitude of these systems is extremely wide—greater than that of film. This means that the CCD-based systems can portray more information, especially at low or high exposures, than can film.

Photometric Accuracy

Because CCD readout of electron information is slower than the image generated by a video camera, each pixel in the array can be digitized with great precision, thus recording the light or x-ray intensity signal accurately. Considering that there are 640×480 (or 307,200) pixels in a standard area array detector, each of which can have a gray-level value between 0 and 255, you can see how precise the image-density information can be in these electronic systems.

High Signal-to-Noise Ratio

Because the image may be enhanced after the exposure (postexposure processing), the CCD has a contrast scale similar to that of sophisticated medical imaging systems such as computed tomography. That is, each pixel can display any one of 256 levels of gray to improve image contrast. This means that a signal, such as an interproximal carious lesion seen as a dark spot on a light enamel background, will be more visible than the surrounding noise (other signals) in this type of imaging system. Such is not the case with dental x-ray film. Once a film is exposed and processed in chemicals, no more information can be retrieved. Box 7-1 outlines the advantages and disadvantages of CCD sensors.

BOX **7-1** ADVANTAGES AND DISADVANTAGES OF CHARGE-COUPLED DEVICE SENSORS

Advantages

1. Instant image viewing
2. Elimination of the darkroom
3. Consistent quality
4. High signal-to-noise ratio (improved detection)
5. Electronic image processing
6. Greater exposure latitude
7. Remote consultation capability
8. Reduced exposure to x rays
9. Elimination of hazardous chemicals

Disadvantages

1. High initial cost
2. Unknown life expectancy of sensor

DIGITAL IMAGING APPLICATIONS

Clinical tasks such as (1) the early detection of carious lesions, oral cancer, and bone loss and (2) the quantification of any changes in the size of soft tissue or bony lesions will become commonplace and simple with the use of digital imaging systems. Better treatment decisions will result, all leading to improved patient care. Box 7-2 outlines some of the potential applications of digital imaging in dentistry. Figures 7-13 and 7-14 show images captured by intraoral direct digital CCD systems.

As you can see from Box 7-2, most of the tasks that a dentist is required to perform for patients on a daily basis require some form of imaging. Clinical decision making is based on disease detection and diagnosis. Detection and diagnosis are based on correlating signs and symptoms with the results of diagnostic tests such as images, biopsies, and laboratory tests. The introduction of solid-state imaging will make these tasks simpler and more accurate for the practitioner and the patient. The sooner dentists adopt this technology into their offices, the more rewarding their practices will become. Your role as a dental hygienist or dental assistant is to be familiar with these imaging systems and be able to generate diagnostically useful images for the oral health care team.

Box **7-2** **Potential Application of Charge-coupled Device Imaging**

1. Improved disease detection
   a. Bone loss
   b. Peripheral lesions
   c. Interproximal caries
2. Quantification of disease change over time
   a. Caries progression or remineralization
   b. Alveolar bone loss or gain using digital subtraction
   c. Peripheral lesion change after endodontic treatment including apical surgery
3. 2D/3D reconstruction of the following:
   a. Bone loss
   b. Implant sites
   c. Pulp canal morphology (anatomy)
   d. Condylar bone changes
4. Improved patient education
5. Remote electronic consultation (teledentistry)

Adapted from Miles DA et al: Imaging using solid-state detectors. *Dent Clin North Am* 37(4):538, 1993.

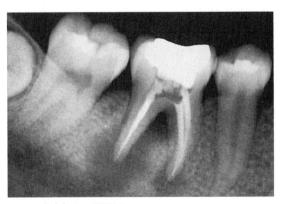

Figure 7-13 Intraoral charge-coupled device (CCD) image.

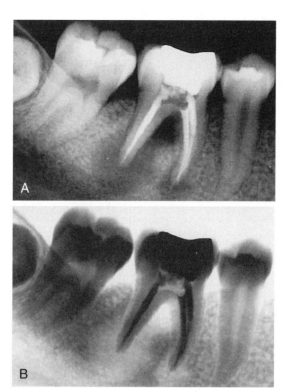

Figure 7-14 Two "processed" images of the original seen in Figure 7-13. **A,** This image has had minor contrast enhancement to see the apical lesions better. **B,** This image has had the contrast inverted by the clinician to evaluate the bone in the furcation area between the roots.

STUDY QUESTIONS

1. Methods for acquiring a digital image include
   A. Direct charge-coupled device (CCD) capture
   B. Photostimulable phosphor plate (PSP) capture
   C. Digitizing or scanning an existing image
   D. A and B
   E. All of the above

2. A CCD is primarily made of which of the following substances?
   A. Silicon
   B. Acetate
   C. Silastic
   D. Phosphor

3. The term *pixel* means
   A. Picture excellence
   B. Picture eliminator
   C. Picture element
   D. Phosphor element
   E. Phosphor eliminator

4. All of the following are imaging properties of a CCD except one. Which one is the exception?
   A. Precise photometric accuracy
   B. High signal-to-noise ratio
   C. Narrow dynamic range
   D. High x-ray sensitivity

5. Applications for CCD imaging include all of the following except one. Which one is the exception?
   A. Video cameras
   B. Telescopes
   C. Microscopes
   D. Laser cameras
   E. Fax machines

6. An x-ray machine that will be used with digital imaging should have all of the following characteristics except one. Which one is the exception?
   A. Low kilovoltage
   B. Low milliamperage
   C. Direct-current circuitry
   D. Accurate timer
   E. Large focal spot

7. Phosphor plate imaging is not quite as rapid as CCD imaging because
   A. The plates must be scanned by a laser before the image can be displayed on a computer
   B. The plates must be erased, or recycled, before using them again
   C. The signal is sent to the computer by radio waves
   D. A and B
   E. All of the above

8. "Processing" a digital image might include which of the following enhancements?
   A. Increased sharpness
   B. Adjusted contrast
   C. Adjusted brightness
   D. Inversion
   E. All of the above are potential enhancements

9. Advantages of digital imaging over film-based imaging include all of the following except one. Which one is the exception?
   A. Reduced exposure times
   B. Elimination of the need for infection control
   C. Instant image viewing
   D. Elimination of developing chemicals
   E. Remote consultation capability

8

Panoramic Imaging

Extraoral (outside the mouth) images, including panoramic images, are taken when large areas of the jaw or skull need to be examined. Small intraoral images cannot adequately capture images of the temporomandibular joint, the maxillary sinuses, or broad areas of the jaws, yet extraoral images taken with radiographic film do not show details as well as intraoral radiographs. Digital extraoral imaging systems, however, have better resolution than the film-based systems.

Extraoral images, including panoramic images, are often used in conjunction with other dental images for patient evaluation. In the past, panoramic images were good for evaluating large areas, but they were not recommended for detecting subtle changes, such as small carious lesions or periodontal defects. This situation has changed somewhat with the introduction of full-featured digital panoramic units with a special C-arm. Panoramic digital images produced with these machines can show details such as small interproximal carious lesions. These digital panoramic units have the capability of "opening up" the interproximal contacts in the premolar regions that traditional panoramic machines show as being overlapped (Fig. 8-1).

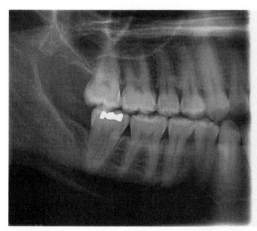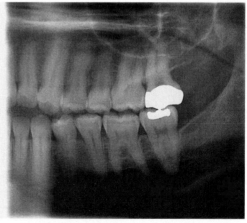

Figure 8-1 A specialized program in the digital software allows this type of "panoramic bitewing" projection. Note that the interproximal contacts are opened. Interestingly, this set of bitewings also displays the periapical regions of all the posterior teeth.

Many different types of extraoral images exist, but this chapter will focus on the panoramic projection. Other extraoral images will be discussed in Chapter 11. First, the equipment necessary to produce film-based panoramic and other extraoral images must be described because it differs from that needed for intraoral images.

EQUIPMENT FOR FILM-BASED EXTRAORAL IMAGING

Cassettes

Extraoral images made with film require special cassettes, which are usually rigid, light-tight devices that hold the film and the intensifying screens (Fig. 8-2, A). Cassettes keep daylight from reaching the film inside, yet they are made of materials that allow x rays to pass through. They come in various sizes to fit large x-ray films, such as 8 × 10 inches. Cassettes for panoramic x-ray machines usually measure about 5 or 6 inches in width and 12 inches in length. Some panoramic cassettes may be flexible instead of rigid, and they may open only at one end, like a manila envelope (Fig. 8-2, B). Cassettes must be marked with leaded letters *L* or *R* to identify the patient's left or right side because no embossed dot is present on extraoral film as it is on intraoral film. Some panoramic units have *L* or *R* markers built into the head positioner or in the cassette itself.

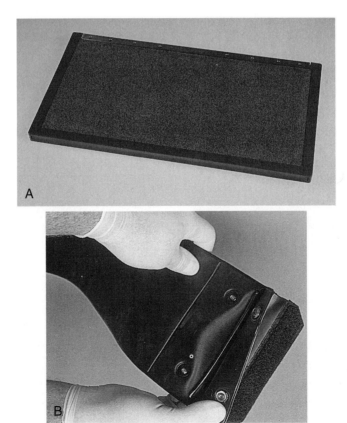

Figure 8-2 **A**, Rigid panoramic cassette. **B**, Flexible 5- × 12-inch panoramic cassette.

Intensifying Screens

Inside the cassette are two intensifying screens; the film is sandwiched between them. These screens contain a layer of material called a **phosphor** that can fluoresce, or emit light, when x rays strike it. This is the same material that is used in digital imaging and is called a *scintillator*. It is primarily the light from the screens that exposes the x-ray film. This process acts to intensify, or amplify, the action of the x rays; hence, fewer x rays are needed to make an image when intensifying screens are used. The process also results in a film with less resolution, or detail, than a periapical film because the light from the screens diffuses (spreads) slightly before exposing the film (Fig. 8-3). The properties of resolution and detail were discussed in Chapter 6.

Some phosphors, such as calcium tungstate, emit blue light. However, many intensifying screens contain other phosphors that emit green light. These rare-earth phosphors are more efficient at converting x rays into light than is calcium tungstate. Therefore, rare-earth screens are "faster" than calcium tungstate screens, and even fewer x rays are needed to make an image with them. The result is less exposure to x radiation for the patient.

As mentioned before, the x-ray film is sandwiched in the cassette between the intensifying screens (Fig. 8-4). The film must be sensitive to the kind of light emitted by the phosphor in the screens for a good image to form. Regular x-ray film is sensitive to blue light emitted by calcium tungstate screens, but special green-sensitive film must be used with the rare-earth screens.

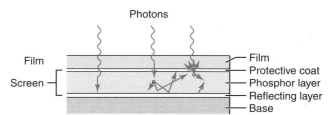

Figure 8-3 One half of a typical screen–film combination. Light striking a phosphor crystal may be scattered or deflected in any direction. Light that misses a crystal on its initial passage may strike another crystal after being bounced backward from the reflecting layer.

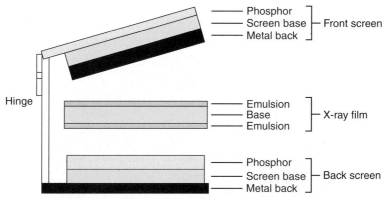

Figure 8-4 A schematic diagram of a typical film–screen combination. Placing the film between two intensifying screens allows for a faster conversion of x-ray photons to light photons. The light exposes the x-ray film much more quickly, and the patient receives less radiation exposure.

EQUIPMENT FOR DIRECT DIGITAL PANORAMIC IMAGING

Several companies manufacture direct digital panoramic units. The main difference between direct digital panoramic imaging and film-based imaging is the image receptor. Digital units use a sensor array rather than film. Table 8-1 lists some digital panoramic systems. The image is produced immediately on a computer screen in the fashion described in Chapter 7 rather than after the film has been processed in chemicals (Fig. 8-5). The image is then available for postacquisition processing in the event that some aspect of the image needs to be enhanced.

PANORAMIC IMAGING PRINCIPLES

When visiting the Grand Canyon, one gets a panoramic, or wide, view of the scenery. In radiography, a panoramic image gives a view of the entire maxilla and mandible on one image. The image is correctly called a **pantomograph** or **panoramic image.** Many people refer to it as a *panorex*. Panorex is actually the brand name of the panoramic x-ray machine first introduced to North America by the S. S. White Company in 1959. Unfortunately, this brand name has stuck in the minds of many clinicians as synonymous with a panoramic image.

Table **8-1** | **Solid-State Panoramic X-Ray Systems**

Company	Product Name	Detector Type
Carestream Health/Onex (formerly Kodak)	Kodak 8000 (formerly TrophyPan)	CMOS*
Danaher (formerly Gendex)	Orthoralix 8500 DDE	CCD*
Instrumentarium (Palodex Group)	Orthopantomograph 200D	CCD
Soredex (Palodex Group)	Cranex D, Cranex Novus	CCD
J. Morita	Veraview Epocs	CCD
Planmeca	ProMax, ProOne	CCD
Schick Technologies Inc.	CDRPan	CCD
Sirona—The Dental Company	Orthophos Plus DS	CCD
Takara Belmont	X-Caliber	CCD

*CMOS, Complementary metal oxide semiconductor; CCD, charge-coupled device.

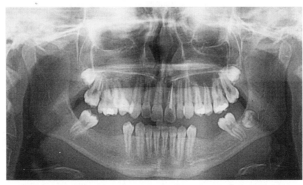

Figure 8-5 Digital panoramic image using charge-coupled device (CCD) acquisition. *(Courtesy of Planmeca Oy, Helsinki, Finland.)*

Today, many types of panoramic x-ray machines are made by many different manufacturers. An example of a film-based machine and a digital machine are seen in Figure 8-6. The basic principles of image formation are the same for most machines whether they are film-based or digital. The x-ray tube and the cassette holder are connected to each other across the top of the unit. These components rotate simultaneously around the patient, and the x-ray beam is always directed at the image receptor. The area where the images are sharp is a three-dimensional horseshoe-shaped zone (like the jaws) called the **focal trough** or *image layer* (Fig. 8-7). Only structures in this zone will be clearly recorded; the rest are blurred out. The result is an image that shows the jaws from one side to the other (Fig. 8-8). The remaining areas of the patient's head are out of focus on the image. The physics of panoramic image formation and the creation of the focal trough are beyond the scope of this textbook.

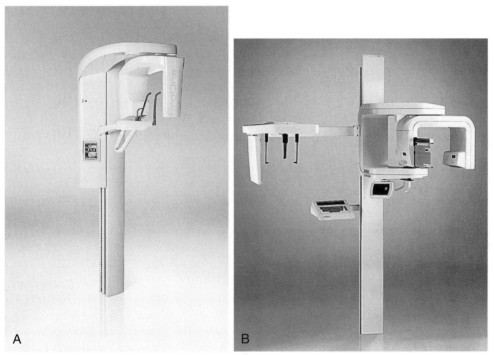

Figure 8-6 A, Digital panoramic machine. **B,** Film-based panoramic machine. *(Courtesy of Planmeca Oy, Helsinki, Finland.)*

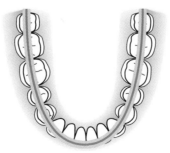

Figure 8-7 Schematic representation of the focal trough, or image layer, of a panoramic machine. Structures in the middle of the layer *(darkest area)* will be sharply depicted; those toward the periphery will be less sharply depicted. All structures outside the layer will be blurred and magnified.

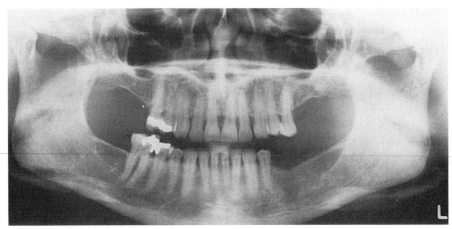

Figure 8-8 Typical film-based panoramic image.

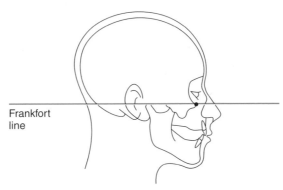

Frankfort
line

Figure 8-9 The Frankfort plane, or Frankfort line, of the skull passes from the floor of the orbit to the external auditory meatus.

Because each panoramic machine is slightly different, the manufacturer's instructions for patient positioning and exposure should be followed carefully. For all machines, the patient should be standing or sitting erect, with the spine as straight as possible. A thyroid collar is not routinely used with panoramic imaging because it interferes with the lower portion of the image. The upward angulation of the x-ray beam in a panoramic unit helps minimize direct exposure of the thyroid gland, a relatively radiosensitive tissue. The most recent NCRP report[*] indicates that the use of a lead apron is not "essential" for panoramic radiography, but because many patients expect its use, it is still "prudent" to use one. Because the rotation of the tubehead is primarily around the *back* of the patient's head, any lead apron that is worn with panoramic imaging must not cover the back of the patient's neck.

The **midsagittal plane** of the patient's face should be *perpendicular* to the floor, and the **Frankfort plane** should be *parallel* to the floor. The Frankfort plane (Fig. 8-9) is the line that passes from the external auditory meatus through the floor of the orbit. This plane is sometimes difficult to visualize on a patient. It may help to visualize a line from the ala of the nose to the tragus of the ear tipped downward about 5°. Additionally, the patient's profile will be straight, without excessive tipping of the chin downward or upward.

---

[*]National Council on Radiation and Measurements (NCRP), *Radiation protection in dentistry,* Bethesda, Md., 2003, NCRP, Report No. 145, p 26.

Some panoramic machines position the Frankfort plane automatically for the operator (Fig. 8-10). Many units have a chin rest and a bite guide for the patient's incisors. Others have only a chin rest for positioning the patient (Fig. 8-11). Because the focal trough is not a very large area, correct patient positioning is critical in panoramic imaging. Incorrect positioning has consequences for the resulting images.

A panoramic image of diagnostic quality can be produced only if several steps are followed precisely. These include (1) machine preparation, (2) patient preparation, (3) proper patient positioning, (4) proper exposure factor selection, and (5) proper film processing if a film-based system is used. If any one of these steps in not performed correctly, the error or errors may lead to a diagnostically unacceptable image.

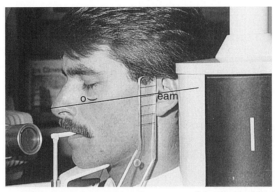

Figure 8-10 The patient's Frankfort plane is correctly and automatically positioned by the downward inclination of the machine chin rest. It is parallel to the linear markings on the head positioner, which are canted downward approximately 5°. The patient is biting correctly on a bite-pin. *o*, Orbit; *eam*, external auditory meatus.

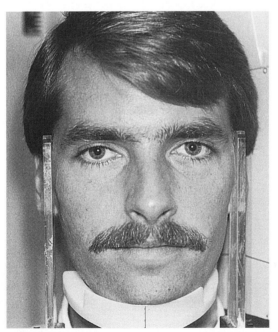

Figure 8-11 A panoramic machine with no bite-pin. A chin rest and head positioners help stabilize the patient's head.

Machine Preparation

The radiographer must prepare the panoramic machine before positioning the patient. Exposure factors should be selected and set (Fig. 8-12), the cassette should be loaded with x-ray film (if a film-based system is used), and the cassette should be positioned in the panoramic machine cassette holder. The height of the machine should be adjusted to the approximate entry position of the patient (Fig. 8-13). The operator also should place a sterile bite-pin in the bite-pin holder if the machine requires one.

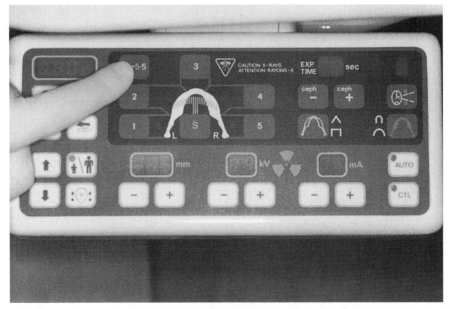

Figure 8-12 The operator selects exposure variables for the patient on a keypad with microelectronic circuitry. Some exposure variables are preprogrammed in the keypad, which reduces the number of buttons that must be pushed.

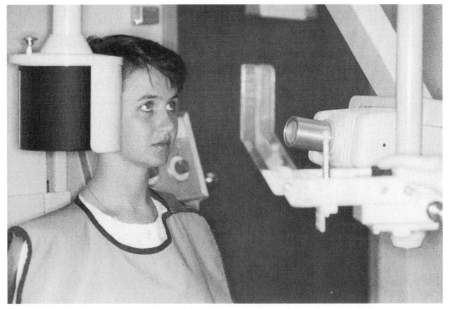

Figure 8-13 The chin rest and head positioner have been opened, or swung away from the chair, to allow the patient to be seated easily. Note there is no thyroid collar on the apron.

Patient Preparation

Eyeglasses, earrings, hearing aids, neck jewelry, hairpins, oral appliances, and any other removable metallic objects between the collar bone and the tops of the ears must be removed by the patient before the exposure of the image. A lead apron, preferably one that covers both the front and back of the patient, *without* a thyroid collar may be placed on the patient (see Fig. 8-13). Instructions to the patient (such as to stand still) or information about the rotational movement of the machine should be given at this time. Note that if the patient is wearing a hearing aid, instructions should be given before having the patient remove the hearing aid.

Failure to remove metallic objects often means that diagnostic information will be lost where the metal prevents x rays from penetrating tissues and reaching the image receptor. Additionally, because of the way the panoramic image is formed, the metal objects often create **ghost images**, or white streaks, on the opposite side of the object (see Fig. 8-22). These streaks also obscure diagnostic information such that a retake is often necessary.

Patient Positioning

Proper patient positioning is probably the most important step in the production of a quality panoramic image. Minor positioning errors can result in artifacts that render the subsequent image at least partially uninterpretable, often in the area of interest. If the exposure must be repeated, the patient's absorbed radiation dose will be doubled. The operator will also have the embarrassment of explaining to the patient why the second exposure is necessary.

Manufacturers have tried to make the positioning of the patient simple and repeatable. As stated earlier, many panoramic machines incorporate a bite-pin to help position the incisal edges of the incisors in a region that will result in a diagnostic image. This optimal region is known by several names, including the *focal trough, the zone of sharpness,* or the *central image layer* (see Fig. 8-7). Some contemporary machines have visible light guidelines that demonstrate the midsagittal plane and the occlusal plane or Frankfort plane. Many also include a visible light guide that indicates the correct position of the incisors in an anteroposterior direction. These light guides assist the operator in centering the patient in the focal trough (Fig. 8-14).

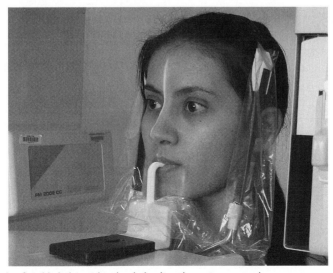

Figure 8-14 Example of visible light guides that help align the patient properly.

Generally, for a standard panoramic image, the patient must be positioned with the Frankfort plane parallel to the floor, the midsagittal plane perpendicular to the floor, and the incisors centered in the zone of sharpness according to the manufacturer's instructions. The patient's tongue should be flat against the hard palate. This avoids an air gap between the dorsum of the tongue and the palate; the air gap shows up as a dark streak over the maxillary teeth (Fig. 8-15). When the patient's tongue is in contact with the palate, the density over the maxilla is more uniform.

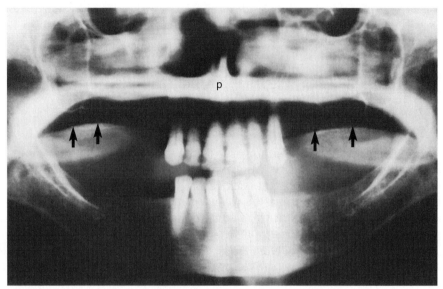

Figure 8-15 An example of an image showing that the patient did not raise the tongue to the roof of the mouth. The black area over the root apices lies between the dorsum of the tongue *(arrows)* and the hard palate *(p)*.

Table **8-2** | **Frequency of Patient Positioning Errors**

Error	Percent
Chin low	31.7
Tongue not raised	25.7
Patient slumped	12.9
Head tilted	9.9
Head rotated	6.9
Lips open	4
Too far forward	2
Bite guide not used	2
Chin high	1
Machine high	1
Prosthesis left in	1
Too far back	0
Chin not in rest	0
Patient movement	0

Adapted from Schiff T et al: Common positioning and technical errors in panoramic radiography, *J Am Dent Assoc* 113(3):422, 1986. Copyright 1986 American Dental Association. Reprinted by permission of ADA Publishing Co, Inc.

Errors in Panoramic Technique

The most common panoramic positioning errors produced are listed in order of frequency of occurrence in Table 8-2. Examples of some patient preparation and positioning errors appear in Figures 8-16 through 8-24. Processing, handling, and other technical errors appear in Chapter 9.

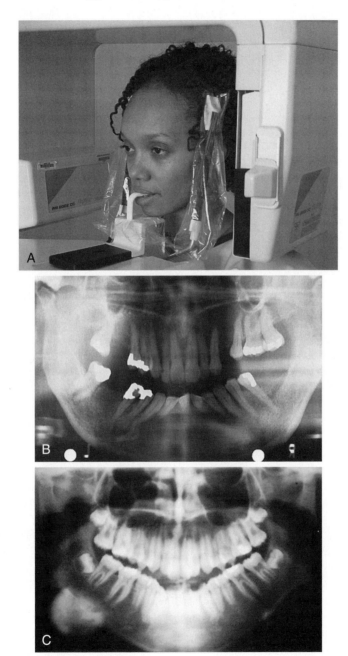

Figure 8-16 **A,** This patient's chin is tipped down too low. This position causes the occlusal plane to become an exaggerated V-shaped curve. **B,** This image demonstrates that the lower anterior teeth are positioned farther away from the image receptor than they should be when the patient's chin is tipped down. The mandibular anterior teeth are thus magnified and distorted, along with the bone of the anterior mandible. **C,** Another example of a patient positioned with the chin too low. Note the V-shaped occlusal plane. The opacity on the patient's right mandibular border is a bony tumor known as an osteoma.

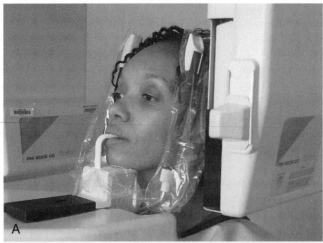

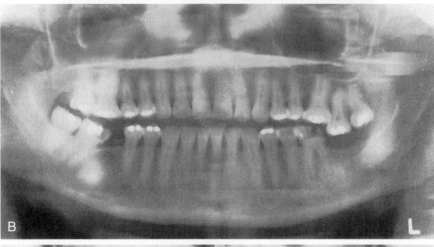

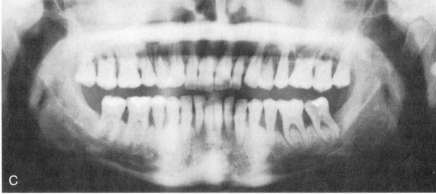

Figure 8-17   A, This patient's chin is tipped up too high. The resulting image will have a flattened or reversed curve of Spee (a frown) and distortion in the maxillary anterior area; sometimes the condyles will be projected off the sides of the image and will not be available for interpretation. **B,** This image shows that the chin is too high. Note the flattened curve of Spee and the loss of information in the anterior area. **C,** Another example of an elevated chin. Note also that the patient's tongue was not contacting the palate, which resulted in the dark streak over the maxillary teeth (see Fig. 8-15).

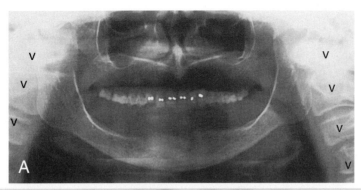

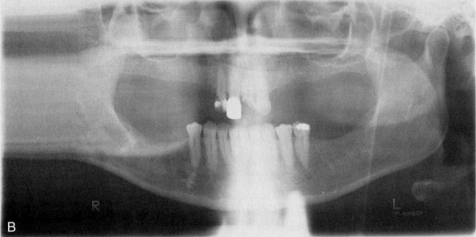

Figure 8-18   A, This patient was slumped too far forward; the neck was not straight. A great deal of the cervical spine is seen (the vertebrae are labeled *v*), and the vertebrae are superimposed over the ramus of the mandible. The patient's upper denture was left in place, possibly to help with positioning. Note also that the patient's tongue was not in contact with the hard palate, which left a dark shadow over the maxillary edentulous alveolar ridge. **B,** This patient was also slumped over. Because the cervical spine is not straight, a white area is seen in the midline of the image extending from the bottom edge to about the level of the hard palate. Some structures (teeth and bone) can still be seen through the white area. This is a typical result when a patient is not sitting or standing up straight in a panoramic unit. The more opaque area just to the patient's left of midline is a bit of the lead apron that was too high on the back of the patient's neck. In addition, the right side of the mandible is smeared due to the machine hitting the patient's right shoulder with resultant patient movement.

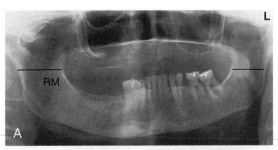

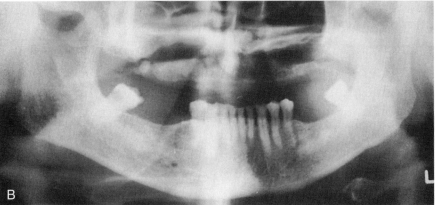

Figure 8-19 A, This patient's midsagittal plane was rotated away from midline. This error caused the right side of the mandible *(RM)* to be farther from the image receptor, more toward the lingual aspect of the focal trough and thus magnified relative to the left side. (Compare the widths of each ramus and see the difference.) The head was also tilted, or canted, upward on the left side. Look at the levels of the left and right angles of the mandible. **B,** This patient's head was rotated away from midline. This position error resulted in magnification of several anatomic structures on the patient's right side.

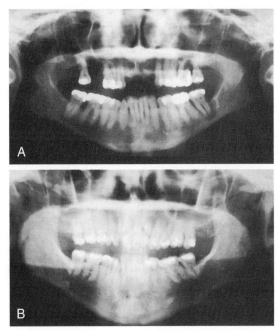

Figure 8-20 A and **B,** These patients were placed too far forward (too close to the image receptor in the anterior part of the mouth). Note the slender appearance of the anterior teeth; they have not been magnified *enough* and therefore appear very narrow.

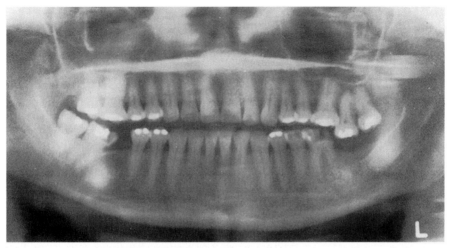

Figure 8-21 This patient was placed too far back. Note that the anterior teeth are now very wide; they are too far away from the image receptor and were magnified too much.

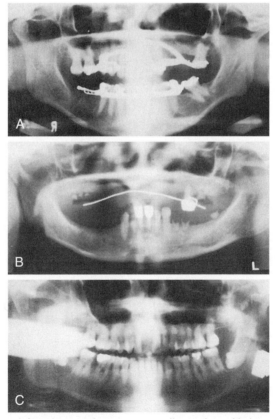

Figure 8-22 Metallic objects left in place. **A,** The patient's maxillary and mandibular removable partial dentures were left in place before exposure. This error caused loss of diagnostic information. **B,** This patient's acrylic partial denture was left in place. The denture contained a thin wire for stabilization and to clasp the remaining maxillary molar. **C,** This patient's hearing aid was left in the patient's left ear. Note the large white streak on the opposite side. This is the ghost image of the hearing aid.

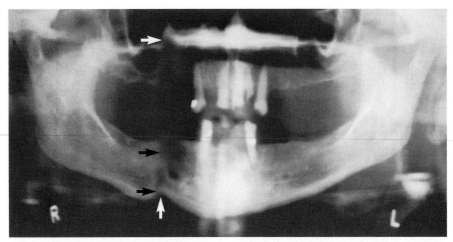

Figure 8-23   The patient moved during the exposure, which resulted in an interruption of the image along the inferior border of the mandible that resembles a fracture. Note, however, that the distortion extends upward through the entire image to the region of the hard palate *(arrows)*.

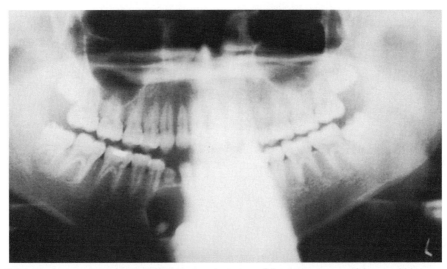

Figure 8-24   The large radiopaque shadow obscuring the image of the anterior parts of the mandible was caused by an improperly placed lead apron. Recall that the beam circles *behind* the patient; therefore it is important that the apron stay low on the back of the neck. Observe that the apron shadow obscures some pathologic condition just to the right of midline on the patient.

Panoramic Anatomic Landmarks

Interpretation of the many normal anatomic structures, artifacts called *ghost images,* and pathologic processes on a panoramic image is complicated because of the complex way the image is produced. As with intraoral images, a sound knowledge of the appearance of normal anatomic structures is mandatory for the operator. Because the production of the panoramic image requires that both the x-ray source and the image receptor rotate around the patient's head, certain anatomic structures, especially those near the center of the patient's head, will be imaged twice. Examples of this include the cervical spine and the hyoid bone. In addition, many of the structures are superimposed over each other. Sometimes one has to look "through" one structure to see another. An example of this is the styloid process, which is frequently seen in the same area as the soft tissue of the ear (Fig. 8-25).

This chapter is limited to the most common anatomic structures seen on most panoramic images. Not all of these structures appear on every panoramic image every time. However, by studying the legends and by practicing finding these structures on actual panoramic images, you will become skilled in identifying these normal features. It is only when you know what is normal that you will be able to determine the abnormal features of pathologic lesions. Figures 8-25 and 8-26 will get you started, and Figure 8-27 has several landmarks labeled.

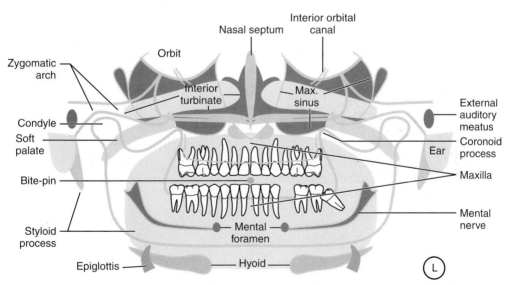

Figure 8-25 This diagram outlines some of the structures that can be visualized on a panoramic image. This example has been labeled with the names of these common structures. Practice naming and identifying these structures before testing yourself with Fig. 8-26.

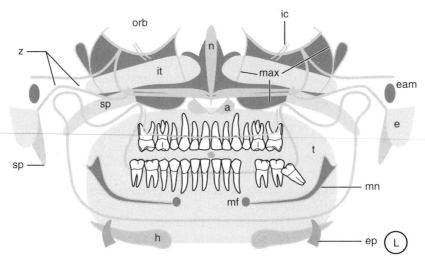

Figure 8-26 See how many structures you can identify without looking at Fig. 8-25. Hint: the initials of the structures are on the diagram.

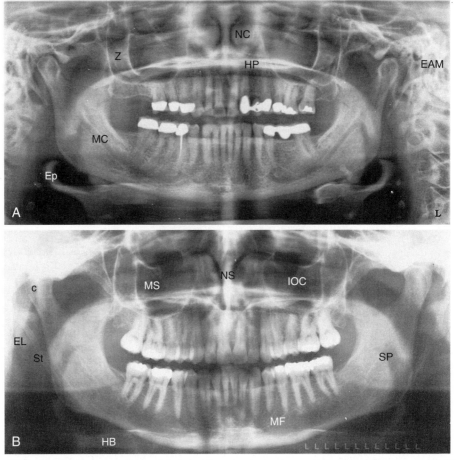

Figure 8-27 **A** and **B,** Panoramic images labeled with anatomic structures. *C,* Condyle; *EAM,* external auditory meatus; *EL,* ear lobe; *Ep,* epiglottis; *HB,* hyoid bone; *HP,* hard palate; *IOC,* infraorbital canal; *MC,* mandibular canal; *MF,* mental foramen; *MS,* maxillary sinus; *NC,* nasal concha; *NS,* nasal septum; *SP,* soft palate; *St,* styloid process; *Z,* zygoma. *(A, Courtesy of Michael J. Murray, DDS, Darien, Conn.)*

CONE BEAM PANORAMIC PROJECTIONS

Cone beam volumetric imaging, discussed more in Chapter 11, is a special kind of digital imaging that is more similar to computed tomography than to conventional radiography. A cone-shaped beam of radiation and a special image detector array rotate around a patient's head. A computer then allows reconstruction of the data recorded by the image detector into many different views, including three-dimensional reconstruction or cross-sectional views. A projection similar to a panoramic projection can be reconstructed by the computer, although the image appears slightly different than a more conventional panoramic image. Interpretation may be somewhat easier for a cone beam panoramic reconstruction because landmarks in the "slice" can be seen more clearly without superimposition of other anatomic structures.

STUDY QUESTIONS

1. The area of the patient that is in focus and thus exhibited on a panoramic image is called the
   A. Latent image
   B. Image layer
   C. Ghost image
   D. Frankfort plane

2. In general, film-based panoramic images have which of the following characteristics compared with film-based intraoral images?
   A. Less contrast
   B. Greater detail or resolution
   C. Greater contrast
   D. Less detail or resolution

3. Which of the following articles would a patient be allowed to wear during a panoramic exposure?
   A. Earrings
   B. Necklace
   C. Wristwatch
   D. Hearing aid

4. You notice a dark streak or band superimposed over the apices of the maxillary teeth on a panoramic image. Which of the following errors occurred during the exposure?
   A. The patient was positioned with the chin too low
   B. The patient was positioned with the chin too high
   C. The patient's head was turned to the side
   D. The patient's tongue was not contacting the hard palate

5. If a patient was positioned in a panoramic unit with his or her chin too high, which of the following would be seen on the resulting image?
   A. Narrow, blurry anterior teeth
   B. Flattened or reversed occlusal plane
   C. Molars on one side more magnified than on the other side
   D. Unusually wide anterior teeth

6. A panoramic image shows very slender (narrow) and blurry anterior teeth. Which of the following errors was made during the exposure?
   A. The patient's chin was too high
   B. The patient's chin was too low
   C. The patient was too far forward in the machine (too close to the image receptor)
   D. The patient was too far back in the machine (too far away from the image receptor)

7. A panoramic image shows an opaque (white) streak in the center of the film, from the bottom edge of the image to the level of the hard palate. You can still make out the teeth and bone in that area, but they are much harder to see than on the rest of the image. What error was made during the exposure?
   A. The patient was not standing/sitting up straight
   B. The patient's chin was too high
   C. The patient's chin was too low
   D. The patient's tongue was not in contact with the hard palate

8. Which of the following anatomic landmarks would you expect to find on a panoramic image but is not normally present on intraoral images?
   A. Mental foramen
   B. Mandibular canal
   C. Maxillary tuberosity
   D. Mandibular condyle

9. Which of the following anatomic landmarks can be seen on both panoramic and intra-oral images?
   A. Coronoid process
   B. Hyoid bone
   C. Floor of the orbit
   D. Styloid process

10. Which of the following anatomic structures is a single structure (there is only one of them) but can be seen more than once on a panoramic image?
    A. Mandibular condyle
    B. Hard palate
    C. Hyoid bone
    D. Mental foramen

9

Trouble-Shooting Technique and Processing Errors

"There is no shortage of errors."* Errors made during either the exposure phase or the processing phase of intraoral radiography often result in excess exposure to ionizing radiation (x rays) for the patient. Images that are undiagnostic are almost always retaken. Each retake of a dental image *doubles* the absorbed x-ray dose to the patient in that particular anatomic region, no matter what image receptor you are using.

Learning the most common radiographic errors and their correction during the preclinical phase of your career will save you embarrassment and save your patient unnecessary radiation exposure. Most errors in intraoral radiographic techniques can be divided into two categories: (1) exposure technique and (2) film processing. The use of digital imaging essentially removes the chemical processing errors, but it is advisable for all operators to be aware of these potential errors in the event that chemical processing is needed for some reason. Before we examine each of these categories let us review the criteria for a diagnostically useful intraoral image. Box 9-1 outlines criteria for both the intraoral periapical and bitewing images.

ERRORS IN EXPOSURE TECHNIQUE

Mistakes in exposure technique can be subdivided into *operator* and *patient* errors. The majority of exposure technique errors are *caused by the operator*. Table 9-1 outlines the most common errors.

Operator Errors

Improper Image-Receptor Positioning

The correct placement of the image receptor is the first and most critical step in good exposure technique. Reviewing the criteria for correct positioning in each anatomic region, as described in Chapter 1, would be helpful before proceeding in this chapter. You will recall that each receptor is placed to image-specific portions of

---

Anonymous—Overheard in all dental radiology training clinics in English-speaking countries.

Box **9-1** CRITERIA FOR A DIAGNOSTICALLY USEFUL RADIOGRAPH

Periapical Image
1. The correct anatomic area should be represented.
2. At least 3 to 4 mm ($^1/_4$ inch) of alveolar bone should be visible beyond the apex.
3. The image should not be elongated or foreshortened.
4. The radiograph should have acceptable density.
5. The radiograph should be free of film handling or processing errors.
6. The interproximal contacts should not overlap.
7. There should be no cone cuts.
8. The embossed (raised) dot should appear at the incisal or the occlusal edge.
9. In a complete mouth radiographic survey, the apex of each tooth should be visible at least once, preferably twice.

Bitewing Image
1. The interproximal contacts should not be overlapped from the distal surface of the canine to the mesial surface of the third molar.
2. The crowns of the maxillary and mandibular teeth should be centered in the image from top to bottom.
3. The crest of the alveolar bone should be visible with *no* superimposition of the crowns of the adjacent teeth.
4. The occlusal plane should be as horizontal as possible.

Table 9-1 | **Exposure Technique Errors**

Common Error	Operator	Patient
Improper film positioning	Improper film-holding	Patient movement
Apical areas missing	instrument assembly	Film movement
Film bending	Improper tubehead angulation	
Film backward	Overlapping	
Improper film selection	Cone cutting	
Double exposure	Overexposure	
	Underexposure	

the teeth and related structures. Three guidelines, if followed closely, will minimize receptor positioning errors:

1. The distal surface of the canine should be visible in the premolar view (periapical *and* bitewing).
2. The third molar region should be visible in the molar periapical view.
3. The tooth/teeth of interest should be centered in the periapical image.

Distal Surface of the Canine Visible in Premolar View. Figure 9-1 reveals that, in most instances, even the ideal positioning of the receptor for the maxillary canine will result in overlap of the lingual cusp of the first premolar onto the distal aspect of the canine (see the diagram of the maxillary canine view in the section on paralleling technique in Chapter 1). This overlap is almost unavoidable. Therefore, the distal surface *must* be visualized on each of the premolar periapical and premolar bitewing views. This visualization is mandatory for the detection of carious lesions on the distal surface of the canine. Figure 9-2 shows both ideal and inadequate premolar views. Missing the distal of the canine in a premolar view is one of the most common, and most critical, positioning errors in intraoral imaging techniques.

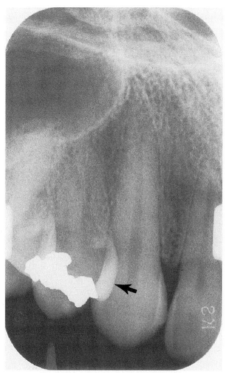

Figure 9-1 Although the maxillary right canine is reasonably well centered in the view, the lingual cusp of the first premolar is superimposed on the distal contact area of the canine *(arrow)*. Any interproximal caries could not be detected in this area.

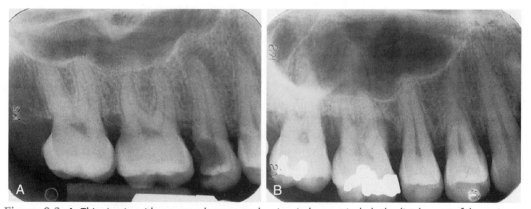

Figure 9-2 **A,** This view is neither a premolar nor a molar view. It does not include the distal aspect of the canine or the entire third molar region. It demonstrates, therefore, incorrect positioning. **B,** This image represents accurate positioning for a maxillary right premolar periapical view.

Third Molar Region Visible. You will note that this guideline reads "third molar *region*" and not just "third molar." The clinical absence of the third molar (in the mouth) does not mean that it is not present in the bone. Unerupted or impacted third molars (wisdom teeth) are very common. If the adult patient states that the wisdom teeth have not been extracted, you must assume that they are present. The molar view you take should extend far enough past the second permanent molar to include the entire third molar, *even if this means excluding the distal surface of the second premolar.*

If the second molar is centered in the film, the third molar region should be seen in the image. This extended view is especially critical in the mandible, where third molars are frequently horizontally impacted and are often larger than maxillary third molars. Figure 9-3 illustrates this point.

Tooth/Teeth of Interest Centered. This concept is simple, but it is crucial to good radiographic technique. With any image-receptor–holding device, if you center the receptor in the bite block and the tooth of interest is on the bite block, there is little chance of incorrect positioning (assuming that you have assembled the instrument correctly to begin with). *Contacting the bite block with the biting surface of the teeth of interest is critical to correct film or image-receptor placement.* For example, in the case of the maxillary premolar view, *if you center the premolar–molar contact in the middle of the bite block, the image will normally extend far enough anteriorly to capture the distal of the canine* (Fig. 9-4).

If you center the maxillary or mandibular second permanent molar in a molar periapical view, you will include the entire third molar region in most cases.

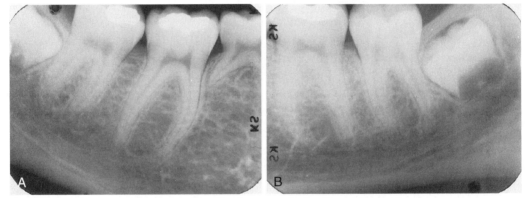

Figure 9-3 **A,** Incorrect positioning: not all of the developing third molar is visible on the image. **B,** Correct positioning.

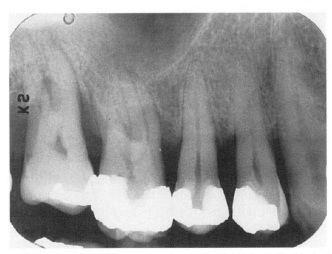

Figure 9-4 If the premolar–molar contact is centered in the middle of the plastic bite block, the image receptor extends far enough anteriorly to include the canine.

Occasionally patient anatomy or tooth position will limit the ideal view. However, if you follow the three guidelines, you will eliminate the positioning errors that are the most commonly made and that require retaking the image. Other positioning errors are included in the section on apical areas missing, which is discussed next.

Apical Areas Missing

One of the most common reasons for the visualization of the apices of the teeth to be missing from the image is that the receptor was not placed high enough in the palate or low enough in the floor of the mouth for adequate coverage of the patient's anatomy. With the paralleling technique, when the operator is using positioning instruments, apical areas are missing because the teeth of interest were not in contact with the bite block (Fig. 9-5).

A patient's inability to completely close on the bite block is often the fault of the operator. If the edge of the film or image receptor is forced into sensitive tissues (often the lingual mucosa or the muscle attachments in the floor of the mouth), the resulting pain will prevent the patient from fully closing on the bite block. The result will look like the image in Figure 9-5.

Patient anatomy usually dictates the orientation of the long axis of the image receptor. If the floor of the mouth is shallow, perfect parallel placement may be impossible. Any receptor in any region of the mouth may be angled up to 15° from parallel and still be reasonably free of significant geometric distortion. Receptor angles steeper than 15° will cause distortion, usually in the form of foreshortening, if the beam is directed perpendicularly to the receptor as indicated by the ring and rod (see also Chapter 10). Improper tubehead angulation can also cause distortion. Remember, however, that failure to show the root apices plus at least a few millimeters of supporting bone at the apices always necessitates a retake (Fig. 9-6). The operator has complete control over the image-receptor placement, including angulation of the receptor.

Film Bending

Sometimes, to make the patient more comfortable, it is appropriate to *gently* curve, or bend, the film. This bending allows the film to follow the contours of the anatomy more readily (Fig. 9-7, A). However, bending a large portion of the film or putting

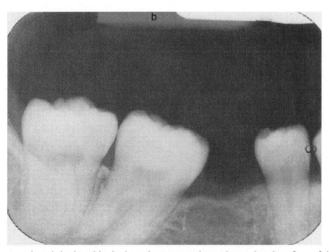

Figure 9-5 The operator placed the bite block *(b)* at least 1 cm above the occlusal surface of the mandibular teeth. The instrument and image receptor may be angled and the tongue gently displaced to allow the bite block to rest against the teeth of interest *before* the patient closes.

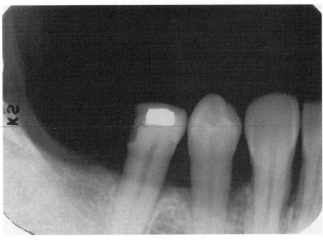

Figure 9-6 Missed apical areas. The patient was uncomfortable and would not close on the instrument. See Chapter 10 for suggestions on how to manage such a patient.

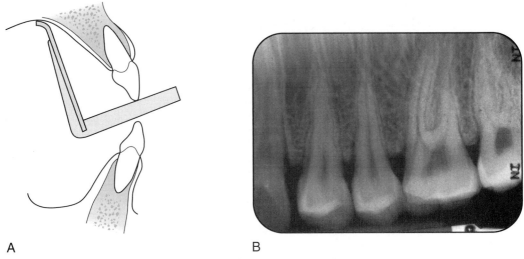

A   B

Figure 9-7 A illustrates bending of the upper edge of the film against the palate. Most of the distortion will be localized to the bent area. **B** illustrates where the film was bent in the floor of the mouth in this mandibular view. The teeth on the right side of the image are not nearly as distorted as those on the left.

a distinct crease in it will result in image distortion (Fig. 9-7, B) or a crease artifact (labeled *c* in Fig. 9-8). Rigid digital imaging receptors cannot be curved or bent, which may be a disadvantage in some patients with restrictive anatomy. Phosphor plates *cannot* be curved or bent because this will ruin the phosphor coating and require replacement of the plate.

Note the difference in the image distortion between Figure 9-7, B (regional distortion) and Figure 9-9 (distortion is seen in all apical areas, but the crowns look proportional). The distortion caused by localized film bending is localized to the bent region. Distortion that is generalized throughout the apical portions of the image was the result of bending the entire bottom edge of the film against the floor of the mouth, probably to make the procedure more comfortable for the child patient.

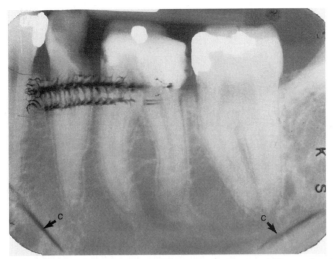

Figure 9-8 The letter *c* designates a crease in the emulsion owing to excessive folding or bending of the film. The artifact that looks like a centipede is due to excessive pressure of a hemostat used to hold the film in place.

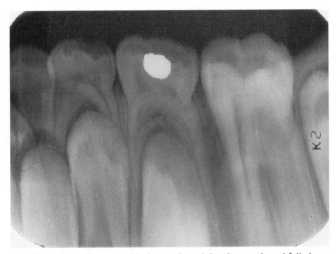

Figure 9-9 Elongation of the apices of the mandibular teeth and developing dental follicles owing to bending of the entire lower edge of the film packet.

Placing the Film Backward

The operator must make sure that the sensitive side of the film or image receptor faces the x-ray beam. If you are in doubt, remember that it is the *white* side of intraoral x-ray film that should be next to the teeth and face the beam. The sensitive side of a charge-coupled device (CCD) digital receptor will not have the wire connector, and the sensitive side of a phosphor storage plate will be identified by the manufacturer.

Note that in Figure 9-10 the image of the teeth and surrounding structures is lighter than normal (underexposed). This is because the lead foil backing in the film packet attenuated (stopped) many of the x rays that would have exposed the film and registered the image. Depending on the film type, a pattern in the lead foil *may* be visible on the image. Films that have been exposed backward also cause confusion when mounting because the embossed dot will be *depressed instead of raised* when looking at the image in its proper anatomic orientation. Therefore, left and right can easily be confused.

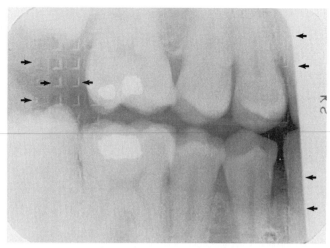

Figure 9-10 This image illustrates many errors. The image is light overall. A cone cut from a rectangular cylinder (see also Fig. 9-22) is visible on the right side of the film *(small arrows)*. Also present is a tire track or pattern from the lead foil *(large arrows)* confirming that this film was placed backward.

Improper Film Selection

Chapter 1 showed several examples of different film sizes (see Fig. 1-16). Improper selection of film size will result in many problems. If the film selected is too small, the region or tooth of interest may not be captured on the image (Fig. 9-11). If the film selected is too large, the patient will not accept the film comfortably. This discomfort can result in errors of distortion, missed apical areas, patient movement, or overlapping of tooth structures.

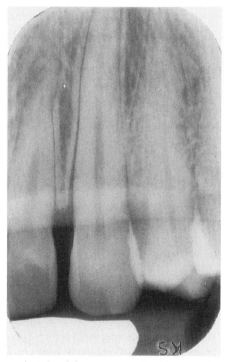

Figure 9-11 A size no. 0 film was selected and the canine apex is not seen. A size no. 1 film should have been used.

Digital imaging receptors, including storage phosphor plates, also come in different sizes, and the principles of proper size selection also apply to digital imaging. Keep in mind that the image will be slightly smaller than the actual receptor size.

Double Exposure

You must be careful to separate exposed and unexposed films to avoid double exposures. There are several ways of doing this, including having unexposed films laid out with the white side up and then placing an exposed film on the tray or counter with the back side showing or placing exposed films into a disposable receptacle before selecting a new, unexposed film. Keeping the films in a disposable receptacle such as a paper cup will also facilitate infection control procedures for film processing, discussed in Chapter 2.

A film that has been exposed twice will (1) be overexposed, (2) be undiagnostic, and (3) result in mandatory retakes (Fig. 9-12). That is correct, *retakes* (plural). A patient will receive *two* times the radiation dose to *two* anatomic areas. For example, if you take a premolar periapical image and then use the same film to take the molar image, that film will be undiagnostic for both areas. Therefore, an image *must be retaken of each area.* This results in lost time because of the necessary two retakes; furthermore, there is the embarrassment of making such an avoidable error. Double exposure of films is easily avoided with attention to detail and a systematic approach to placement and exposure.

It is also possible to doubly expose a panoramic image (Fig. 9-13). Being organized in the darkroom will help prevent this error.

Improper Instrument Assembly

When preparing image-receptor holders that come in separate pieces, you should always look through the indicator ring to ensure that the image receptor is centered in the ring. If it is not, reassemble the instrument correctly. Figure 9-14 shows this simple check for proper assembly. If the instrument assembly is *not* checked, and the ring happens to be misaligned, you will not be able to see the bite block once the patient's mouth is closed. You will undoubtedly align the x-ray beam with the ring, which is not pointing at the bite block. The result will be a significant "cone cut" that may result in a retake.

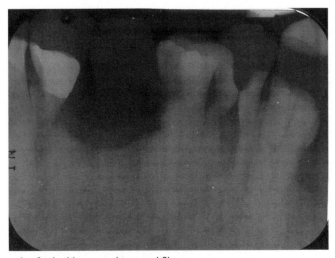

Figure 9-12 An example of a doubly exposed intraoral film.

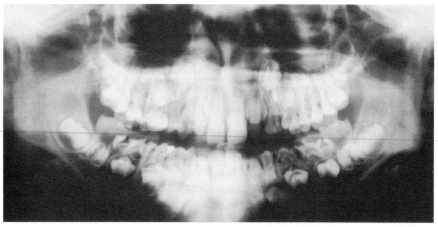

Figure 9-13 This unusual panoramic image is the result of a double exposure. The film was exposed twice in the cassette before processing.

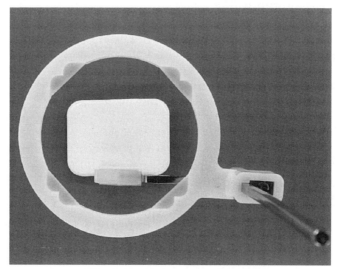

Figure 9-14 Proper instrument assembly. The bite block is centered in the ring.

Improper Beam Angulation (Vertical)

The proper image receptor has been selected. The receptor holder is correctly assembled, and the receptor is placed correctly in the patient's mouth. The patient is comfortable. Nonetheless, various errors can occur subsequent to all these steps. Aligning the face of the tubehead cylinder with the indicator ring and paralleling the length of the cylinder with the indicator rod will ensure correct x-ray beam alignment in the vertical dimension (Fig. 9-15).

Figures 9-16 and 9-17 show what happens to the radiographic image when the vertical angulation is too steep, either positively or negatively (causing foreshortening), or too shallow (causing elongation). The use of the paralleling technique with positioning devices minimizes these errors significantly.

Patient anatomy can also cause problems. Knowing a patient's anatomic variations by thoroughly inspecting the patient's mouth clinically will help you reduce the number of undiagnostic images. Figure 9-18, A, shows a correctly positioned cylinder and the image receptor correctly placed in a shallow palate. Note how the receptor

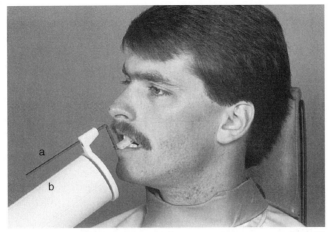

Figure 9-15 The cone is properly aligned with the ring. This proper alignment is confirmed by the orientation of the indicator rod *(a)* parallel to the top of the cylinder and to the indented linear markings *(b)* on the cylinder surface.

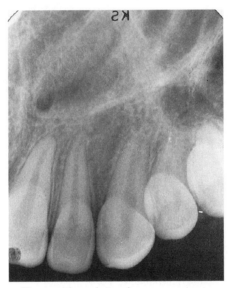

Figure 9-16 Foreshortening caused by vertical angulation that was too steep.

position has changed from a preferred parallel position to a more horizontally tipped position. The instrument is indicating to you to use a very steep angulation, but this would foreshorten the teeth *(arrows,* Fig. 9-18, B) and cast the shadow of the zygoma *(z)* onto the teeth apices. Your prior awareness of these potential problems would alert you to "cheat" the instrument, that is, select a slightly shallower vertical angulation, thus minimizing the potential problems described. The film holder is an *indicating* device, not a *dictating* one.

Improper Beam Angulation (Horizontal)

Errors in beam angulation can occur in the horizontal, as well as the vertical, direction. Improper selection of the horizontal angulation will result in *overlapping* of interproximal contact areas of proximal enamel surfaces (as in Figs. 9-19, 9-20, A, and 9-21, A). This error is especially critical in interproximal bitewing imaging. Because many periapical views also afford the clinician another look at the

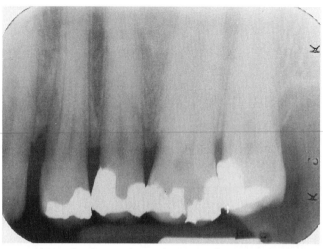

Figure 9-17 Maxillary premolars and molars are distorted owing to elongation (too shallow vertical angulation).

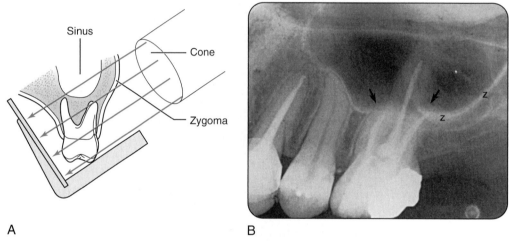

A   B

Figure 9-18 A, The shallow palate causes the image receptor to be inclined away from the long axis of the molar. As a result, the zygoma may be superimposed over the tooth, and the buccal roots will appear much shorter than the palatal root of the molar. **B,** Image demonstrating superimposition of the zygoma *(z)* and short buccal roots *(arrows).* The opacity at the top edge of the image is a palatal torus, which probably contributed to the compromised film position.

proximal surfaces and alveolar bone levels, the operator should always try to open contacts (as in Fig. 9-20, B) on these views as well. Additional bitewing views may also be needed to open all contact areas (Fig. 9-21, B).

It is generally accepted that two bitewing views, a premolar and a molar, are necessary to demonstrate correctly all contact areas when the patient has complete adult dentition. This is because the arch curvature from canine to third molar rarely allows one film to demonstrate open contacts of the entire region (see Fig. 9-21, B). For this reason we discourage the use of the no. 3 size bitewing film and suggest that two no. 2 size image receptors are usually necessary to adequately open all contact areas.

Cone Cutting

The term *cone cutting* is an unusual phrase but one that is commonly used in intra-oral radiography to describe an area of the image receptor that was not exposed. The cone is really an open-ended cylinder, usually round, but the beam-indicating device

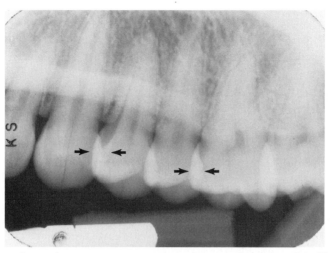

Figure 9-19 Overlapped enamel areas *(arrows)*. Here the patient opened slightly, and the film shifted. The shift changed the horizontal angulation of the beam in relationship to the teeth.

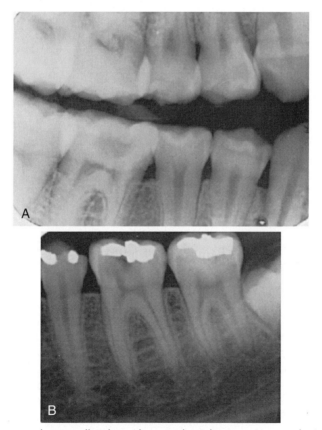

Figure 9-20 **A,** The contacts between all molar teeth are overlapped owing to improper horizontal angulation. **B,** "Open" contacts on a periapical image with correct horizontal angulation.

may also be an open-ended rectangle, not a cylinder. *Cone* is used as a generic term for them all.

Figure 9-22 illustrates what happens if a round cylinder does not cover the image receptor correctly. A rectangular cone cut was shown in Figure 9-10. One region in which cone cutting commonly occurs is the molar view. Operators may be so

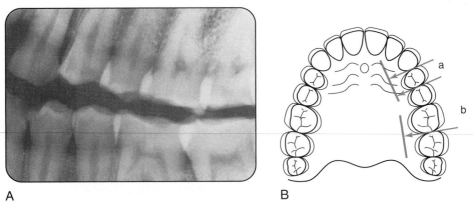

A   B

Figure 9-21   **A,** This image illustrates an "open" contact area on the distal surface of the canines, but the posterior contacts are "closed" or overlapped. Additional views are required to image all interproximal areas. **B,** The *arrows* show the different directions from which the central ray *(CR)* must enter to minimize or eliminate overlap; *a* is the premolar view and *b* the molar view.

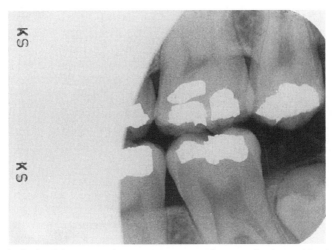

Figure 9-22   A round cylinder did not cover the image-receptor surface completely, resulting in a cone cut.

concerned with covering the distal region of the third molar or with showing all the contacts on the bitewing image that they move the tubehead too far posterior. This results in a cone cut in the premolar region. Remember that the molar *bitewing* image needs to cover only the contact between the second and third molars; extending past the distal surface of the third molar is not necessary.

Figure 9-23 shows both the correct and incorrect versions of beam alignment. To help with alignment if you are not using a positioning instrument, ask the patient to part his or her lips or "grin at you" with the teeth closed (Fig. 9-24). You can often see the most anterior edge of the image receptor, and you can extend the anterior edge of the cylinder or cone just slightly beyond this point (anteriorly) to ensure total exposure of the image receptor.

Overexposure or Underexposure

Overexposed (dark) films can occur in several ways. One way was discussed in this chapter's section on double exposure. In addition, one can overexpose an image by improper selection of (1) the exposure time (too long), (2) the kilovoltage peak

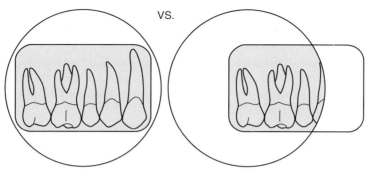

Figure 9-23 Correct beam position *(left)* versus incorrect beam position *(right)*.

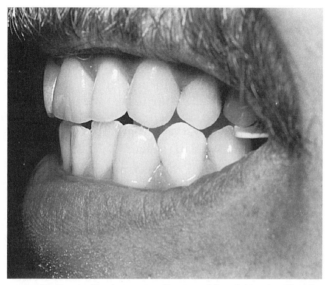

Figure 9-24 Patient parting his lips to allow better visualization of the tab bitewing film placement to assist in positioning the cone. Note that you can see the anterior edge of the film near his canines.

(too high), or (3) the milliamperage (too high). However, most modern dental x-ray machines have a fixed milliamperage and kilovoltage. Therefore, the most common overexposure error is due to improper exposure time selection. Keep in mind, too, that the distance of the x-ray source to the image receptor also affects film density. A shorter-than-normal distance will result in an overexposed, dark image.

A list of exposure factors in the form of a chart should be posted in all operatories to ensure proper time of exposure. Attention to this chart will help eliminate overexposure of dental images. However, be prepared to use longer times on larger-than-average patients and shorter times on smaller-than-average patients. This rule applies to both adults and children.

Underexposed images can also occur in several ways. If routine or average exposure factors are selected for the larger-than-average patient, it may be difficult to penetrate the tissues; that is, the thickness of the patient's tissues may not allow the x rays to reach the film. A film placed backward, with the lead foil between the tubehead and the film, will also be underexposed (see Fig. 9-10). Not moving the indicator ring close enough to the patient may also result in an underexposed image; the inverse square law dictates that if the x-ray source is too far away from the patient, the beam will not be as intense.

Just as you can select too long an exposure time, you can also select too short an exposure time. If you have exposed a mandibular central incisor region for 0.1 second and you forget to *change the time* for a maxillary molar periapical view, which should be 0.2 second, the molar periapical image will be underexposed and possibly undiagnostic. Remember that a digital image receptor may be underexposed just as film may be underexposed. This error may require a retake. Figure 9-25 demonstrates an underexposed image.

Digital receptors offer a unique advantage here because it is almost impossible to overexpose or underexpose them. In addition, if an improper time was selected, the information is often recoverable by using the image processing software of the imaging system or perhaps the practice management system.

Patient Errors

Patient Movement

Just about the only retake that can be blamed on the patient is that resulting from patient movement. However, the operator can *control or minimize this problem*. Patient movement usually arises from discomfort (for example, because of improper image-receptor placement, failure to take anatomic restrictions into account, or an unsupported patient head position). These are really operator errors. Patient movement resulting from gagging or swallowing or both can also largely be prevented but is sometimes unavoidable. Figure 9-26 demonstrates images with *(A)* and without *(B)* patient movement. Figure 9-27 demonstrates patient movement, as well as film creases. See Chapter 8 for an example of patient movement during a panoramic exposure.

Film or Image-Receptor Movement

An image receptor may move in the bite block because the plastic holder is worn out from bending the backing plate too much or too often (Fig. 9-28).

Image receptors can also move if patients move their tongues or swallow. It is sometimes difficult to separate patient and film movement: one is often the result of the other. The results are the same: a blurred image. Some patients will move their heads (thus moving the image receptor) in response to your directions; patients

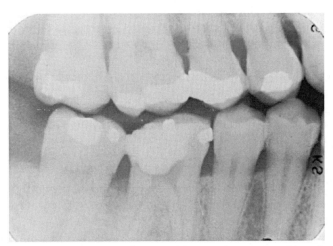

Figure 9-25 This molar bitewing image is so underexposed that it is almost impossible to distinguish enamel from dentin. Caries would be impossible to detect in this image.

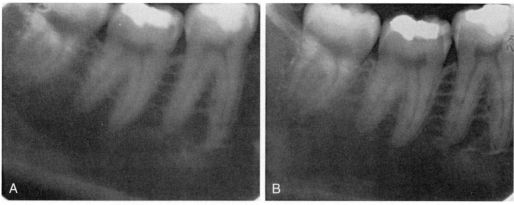

Figure 9-26 Images with **(A)** and without **(B)** patient movement.

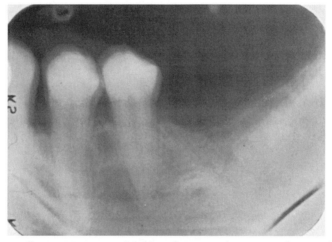

Figure 9-27 This image illustrates patient motion (blurred image) and a crease artifact (see also Fig. 9-8).

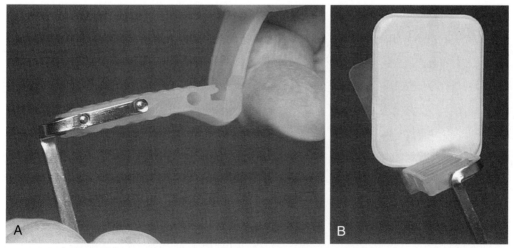

Figure 9-28 **A,** Operator bending backing plate. **B,** Film dislodges easily and would be incorrectly positioned in the patient's mouth.

often nod in agreement. The best results come from direct observation of the patient at the moment of exposure. If any movement is seen, do not continue. Reinstruct the patient and/or reposition the image receptor as necessary.

PROCESSING ERRORS

Successfully exposing the image receptor is only half of the radiographic imaging process. Many films are rendered undiagnostic because of improper film processing. Dental x-ray films, as discussed in Chapter 2, must be processed carefully, with attention to detail, under good safelight conditions, and in a clean environment. Poor chemicals, inadequate development time or temperature, and improper darkroom safelighting are but a few examples of how a quality film can be ruined. Box 9-2 outlines the major processing errors that the operator must avoid.

Stained Films

Any fluid can stain a dental x-ray film. If drops of water on a film are left in contact long enough, they will dissolve the emulsion in the area and leave a clear spot (Fig. 9-29). Some water stains will be dark but translucent because they only dilute the film emulsion and allow it to run (Fig. 9-30). Yellow or brown stains on a radiograph are usually a sign of improper washing or clearing of the fixer solution from the film. The excess fixer oxidizes with age and discolors, leaving a yellow or brown stain. Fixer dropped onto an unprocessed film will cause a white spot, usually in a round or ovoid shape (Fig. 9-31).

Box **9-2** **Processing Errors**

Stained Films

- Fixer artifact
- Developer artifact
- Water stains
- Fluoride stains

Dark Films

- Light leaks
- Development time too long
- Developer concentration high
- Paper stuck to film
- Improper fixation
- Temperature too high

Fogged Films

- Safelight problems
- Improper film storage

Light Films

- Development time too short
- Developer concentration low
- Contaminated developer
- Excess fixer
- Temperature too low

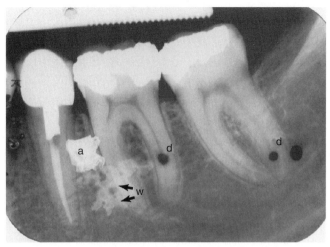

Figure 9-29 Water *(w)* dropped on film; developer spots *(d)* on film; artifact *(a)*.

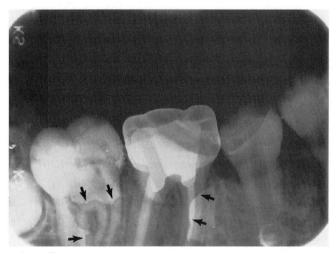

Figure 9-30 Water marks on film *(arrows)*.

If developer is dropped or spilled onto a film, the resulting artifact will be dark or black. Other black marks on radiographs can occur if the films were handled by operators with developer solution or fluoride on their fingers. These artifacts appear as fingerprints (Fig. 9-32).

Fogged Films

We have distinguished fogged films from dark films because, although fogged films are dark, they still appear to be relatively normal. Fog may be caused by improper safelighting in the darkroom (light leaks), storage in a warm-to-hot environment, or out-of-date film. The changes in film density as a result of fog are subtle. Fogged films usually appear almost uniformly gray. This uniformity reduces the film's contrast; enamel, dentin, and bone all start to appear to be the same density, and dental problems such as early carious lesions in enamel may be obscured. If contrast (black/white) is insufficient, the gray cavity may just blend into the gray background. Figure 9-33 is an example of a fogged film.

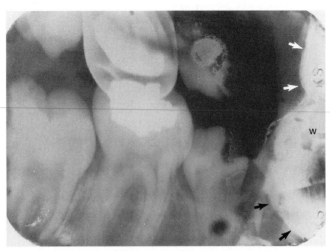

Figure 9-31 This film has multiple processing and handling artifacts. The fixer stain is the white region on the right side of the film *(arrows)*. Water marks *(w)* are also seen.

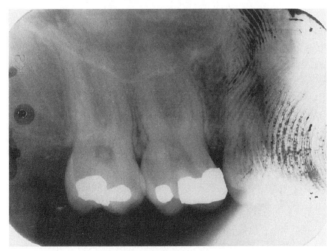

Figure 9-32 Fingerprints are obvious on the right side of the film. Can you name two other errors that are present? Hint: One is a technique error, and the other is a processing error.

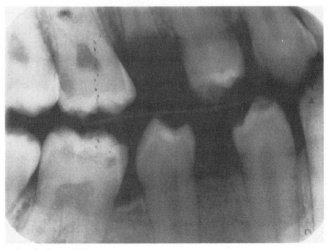

Figure 9-33 An example of a fogged film.

Dark Films

Many causes of dark films exist. You saw in the section on technique errors earlier in this chapter that overexposure leads to an overall dark film because far more x rays reached the image receptor to expose it. Similarly, light photons (like x-ray photons) striking radiographic film will cause the formation of a latent image center that, when subjected to the developing process, will turn black. Thus stray light can expose a dental x-ray film unnecessarily. After all, light is electromagnetic radiation, just as x rays are.

One of the more common processing errors in which stray light exposes the undeveloped film is caused by loose-fitting fabric openings on the daylight hoods or loaders of automatic developers (Fig. 9-34). The quick removal of your hands from these openings could also allow light to expose the film before it has fully entered the developing tank. These errors are easily avoided.

Figure 9-35 shows a panoramic image with a very dark area on one side. This was caused by a light leak in the cassette that allowed white light to reach the film inside. Extraoral film is extremely sensitive to light, even in darkroom settings. Therefore, it is essential that darkrooms that process extraoral films are light tight and that safelighting is correct. Darkroom safelight filters for extraoral films must be deep red (not orange or yellow) and must be placed at least 4 feet from the work surfaces or automatic processors. Cracked or incorrect safelight filters may result in fogged films. Additionally, "unsafe" safelights may cause panoramic images to be darker

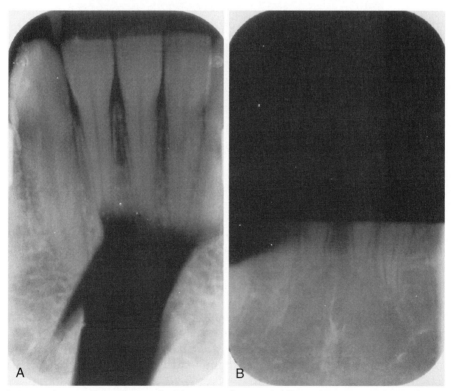

Figure 9-34 **A,** The irregular artifact resulted from a small tear in the film packet, exposing the emulsion to light. **B,** The black area resulted from exposure to overhead white light before the film was all the way in the automatic processor.

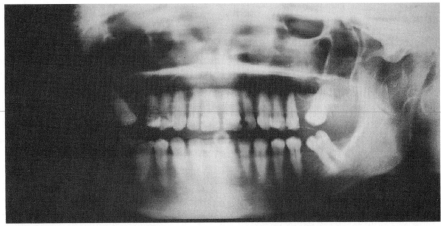

Figure 9-35 The black area on the left side of the film was caused by a light leak in the panoramic cassette.

Figure 9-36 Overdevelopment. The details, seen here as dots, are not readily discernable.

on one side than the other because of the time it takes for the film to enter the automatic processor. The end of the film that is exposed to the unsafe darkroom conditions the longest will be dark and fogged.

Overdevelopment of a film because of an overly long development time (usually during manual processing) or an overly strong developer concentration (owing to overreplenishment or incorrect mixing) will result in films that are dark. Additionally, if the fixer concentration is weak, it cannot remove all of the excess developer from the film, and the image will be darker (Fig. 9-36).

Finally, if the operator is in a rush or is not paying proper attention, the wrapping paper from inside the film packet may be placed into the solution along with the film. The paper sticks to the film surface and is developed, fixed, and subsequently "baked" onto the film in the dryer. This results in an unsalvageable film, a retake, and undue patient exposure. Proper maintenance of processing chemicals and care in film developing (as discussed in Chapter 2) are mandatory to reduce these errors. One positive note is that overexposed or dark films (with the exception of chemical stains, light-leak problems, or paper stuck on the film) can often be viewed under a "hot light" (a bright light source) to retrieve some information. Furthermore,

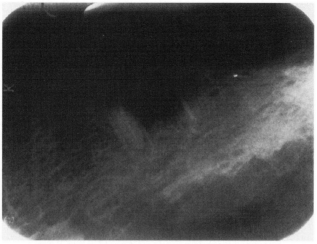

Figure 9-37 The bone around these root tips is not interpretable. See Figure 9-38.

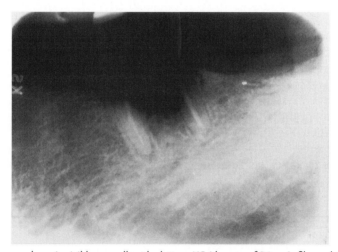

Figure 9-38 Here, more bone is visible, as well as the letters *KS* (the manufacturer's film code). This image was produced through duplication of the one in Figure 9-37. Using increased exposure time for the duplicate allows more information to be seen.

duplication of the dark film with the use of overexposure of the direct positive film may also salvage some information (Figures 9-37 and 9-38), thus saving the patient additional x-ray exposure.

Light Films

Unfortunately, underexposed, or light, films caused by the following errors are, for the most part, undiagnostic; that is, they will require a retake. Even if you have properly exposed a film, if your development time is too short or your developer concentration is too weak (exhausted), you may be left with a light film with insufficient contrast or detail for diagnostic interpretation (Fig. 9-39). Other causes of light films are excess fixation, inadequate (too low) developing temperature, and films placed backward. With the advent of automatic processors, an additional cause for light films exists: the operator may forget to separate the two films in a double-film packet, or one film might be fed into the processor too soon after the first one. In

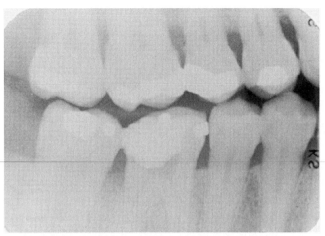

Figure 9-39 A light image with little contrast. This could be the result of underexposure or short development time or weak developer solution.

both instances, the films stick together either wholly or partially. After they are re-trieved, the only corrective measure is to peel them apart and place them back into the *fixer* section for reprocessing before bringing them out of the darkroom. Even after reprocessing, part or all of the emulsion on one side of the films will not get developed, and the resultant films will have light areas.

Films that have stuck together in an automatic processor and that are brought out of the darkroom into the white light cannot be salvaged. If they are peeled apart and not reprocessed, the undeveloped areas (the areas that were stuck together) will look opaque and green. If they are redeveloped, the original undeveloped portions will turn completely black because they were exposed to the light outside the darkroom; therefore, it is pointless to try to salvage them. Films like these are undiagnostic and will need to be retaken.

Overlapped Films

When using an automatic processor, it is important to wait until a film is completely taken into the developer by the roller system before inserting another film. It is tempting to insert another film after the first film has disappeared from the intake tray, but it is most likely still on the intake rollers. Placing another film in the proces-sor too quickly may result in overlapped films (Fig. 9-40). As the emulsion softens, the films stick together and the processing chemicals cannot fully reach the silver halide crystals in the emulsion. Resulting images may have the outline of the other film on them, or if they are stuck together completely, the films may have a green-ish color and be undiagnostic in the overlapped areas. If the error is noticed before taking the films out of the darkroom, they may be reprocessed with relatively reason-able results. However, once the films are exposed to daylight, any undeveloped areas will become completely undiagnostic.

Static Electricity

Extraoral films in particular are subject to static electricity artifacts (Fig. 9-41) because they are so light sensitive; however, static can also been seen on intraoral films. Static discharge builds up in environments with low humidity when film is rubbed over other films when taking it out of the box, putting it in the cassette, and taking

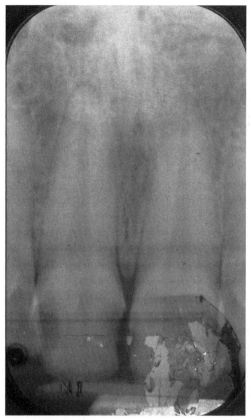

Figure 9-40 Overlapped films.

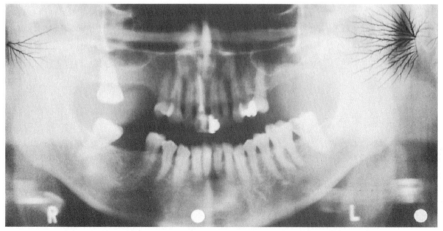

Figure 9-41 These black streaks resembling tree branches were caused by static electricity discharge before processing the film.

it out of the cassette. Clothing choice can also affect the amount of static buildup; nylon-based uniform tops and slacks may create more static buildup than natural fibers such as cotton.

ADDITIONAL MISCELLANEOUS ERRORS

- A maxillary complete denture left in the mouth (Fig. 9-42)
- A cast metal maxillary partial denture left in the mouth (Fig. 9-43)
- An acrylic orthodontic appliance left in the mouth, of which only the retentive clasp can be seen (Fig. 9-44)
- Chewing gum left in the mouth (Fig. 9-45)
- A finger superimposed over the mouth (Fig. 9-46)
- A "crimping" artifact (Fig. 9-47)

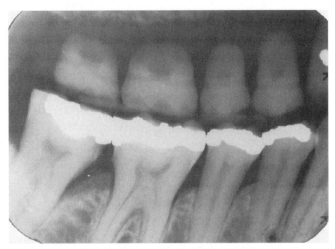

Figure 9-42 It is sometimes beneficial to leave a prosthesis in the patient's mouth to assist with correct image-receptor placement. Here the bitewing is stabilized by the denture; without it, placement would be much more difficult.

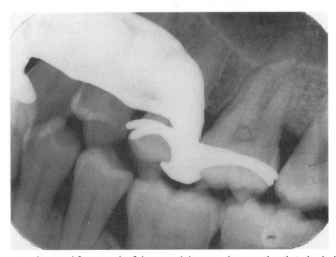

Figure 9-43 In this case, the metal framework of the partial denture obscures details in both the teeth and the alveolar bone.

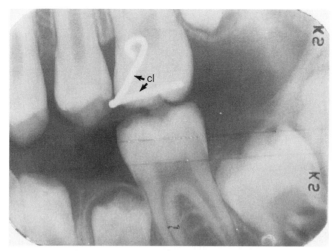

Figure 9-44 Because the retainer is made of acrylic (plastic), it is not visible on the image. Only the wire clasp *(cl)* used for retention is visible.

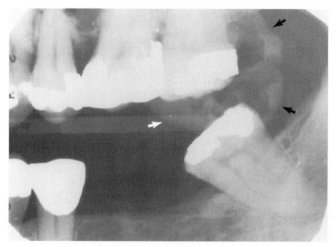

Figure 9-45 Chewing gum *(arrows)*. Note the indentations (bite marks) present.

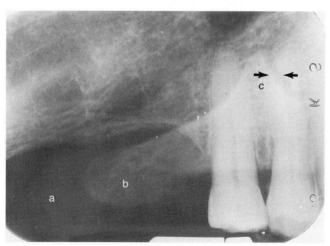

Figure 9-46 This patient was holding a film in the mouth during a radiographic procedure. The index finger was behind the film on the palate, and the thumb was outside the dental arch between the film and the x-ray beam. Thus, *a* is the soft tissue of the end of the finger, *b* is the finger bone, and *c* is the interphalangeal joint. This type of artifact has been facetiously called a *phalangioma*.

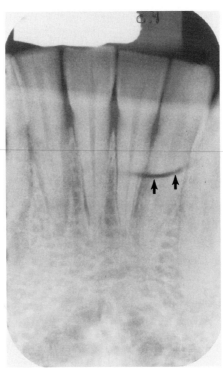

Figure 9-47 If operators have difficulty inserting the film into the film holder, removing the film from the film holder, or removing the film from the packet, they may create this semilunar "crimp" artifact in the emulsion. This is sometimes called a fingernail artifact, but it is not caused by the fingernail but by grasping the film too tightly. These crimps can also be seen on panoramic radiographs.

STUDY QUESTIONS

1. You develop a set of bitewings in an automatic process; three are fine, but one is totally blank (clear), with no hint of an image. What can you assume about the blank film?
   A. It was accidentally exposed to light
   B. It was put in the fixer solution first
   C. It was not exposed to radiation
   D. It was double-exposed

2. You look at the bitewings you took during Mrs. Jones's last appointment 1 year ago. They are brownish and somewhat opaque—not interpretable. What might be the cause of the discoloration? The films were
   A. Not developed long enough
   B. Not fixed or washed long enough
   C. Exposed to light leaks in the darkroom
   D. Developed too long

3. You turn on the water in the manual developing tanks at the beginning of the day, stir the solutions, check the temperature, and set the timer to go with the temperature. You develop a set of films at 9 AM that appear fine. Around 4 PM, you process another set of films that are so dark that you can barely see images on them. What was the most likely cause of the appearance of the second set of films?
   A. The exposure time was too long
   B. The darkroom has a light leak
   C. The water temperature changed
   D. The chemicals are contaminated

4. You take a set of bitewings, and they all have a few little black spots on them. The most likely cause is
   A. Developer splash
   B. Fixer splash
   C. Water splash
   D. Light leaks

5. You notice that over the past few weeks the films have been getting lighter and lighter. No difference is noticeable from one day to the next, but there is a big difference between a periapical you took today and one that was taken 2 weeks ago. What is the most likely cause of this problem?
   A. Light leaks
   B. Weak or contaminated developer
   C. Weak or contaminated fixer
   D. Processing temperature too high

6. You have unwrapped a set of bitewing films in the darkroom with gloves on, disposed of the wrappings and the gloves, and washed your hands. You then notice a puddle on the counter near the automatic processor and you wipe it up with a paper towel, but do not rewash your hands. You then load the bitewings into the automatic processor without gloves on. When the films are processed, there are dark fingerprints on them. What was the most likely cause?
   A. The emulsion began to soften while the unwrapped films sat on the counter while you were wiping up the spill
   B. There was a light leak in the darkroom that recorded the image of your fingers on the films
   C. The fingerprints were left from someone in the film manufacturing plant
   D. The spill on the counter was developing solution, which got on your fingers from the paper towel, and then onto the films as you processed them

7. You are preparing to mount the complete mouth radiographic survey that you have laid out on the view box in front of you. You notice that one film is blank. The other films look normal except for one that seems darker than the others and has a rather peculiar-looking image on it. What is the most likely cause of this situation?
   A. The x-ray machine malfunctioned
   B. The films were stuck together in the automatic processor
   C. The film-holding device was incorrectly assembled
   D. The dark film was double-exposed, and the blank one was unexposed

8. A patient has a very shallow palate and you are using the paralleling technique. You find you must tip the maxillary posterior periapical image receptors off parallel to get them into position. If the cone is aligned exactly with the indicator ring, what will the resulting images look like?
   A. They will be elongated
   B. The apices will be missing
   C. They will be foreshortened
   D. They will be too light

9. You notice that a maxillary premolar periapical view looks rather odd at its anterior aspect. The most apical portion of the canine root and the first premolar root look stretched out, like they were made of rubber and you pulled on them. The second premolar and the first molar look fine, as do *all* the crowns of the teeth. What happened?
   A. The anterior corner of the film bent against the palate
   B. The anterior portion of the film got stuck in the rollers of the automatic processor
   C. The anterior corner of the film was stuck to another film in the automatic processor
   D. The patient moved

10. How will you know if you positioned a film backward (white side *away* from the x-ray beam)?
    A. It will be lighter than normal
    B. The embossed dot will be depressed (not raised) when the film is looked at in the correct anatomic orientation
    C. There will be a pattern of the lead foil on the image
    D. All of the above

Accessory Radiographic Techniques and Patient Management

BISECTING-ANGLE TECHNIQUE

The bisecting-angle technique is based on a geometric principle of dividing a triangle into equal halves. This technique differs from the paralleling technique in that instead of moving the image receptor away from the teeth to achieve parallelism, the operator places the image receptor directly against the teeth to be imaged (Fig. 10-1).

You will notice in Figure 10-1 that the image receptor touches the teeth at the incisal edges, or lingual/occlusal surfaces. The apical portion of the image receptor is held away from the teeth at a distance determined by the patient's anatomy. Thus, the image receptor is not parallel to the long axes of the teeth but meets the teeth at an angle.

If you direct the x-ray beam at a right angle to the image receptor, the image produced will be much shorter than the actual structure: the image will be foreshortened (see Fig. 9-16). If you direct the x-ray beam perpendicular to the long axes of

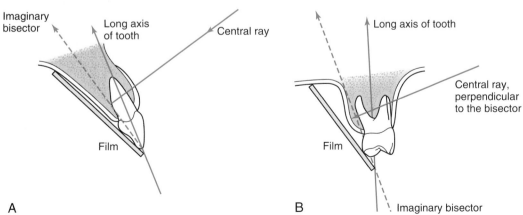

A

B

Imaginary bisector
Long axis of tooth
Central ray
Film

Long axis of tooth
Central ray, perpendicular to the bisector
Film
Imaginary bisector

Figure 10-1 **A,** A diagram of an anterior tooth with the central ray perpendicular to the imaginary bisector of the angle between the long axis of the tooth and the film plane. **B,** A posterior tooth with the bisecting-angle concept.

the teeth, the image will be much longer than the actual structure: the image will be elongated (see Fig. 9-17). The bisecting-angle technique combines these positions to obtain a reasonably accurate image.

With this technique, the angle formed by the long axes of the teeth and the film is bisected into two equal parts, and the x-ray beam is directed perpendicular to the bisecting line (see Fig. 10-1). This concept is often difficult to visualize; therefore it is often difficult to obtain a quality image with the use of this technique. Problems are posed by the fact that (1) the operator cannot see the long axes of the teeth and therefore must estimate their correct orientation; (2) the operator must imagine the line that bisects the angle; it cannot be seen; (3) the operator cannot see exactly where the film is and thus cannot be certain that the beam will cover the entire area of the image receptor; and (4) the patient, in many instances, must hold the image receptor in place, which may result in improper receptor placement. Image-receptor holders are commercially available for use with the bisecting-angle technique, but some do not have beam alignment guides. Consequently, this technique may result in more operator and patient errors than the paralleling technique, which uses positioning devices that assist the operator in beam alignment.

Uses

Because of the increased risk of operator error and greater image distortion, the bisecting-angle technique is not recommended as a standard technique for obtaining diagnostic images. However, the technique provides an alternative way of obtaining an image when the paralleling technique cannot be used effectively. Examples of such situations include the presence of a shallow palate or floor of the mouth, a large palatal torus or mandibular tori, or a short lingual frenum. Additionally, the technique may be useful with some patients who cannot cooperate with the paralleling technique, such as children. It may also be useful with certain endodontic procedures when the patient cannot bite on a biteblock.

Image-Receptor Placement

The number of images used and the anatomic areas covered in the bisecting-angle technique (image-receptor placement) are similar to the paralleling technique. The anterior-posterior placement and the **horizontal angulation** are determined similarly to the paralleling technique except that a positioning instrument may not be present as a visual guide. Vertical placement of the image receptor should allow for approximately $^1/_8$ to $^1/_4$ inch (3 to 6 mm) of space beyond the occlusal plane. The **vertical angulation** is determined by the bisector line, as described previously. However, if the patient's occlusal plane is parallel to the floor, the following vertical angles may be used as a rough estimate of those needed for diagnostic images:

Views	*Maxilla*	*Mandible*
Incisors	+40° to 50°	−5° to 15°
Canines	+45° to 55°	−5° to 15°
Premolars	+30° to 40°	−10° to 15°
Molars	+20° to 30°	−5° to +5°

OCCLUSAL IMAGING

A supplementary technique to periapical and bitewing imaging is occlusal imaging. This technique uses a larger film that can be placed in the mouth as if the patient were biting a sandwich (Fig. 10-2). See Figure 1-16, A, for a comparison of various film sizes.

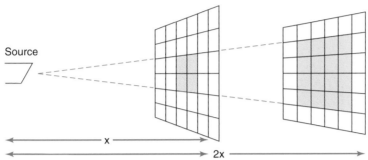

Figure 10-2 A shorter source-to-receptor distance creates greater magnification of the entire image on the receptor.

Uses

Occlusal imaging can be used in the following situations:
1. To determine the location of objects in all three dimensions
2. To locate roots, as well as supernumerary, unerupted, and impacted teeth
3. To localize foreign objects in the jaws and stones in the salivary gland ducts
4. To visualize and evaluate the integrity of the anterior, medial, and lateral outlines of the maxillary sinus
5. To determine the nature, extent, and displacement of fractures of the mandible or maxilla
6. To determine the presence and extent of pathoses such as cysts, tumors, or osteomyelitis
7. To demonstrate bony expansion of either jaw
8. To examine larger segments of the jaws than can be seen on a periapical view
9. To capture an image for a patient who is unable to open the mouth wide enough for periapical imaging because of such problems as trismus or pain
10. To capture an image for pediatric patients who cannot tolerate or cooperate with the procedure for periapical imaging

With pediatric patients, occlusal images can be used for localization of developing teeth, that is, to help determine whether an object is positioned buccally or lingually to the other teeth in the jaws. Occlusal images can also be used to evaluate dental arch symmetry.

Two standard techniques can be used to obtain occlusal images, each giving a slightly different view. The first technique renders a *maxillary topographic view* (Figs. 10-3, B, and 10-4, B) and uses a technique that is somewhat similar to the bisecting-angle technique. The dental arch to be examined is positioned parallel to the floor, and the film is placed in the patient's mouth. The central ray is directed perpendicular to the line that bisects the angle formed by the long axes of the teeth being examined and the plane of the image receptor. The vertical angulation will be approximately +60° (Fig. 10-3, A). The horizontal angulation will be determined by the area being examined. If an anterior view is desired, the beam is aimed over the patient's nose; if a lateral view is desired, the beam is aimed over the patient's cheekbone (Fig. 10-4, A). The topographic *maxillary anterior occlusal view* affords an excellent view of the palate and incisors. The topographic *maxillary lateral occlusal*

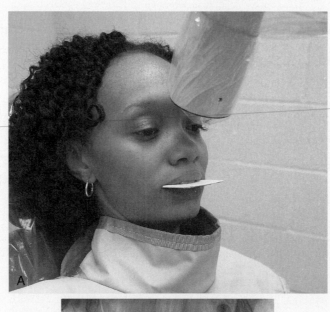

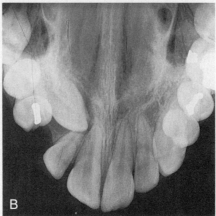

Figure 10-3 **A,** The patient positioned for a topographic maxillary occlusal view. **B,** The topographic maxillary occlusal view affords an excellent view of the palate.

Head Position
Occlusal plane parallel to the floor.

Image-Receptor Placement
Sensitive side up. Long or short side of the receptor may be placed into the mouth with approximately ¼ inch extending beyond the central incisor incisal edges. Patient should gently close on receptor.

Vertical Angulation
+60° to 70° downward.

Horizontal Angulation
Along the midsagittal plane.

Point of Entry of Central Ray
At the bridge of the nose.

Pediatric Patient

Use the size no. 2 receptor, because children may not be able to accommodate the larger occlusal film in their mouths.

Approximate Exposure

Roughly the same exposure as a maxillary central incisor view.

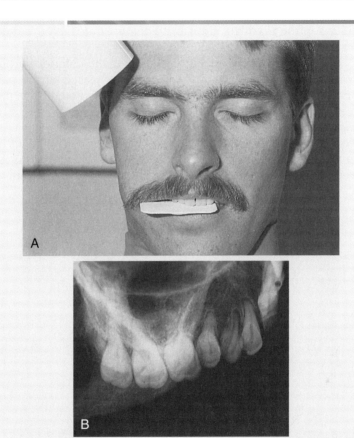

Figure 10-4 **A,** Occlusal film placed to the right side of the arch for examination of that area. **B,** Resulting image.

Head Position

Occlusal plane parallel to the floor.

Image-Receptor Placement

Sensitive side up, positioned in the mouth with one of the long edges lying parallel to and extending ¼ inch (6 to 7 mm) beyond the buccal cusps of the posterior teeth. Patient should gently close on the receptor.

Vertical Angulation

+60° downward.

Horizontal Angulation

Depending on the view required, the beam should be aligned between the contacts of the premolars and molars.

Continued

Point of Entry of Central Ray
The contact between the second premolar and the first molar.

Approximate Exposure
Roughly the same exposure as a maxillary molar view.

view depicts the roots of the molars and premolars. This view may be used to locate foreign objects in the maxillary sinus or to demonstrate larger portions of the maxilla than can be seen on periapical views.

The *mandibular anterior topographic view* shows the anterior portion of the mandibular bone and incisors. The image receptor is placed in the patient's mouth, and the sensitive side is in contact with the mandibular teeth. The patient's head is tipped back approximately 45°, and the vertical angulation of the beam will be –55° to the image receptor (Fig. 10-5).

The second standard technique is the *mandibular cross-sectional view,* in which the image receptor is placed between the teeth, and the central ray is angled at 90° to the receptor (Figs. 10-6 and 10-7). This view is especially helpful when trying to

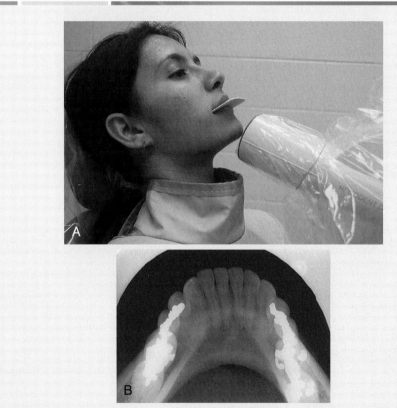

Figure 10-5 A, Topographic mandibular occlusal view. **B,** Topographic mandibular occlusal image. Note the impacted premolar.

Head Position
Tipped back to a comfortable position, approximating having the occlusal plane at a 45° angle to the floor.

Image-Receptor Placement

Sensitive side down (facing mandibular teeth). Long or short side of the receptor may be placed into the mouth with approximately ¼ inch extending beyond the central incisor incisal edges. Patient should gently close on the receptor.

Vertical Angulation

As determined by bisecting-angle principles. If occlusal plane is approximately 45° to the floor, angulation will be approximately −15° to −20° upward.

Horizontal Angulation

Along the midsagittal plane.

Point of Entry of Central Ray

Approximately the indentation between the lip and the chin point (just below the apices of the mandibular incisors).

Approximate Exposure

Roughly the same exposure as a mandibular canine view.

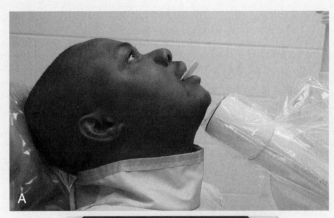

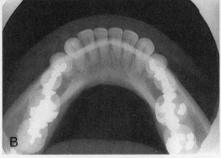

Figure 10-6 **A,** Cross-sectional mandibular occlusal view. **B,** Resulting image.

Head Position

Tipped back as far as comfortably possible.

Continued

Image-Receptor Placement

Sensitive side down (facing mandibular teeth). Long or short side of the receptor may be placed into the mouth with approximately ¼ inch extending beyond the central incisor incisal edges. Patient should gently close on the receptor.

Vertical Angulation

Perpendicular to the plane of the image receptor.

Horizontal Angulation

Along the midsagittal plane.

Point of Entry of Central Ray

Under the chin, aimed at the floor of the mouth.

Approximate Exposure

Roughly the same exposure as a mandibular canine view.

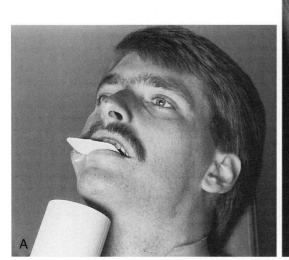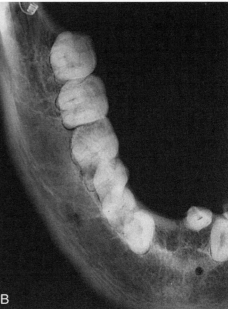

Figure 10-7   **A,** A variation of the cross-sectional technique, offset to one side. **B,** The resulting image.

localize an object within the floor of the mouth or when evaluating the buccal and lingual aspects of the mandible. As with the topographic view, the mandibular cross-sectional view can be positioned over either side of the mandible rather than in the anterior portion.

The cross-sectional technique is not often used in the maxilla because it is difficult for most dental x-ray machines to generate enough radiation to penetrate the skull without long exposures (e.g., greater than 2 seconds).

PEDIATRIC IMAGING TECHNIQUES

Management of the behavior of the pediatric patient is the key to successful technique. With children, you have to be imaginative, creative, entertaining, quick-witted, and patient. Here are some basic guidelines to consider when your patient is a child:

1. *Show the child what you are going to do* every chance you get. Talk about the "pictures" you are going to take and the "camera" you are going to use. Let the child touch the equipment, push the exposure button (with the unit *turned off*), touch the film packet or digital sensor, and see what an image looks like. You might even bring in an extra image receptor and holding device to demonstrate on yourself. Show the child that you are comfortable with the device in place.
2. *Work quickly but accurately.* Remember that many children move continually. Tell the child the importance of staying perfectly still. Reinforce any positive behavior with praise.
3. *Be creative.* If your regular technique does not work, improvise. Be prepared to substitute a smaller image receptor, use a different kind of film holder, or use the occlusal technique. In some situations it might be possible to obtain adequate diagnostic information from a panoramic image and bitewings alone.

Radiation Protection

Because children are growing and developing, their tissues are generally more sensitive to radiation than many adult tissues. It is imperative to follow good patient protection procedures. Because a child's thyroid gland is particularly sensitive to radiation, the use of a leaded thyroid collar is especially critical with children, and the most recent NCRP report[*] mandates the use of a thyroid shield in children.

Type of Radiographic Survey

The need for a complete mouth radiographic survey (CMRS) for children is variable. Selection of the number, size, and type of images depends on the child's age, dental development, and the ability of the patient to cooperate with radiographic procedures. Figure 10-8 shows examples of some pediatric surveys with different film sizes and types of projections used. Selection criteria guidelines should be closely followed when choosing radiographic surveys for children.

Alterations in Exposure Time

Exposure times are generally reduced for children because their tissues are often not as thick as adults' tissues; thus children require less radiation for an adequate image. The amount of time reduction depends on the size of the child; however, some x-ray machines allow the operator to choose a "child" setting. The machine's "child setting" is a good place to start, but the actual exposure time may need to be adjusted slightly upward or downward, depending·on the size of the child. Additionally, if a child is very small, a booster seat may be necessary for proper x-ray beam alignment.

*Radiation Protection in Dentistry, National Council on Radiation Protection and Measurements (NCRP) Report No. 145, 2003.

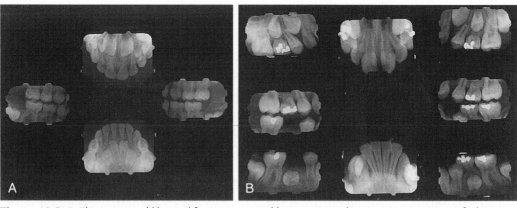

Figure 10-8 **A,** This survey could be used for a 3- to 5-year-old patient. It employs two size no. 1 images for bitewings and two size no. 2 images for maxillary and mandibular occlusal views. **B,** This survey could be used for a child with a mixed dentition (ages 6 to 10 years). It uses four size no. 1 periapical images in addition to the images described in **A.**

Image-Receptor Size

Use the smallest image-receptor size that is compatible with the patient's anatomy. The use of oversized film will cause discomfort and loss of cooperation. For a primary dentition, size no. 0 film is recommended. Size no. 0 or 1 may be used for a child with mixed dentition. Sizes no. 1 and 2 may be used for preadolescent and adolescent dentitions.

Bitewings

In a child without second molars, usually only two bitewings (one on each side) are necessary because all erupted posterior teeth will most often fit onto one image.

EDENTULOUS RADIOGRAPHIC TECHNIQUES

Evaluation of the bone in the jaws is important when considering patient treatment options such as denture fabrication or implant placement. Additionally, periodic radiographic evaluation of edentulous patients is important when the possibility of pathologic conditions within the jaws exist. Following established selection criteria when deciding when to image an edentulous patient will be helpful.

Although a **panoramic image** may not provide all the necessary information required for patient diagnosis and treatment, it can be an effective and efficient way to image edentulous jaws and the maxillary sinuses and condyles. If a panoramic x-ray machine is not available, it is possible to obtain intraoral images of edentulous ridges.

Intraoral Images

A typical edentulous intraoral radiographic survey may contain as many as 14 images (six anterior and eight posterior) or as few as 10 images (two anterior and eight posterior). Figure 10-9 demonstrates an edentulous survey. No bitewing images are obtained because no posterior teeth are in contact. Obtaining topographic occlusal

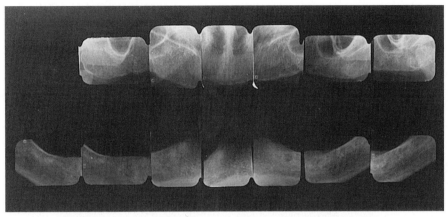

Figure 10-9 This series of 13 images was taken in a completely edentulous patient.

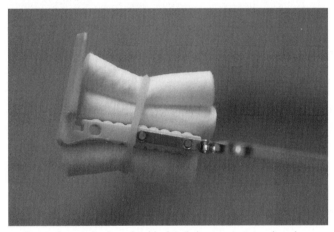

Figure 10-10 Cotton rolls may be attached to a biteblock to help support it in edentulous areas. More than one roll may be needed.

images along with posterior periapical views is an acceptable alternative to a CMRS in an edentulous patient.

Technique

Either the paralleling technique or the bisecting-angle technique may be used for edentulous images. If the paralleling technique is used with paralleling instruments, cotton rolls may be attached to the under surface of the biteblock with rubber bands for support (Fig. 10-10) or even to both sides of the biteblock to substitute for the height of the teeth. If the bisecting-angle technique is chosen, image receptors should be placed so that about ¼ inch of the receptor extends beyond the edentulous ridge. Because of the absence of teeth, the distortion inherent in the bisecting-angle technique does not interfere with diagnosis of bony conditions.

Exposure Factors

The exposure time for each region in an edentulous intraoral survey should be reduced by approximately one fourth of the normal time to avoid overexposure. The edentulous ridge is often thinner and less dense owing to the lack of teeth.

ENDODONTIC IMAGING TECHNIQUES

Accurate images are essential for diagnosis, treatment, and follow-up care in patients who require endodontic (root canal) treatment. Endodontic images are difficult to obtain during treatment because of rubber dam clamps, endodontic files, or obturating material extending from the tooth (Fig. 10-11). In addition to these physical challenges, visualization of correct film placement is compromised because the rubber dam obstructs the view. A diagnostic endodontic image should ensure that

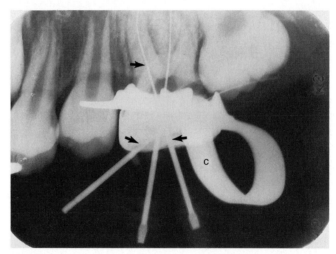

Figure 10-11 This radiograph demonstrates an attempt to image the apices of the maxillary left first molar. The rubber dam clamp *(c)* and gutta percha points *(arrows)* make image-receptor placement difficult. The apex of the molar is not visible; a retake is needed.

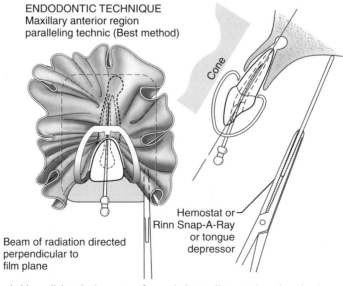

ENDODONTIC TECHNIQUE
Maxillary anterior region
paralleling technic (Best method)

Cone

Beam of radiation directed
perpendicular to
film plane

Hemostat or
Rinn Snap-A-Ray
or tongue
depressor

Figure 10-12 Film held parallel to the long axis of an endodontically treated tooth with a hemostat clamp. *(Courtesy of Dr. John Preece, University of Texas Health Science Center, San Antonio, Tex.)*

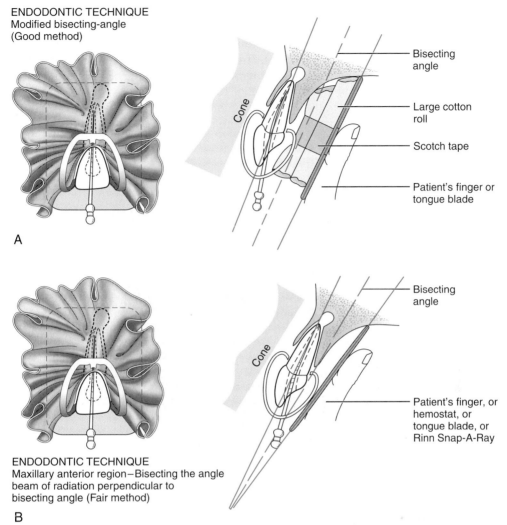

ENDODONTIC TECHNIQUE
Modified bisecting-angle
(Good method)

Bisecting
angle

Large cotton
roll

Scotch tape

Patient's finger or
tongue blade

Cone

A

ENDODONTIC TECHNIQUE
Maxillary anterior region – Bisecting the angle
beam of radiation perpendicular to
bisecting angle (Fair method)

Bisecting
angle

Patient's finger, or
hemostat, or
tongue blade, or
Rinn Snap-A-Ray

Cone

B

Figure 10-13   **A,** An alternative technique using a tongue blade and cotton rolls. **B,** A bisecting alternative. This technique results in more distortion. *(Courtesy of Dr. John Preece, University of Texas Health Science Center, San Antonio, Tex.)*

(1) the tooth is centered on the image, (2) at least 5 mm of bone beyond the apex of the tooth is visible, and (3) the image is as anatomically correct as possible.

The preoperative diagnostic image and the postoperative follow-up image should be taken with the use of the standard paralleling technique. The bisecting-angle technique is not recommended because of the inherent dimensional distortion.

Anterior Views

Image receptors may be held parallel to the long axis of the tooth by means of a hemostat, an alligator-clamp instrument, a tongue depressor, or the patient's finger (Fig. 10-12). If this approach cannot be used, cotton rolls may be taped to the image receptor to hold it away from the tooth so that the most parallel relationship possible can be obtained (Fig. 10-13). If neither of these methods seems to work, the bisecting-angle technique can be used as long as the clinician is aware of the geometric distortion that will result.

Posterior Views

The paralleling technique is superior to the bisecting-angle technique for posterior images, as well as for anterior views. If image receptors can be held parallel to the long axis of the tooth by the use of a hemostat or Snap-a-Ray instrument, the accuracy of the image will be maximized (Fig. 10-14). If this approach is not possible, a cotton roll may be taped to the image receptor to hold it farther away from the tooth, which will make it more parallel to the tooth's long axis.

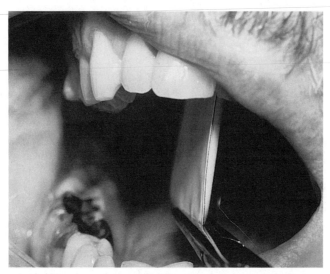

Figure 10-14 Film packet held by a hemostat in a parallel position. Care must be taken to ensure that the apices of the teeth in question are included on the image.

LOCALIZATION TECHNIQUES

Sometimes the operator needs to know whether an object is located toward the buccal (facial) or lingual portion of the jaw. The object of interest might be an impacted tooth, a pin retaining a large restoration in a tooth, or a foreign object. Two common methods exist for determining the facial/lingual position of an object in the jaws.

Right-Angle Technique

The right-angle technique (also called Miller's technique) is a simple method for determining the facial/lingual position of teeth or foreign objects. Two images are taken at right angles to each other. The first image may be a periapical or bitewing already available in a CMRS. This image will show the position of the object in an *inferior/superior* and *anteroposterior* direction. That is, the clinician will be able to tell how high or low the object is and its mesial-distal position. A second image is needed to show the third dimension, and a cross-sectional occlusal projection will show the *facial/lingual* and *anteroposterior* position. Using the differing views of the two types of images, the clinician can pinpoint the object in three dimensions. This technique is used primarily for locating objects in the mandibular arch (Fig. 10-15).

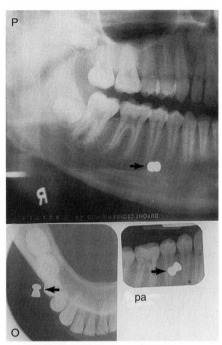

Figure 10-15 The initial radiographs were the panoramic view *(P)* and the periapical view *(pa)*. These views give the impression that the radiopaque object *(arrow)* is in the bone. A third image, the occlusal view *(O)*, reveals that the object is actually in the soft tissue on the outside, buccal to the mandible.

Buccal Object Rule

The **buccal object rule** (also known as Clark's rule or the **same/lingual-opposite/buccal [SLOB] rule**) can be used if two images are already available with slightly different angulations or positions. The principle of the buccal object rule states that the object closest to the buccal surface will appear to move in the opposite direction relative to the movement of the tubehead when a second image is taken (Fig. 10-16). An additional illustration of the SLOB rule is found in Chapter 12, Fig. 12-38.

To grasp this concept, consider the following example. If you stand directly in line with two trees such that one is exactly behind the other, the tree that is farthest away from you will be blocked from your vision by the tree in front. If you move to the side, you will be able to see both trees. If you move to your *right,* the tree in front (the one closest to you, the "buccal" one) will appear to move to the *left* relative to the tree that is farther away from you (the "lingual" one). If you move to the left, the tree in front will appear to move to the right relative to the tree that is farther away.

In radiography, *near objects* (those that are **buccal**) appear to move in the *opposite* direction relative to the direction that the tubehead moved. *Far objects* (which would be **lingual**) appear to move in the *same* direction as the tubehead. Consider an image in which a round opacity is seen in the crown of a maxillary molar. It is most likely to be an amalgam restoration on either the buccal or lingual surface. In the maxillary molar periapical, it is seen approximately in the middle of the crown. In the molar bitewing view, it appears closer to the occlusal surface. Therefore, when the round restoration from the maxillary periapical view is compared with the bitewing, the restoration appears to have moved *downward.*

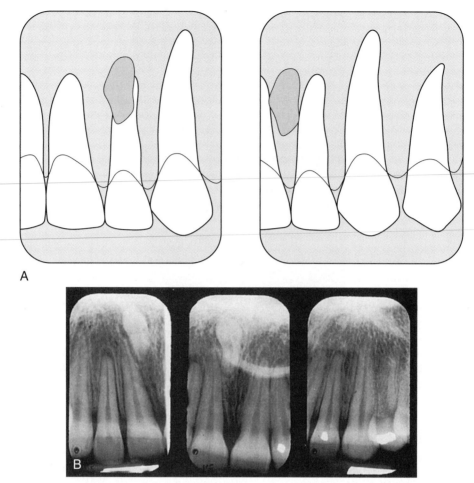

Figure 10-16 **A,** As the operator shifted the tubehead posteriorly to move from a lateral incisor view to a canine view, the object above the apices moved anteriorly (opposite to the tube shift). Therefore when the buccal object rule is applied, the object is located to the buccal aspect. **B,** As the operator shifted the tubehead posteriorly to move from a central incisor view to a lateral incisor view, the object (a supernumerary tooth) appears to move from the midline (on the central view) closer to the apex of the central incisor (on the lateral view). Therefore the object appears to move in the same direction as the tubehead moved; therefore the object is lingual to the teeth. The same principle applies to the metallic restoration in the lingual pit of the left lateral incisor. *(B: From Razmus TF, Williamson GF:* Current oral and maxillofacial imaging, *ed 1, Philadelphia, 1996, Saunders).*

When a maxillary molar periapical image is taken, the tubehead is often positioned over the patient's cheekbone. When the bitewing image is taken, the tubehead is positioned lower, directly toward the side of the patient's face. Therefore the tubehead moves *downward* from a maxillary molar periapical to a molar bitewing view. With the use of the SLOB rule, the object (the round restoration) moved in the *same* direction as the tubehead moved when the maxillary molar periapical view was compared with the molar bitewing view. Therefore that round restoration is on the *lingual* surface of the molar.

PATIENT MANAGEMENT

Many patients consider radiographic procedures to be unpleasant, especially if the patients have had previous negative experiences. Without patient cooperation the radiographer is greatly handicapped in the attempt to produce quality images.

Additionally, patients often transfer their previous negative feelings about the procedure to the current operator. This section of the chapter suggests ways to make the experience more acceptable to the patient and less stressful for the operator.

Operator Attitude

In your initial attempts at radiography, you may be unsure of yourself. Patients are often aware of this, and you may believe your confidence to be undermined, especially when the patient questions the procedure.

The first requirement for your success and for a less stressful experience is to maintain an air of confidence and authority, regardless of whether you believe it. Remember, if you were not capable of exposing images on a patient successfully, your instructor would not let you begin. Have faith that you have the proper skills and be confident. You should also be familiar with potential problems and how to deal with them.

Just as important as confidence is the knowledge that, between you and the patient, you are the expert. If image-receptor placement is uncomfortable, the patient might try to dictate what you should do. If so, remember that you have been taught how to produce quality images, and the patient usually has not. You, therefore, are the one who should control the situation. Following are some useful tips to increase your success:

1. *Try to relax the patient.* Chat with the patient. Explain what you are about to do. Be prepared to answer questions about the hazards of radiation, such as how much exposure will be received and the need for the images.
2. *Be as gentle as possible, and place films quickly and precisely.* Describe as clearly as possible what you want patients to do and let them know when it is being done correctly. Praise and encouragement will help make patients cooperative. If patients are not following instructions correctly, keep working with them until receptor placement is correct. You may need to reword your instructions to patients.

Gagging

One of the more common problems is the patient who gags. Gagging is a physiologic reaction greatly influenced by psychological factors. If you can overcome the psychological barriers, you will increase your chances for a successful experience. The following tips may be useful.

1. *Do not discuss gagging with patients in advance.* This discussion would just reinforce any thought about gagging that patients may be having. If patients bring it up, stating that they are notorious gaggers, just smile and say that you have a few tricks to deal with it.
2. *Start with images that do not normally trigger the gag reflex,* such as the maxillary incisor views. If you start with anterior images and are successful, you will show patients that you have the ability and skill to place image receptors and that they can tolerate them. If patients gag with more posterior views later in the procedure, they must assume some of the responsibility. You have already demonstrated that you can do your part of the procedure.
3. *Do as much as you can in preparation for the exposure before placing an image receptor in the patient's mouth.* Turn the unit on, select the appropriate exposure factors, and position the tubehead and the chair as close to the final position as possible before you place the image receptor in the patient's mouth. Use quick, precise movements to place the receptor. If you try to coax the receptor into the mouth slowly, you may trigger the gag reflex before the

patient begins to close on the biteblock. This is especially true in the maxillary molar area; try to avoid slowly dragging the image receptor over the soft palate or wiggling it around after it is in contact with the palate or floor of the mouth.

4. *Have patients begin to take deep breaths before you place the receptor.* Then have them *breathe through their mouths* while you are placing the receptor. Tell patients that this should keep them from gagging. This gives patients something to concentrate on other than gagging and reinforces the thought that they will not gag, and it is much easier to breathe through the mouth than the nose. With some patients, having the mouth open and trying to breathe through the nose may actually trigger palatal reflexes and cause them to gag.

5. *If the patient gags anyway, do not panic.* Simply remove the receptor and try something else. Distraction techniques (such as asking the patient to lift one leg slightly) may be useful.

6. *You may choose to mildly anesthetize the oral cavity.* Some mouthwashes or throat lozenges contain a mild anesthetic. These work best if patients are made to believe that they will stop the gag reflex. (Remember, the psychological factor has a big influence on gagging.) A topical anesthetic should be considered only in extreme cases, after all other techniques have failed. Definite risks are involved in administering topical anesthetics for radiographic procedures. Spray anesthetics might be inhaled into the lungs and cause a toxic reaction. Liquid or gel anesthetics might anesthetize the throat, causing patients to have difficulty swallowing. This might lead to aspiration of the patients' own saliva into their lungs.

7. *In a few instances (but only a very few), a patient's gag reflex will be so severe that intraoral images are just not possible.* If none of the techniques described here work, you may consider alternative projections such as panoramic, lateral jaw, or other extraoral views.

PATIENTS WITH DISABILITIES

The problems associated with disabled patients vary with the disability and with its degree of severity. A problem frequently encountered with wheelchair patients is getting them close enough to the x-ray unit to properly align the beam. If the patient chooses to or must remain in the wheelchair, the arm of the x-ray unit may be able to be extended to accommodate radiographic procedures. You should be prepared for this necessity in advance. X-ray operatories may have to be arranged to make the necessary accommodations.

A patient who experiences spastic movements may also make radiography difficult. The patient may be unable to hold image receptors or to bite properly on biteblocks. In such cases, the parent, guardian, or aide accompanying the patient can be asked to hold the image receptors during the procedure. This assisting person should wear a lead apron; thyroid shield; and, if possible, leaded gloves for radiation protection. Extraoral images may be indicated for patients who have uncontrolled movements. However, it may not be possible to obtain a diagnostic panoramic image of a patient who cannot hold still for approximately 15 to 20 seconds while the tubehead rotates around the patient.

ANATOMIC CONSIDERATIONS

Palatal Torus

Patients may present a variety of anatomic variations that require a compromise of normal radiographic technique. A palatal torus is not difficult to work around. The largest part of the bony structure is often directly in the center of the palate, where the vault is the highest and the image receptor is usually placed. The torus may prevent receptor placement high enough in the palate to capture the image of the molar apices. In this situation, the image receptor can be placed on the opposite side of the torus from the teeth to be imaged. The added distance from the receptor to the teeth being imaged might cause the receptor to lie at a slightly greater angle to the teeth than usual. This angle could result in foreshortening, although the apices will be imaged with little loss of quality. If the image of the torus is superimposed over the apices, the angulation of the receptor and/or x-ray beam may be adjusted. *Care must be used to avoid scraping the thin, sensitive mucosa covering the torus.*

Mandibular Tori

Mandibular tori may pose more of a challenge than a palatal torus, depending on their size. The space between the teeth and the tongue is smaller than that in the palatal vault. You should move the image receptor away from the torus and toward the tongue. If you place your finger between the torus and the image receptor, you can then slide the receptor into place without scraping the overlying mucosa. Moving the receptor toward the tongue allows it to seat into the floor of the mouth, away from the torus.

Ankyloglossia: the "Tongue-Tied" Patient

When the lingual frenum is attached high on the lingual surface of the mandible and/or close to the tip of the tongue, the patient has restricted movement of the tongue, and there is little room to place the image receptor (Fig. 10-17). The receptor will still be held in place by the patient closing on the biteblock; the vertical angle of the receptor may not be parallel to the long axis of the tooth, but this is acceptable under the circumstances. The vertical angulation of the x-ray beam can be adjusted accordingly. The soft tissue shadow of the tongue might be present on the image but should not interfere with its diagnostic quality.

Narrow Palatal Vault

When the arch is extremely narrow, some slight change in normal technique may help. The most important factor is to be sure that a narrow image receptor (no. 1 size) is used for anterior projections. You may have to image each tooth individually to obtain quality films without excessive overlap or film bending. Film packet bending is the most common error associated with this condition. Some people recommend curling the film to get it into the narrow arch (Fig. 10-18). However, curling will distort the entire image, reduce diagnostic quality, and possibly lead to a retake. Therefore this technique is not recommended.

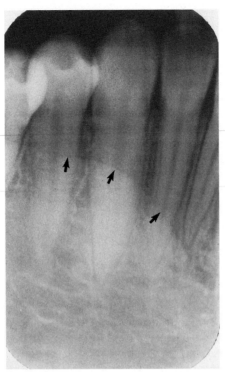

Figure 10-17 Soft tissue shadow of the tongue *(arrows)*. Note that its superimposition makes the root appear more radiopaque (lighter) than it normally would be. The image, however, is still diagnostic.

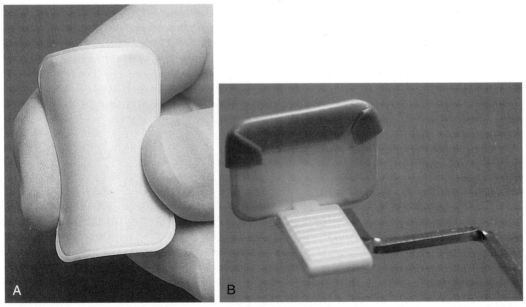

Figure 10-18 **A,** Curving or bending a film packet is *not* recommended. It often results in extreme distortion of the image. If proper placement is not possible, select a smaller image receptor. **B,** If the patient complains of sharp edges on the image receptor, there are commercially available foam cushions that can be applied.

Misaligned Teeth

When the patient's teeth are misaligned, you must use your judgment to determine the correct horizontal angulation. Most often, misaligned teeth dictate the need for an extra image or two. The rotated or malpositioned tooth must be imaged separately to obtain open contacts or a clear view of the roots.

Study Questions

1. In the bisecting-angle technique, the vertical angle of the central ray is directed
   A. Perpendicular to the long axis of the tooth
   B. Perpendicular to the image receptor
   C. Perpendicular to a line bisecting the angle made by the long axis of the tooth and the image receptor
   D. Parallel to a line bisecting the angle made by the long axis of the tooth and the image receptor

2. As you view a full mouth survey of radiographs, you notice a well-defined radiopaque object on the image that is obviously not part of the dentition. The object is superimposed over the mesial root of the mandibular first molar in the molar periapical view. As you then look at the premolar periapical view, you notice that the opaque object appears to have moved distally and is now closer to the distal root of the first molar. Which of the following statements is true?
   A. The object is in a lingual position to the teeth
   B. The object is in a buccal (facial) position to the teeth
   C. As the image receptor was moved more posteriorly, the object was pushed distally
   D. You cannot tell from these images where the object is located

3. To localize the posteroanterior position of a broken instrument tip in the mandibular premolar area, you would take a standard periapical image. To localize the precise facial/lingual position for its removal, which of the following views would be the best choice?
   A. Cross-sectional occlusal
   B. Topographic occlusal
   C. Bitewing
   D. Panoramic

4. A mandibular cross-sectional occlusal image requires
   A. A size no. 3 image receptor
   B. A hemostat or other receptor-holding device
   C. A vertical angle of at least 70° to 75°
   D. Alignment of the x-ray beam perpendicular to the image receptor

5. If a patient is suspected of having a bone lesion, such as a cyst, in the posterior area of the mandible, which of the following views would give the best indication of any facial or lingual bony expansion?
   A. Mandibular cross-sectional occlusal image
   B. Molar periapical with the use of the bisecting-angle technique
   C. Molar periapical with the use of a hemostat or tongue blade to hold the film in place
   D. Standard molar periapical image

6. A patient has an extremely large maxillary torus. You are not able to place the periapical image receptors as you usually would. What should you do?
   A. Place the image receptor on the opposite side of the torus (farther away from the teeth being imaged)
   B. Increase the vertical angle of the x-ray beam
   C. Use a hemostat to hold the image receptor closer to the teeth being imaged
   D. Use a no. o size image receptor, but take two additional exposures to image all posterior teeth

7. To help facilitate correct image-receptor placement when the patient has large mandibular tori, the operator should
   A. Use a no. 1 size image receptor
   B. Place the image receptor less deeply into the floor of the mouth
   C. Place a finger between the torus and the image receptor while sliding it into place
   D. Place the image receptor on top of the tongue for cushioning

8. If a disabled patient is unable to successfully hold an image receptor in the mouth either with a receptor-holding device or manually, what can the operator do?
   A. Hold the image receptor in the patient's mouth for the patient
   B. Attach the image receptor to the outside of the patient's cheek with adhesive and take the exposure from the opposite side of the patient's face
   C. Have the patient's parent, guardian, or attendant hold the image receptor after supplying that person with appropriate protective gear
   D. Eliminate the radiographic survey and collect all patient information through a clinical examination

9. When taking radiographs of children, the operator must remember that
   A. Shielding from radiation is not necessary for children
   B. Exposure factors may need to be reduced from adult settings
   C. It is best to work slowly and cautiously
   D. Children may refuse to cooperate if you explain procedures to them ahead of time

10. The best method to obtain the most accurate endodontic image is to use
    A. A topographic occlusal view
    B. The paralleling technique with an image-receptor holder such as a hemostat or tongue blade
    C. The bisecting-angle technique with the patient holding the image receptor
    D. The bisecting-angle technique with an image-receptor holder such as a hemostat or tongue blade

11

Extraoral, Specialized, and Implant Imaging

M aking a diagnosis, or assessing a patient's problem, may require information that is not available on standard intraoral or panoramic images. Various extraoral radiographic views allow the clinician to evaluate specific areas of the skull and jaws that are not included in other types of dental images. This chapter discusses views that are needed for a cephalometric analysis and imaging of the maxillary sinuses, temporomandibular joints (TMJs), or other large portions of the jaws. For film-based imaging, these radiographic techniques require rigid cassettes equipped with intensifying screens, such as those discussed in Chapter 8 (Fig. 11-1). Keep in mind that it is primarily the light from the intensifying screens that exposes the film. As a result, film-based extraoral images do not have the resolution or detail that an intraoral image will have because the light spreads out slightly. Additionally, the film is exquisitely sensitive to light, so darkroom conditions must be ideal. Digital extraoral images often have better resolution than film-based extraoral images.

It is a good idea to label film cassettes with an *L* or an *R* so that interpreters know the orientation of the images in relation to the patient. Some views, such as the cephalometric projection, require the use of a special cassette holder and cephalostat to hold the patient's head in place (Fig. 11-2).

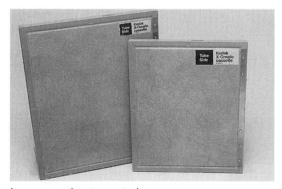

Figure 11-1 A 10- × 14-inch cassette and an 8- × 10-inch cassette.

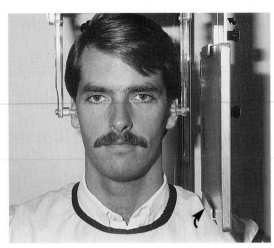

Figure 11-2 The cephalostat holds the patient's head in proper alignment.

LATERAL OBLIQUE JAW PROJECTIONS

Although many dental practices have a panoramic x-ray machine, there may be times when such a machine is not available. Large areas of the mandible can be visualized with an extraoral view called the lateral oblique jaw technique. To perform this technique, operators should seat patients with their occlusal plane parallel to the floor and the midsagittal plane perpendicular to the floor. A 5- × 7-inch or 8- × 10-inch cassette is used; it can be placed in a cassette holder, or the patient can hold it between the palm of the hand and cheekbone, with the cassette resting on the shoulder for stability. The cassette is positioned on the side of the patient's face that is to be examined and should contact the cheekbone, ear, and mandible. At least 1 inch of the cassette should extend below the inferior border of the mandible.

Once the cassette has been positioned, the patient should tip the chin up to move the mandible away from the cervical spine. The operator should then tilt the long axis of the patient's head about 15° toward the cassette. This elevates the opposite side of the mandible so that its superimposition over the opposite side will be minimized. If the *body of the mandible* is the area of interest, the cassette should be in contact with the mandible. The central ray of the x-ray beam is directed from beneath the opposite side of the jaw at a vertical angle of approximately −10° to −15°. The beam should be as perpendicular to the cassette as possible, entering in the area of the premolars and first molar (Fig. 11-3).

If the *ramus of the mandible* is the area of interest, the cassette should rest along the cheekbone and ear. The central ray should be at a vertical angle of approximately −15° to −20°. It should be as perpendicular to the cassette as possible, and it should enter distal to the third molar (Fig. 11-4). Images produced with the use of these techniques should resemble those in Figure 11-5.

CEPHALOMETRIC PROJECTIONS

Some dentists (orthodontists in particular) use a lateral view of the entire skull to assess a patient's profile and to assist in predicting growth patterns of the jaws. The technique is called **cephalometric imaging** (*cephalo* refers to the head, and

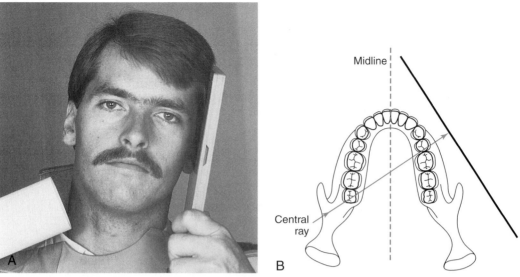

Figure 11-3 A, The patient's head and the cassette are angled about 15° from the midsagittal plane. With a negative tubehead angulation of 10° to 15°, the total angle is close to –25°. The thyroid collar has been lowered to prevent its superimposition on the image. **B,** The central ray enters near the first molar for a view of the body of the mandible.

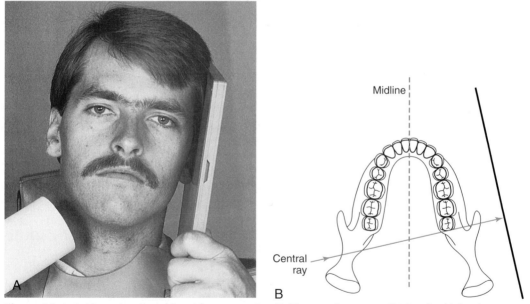

Figure 11-4 A, The patient is positioned for a ramus view. **B,** The central ray enters distal to the third molar.

metric means measurement). Because the image is used for measuring arch sizes, it must be taken in a precise manner that can be repeated at a later date to determine size change.

An 8- × 10-inch cassette is inserted into a cassette holder. The patient's midsagittal plane should be parallel to the cassette, and in North America it is customary for the left side of patient's head to be positioned against the cassette. A cephalostat, or head-holding device, helps position the patient by employing rods that fit into the patient's ears. The patient's Frankfort plane should be parallel to the floor. Some

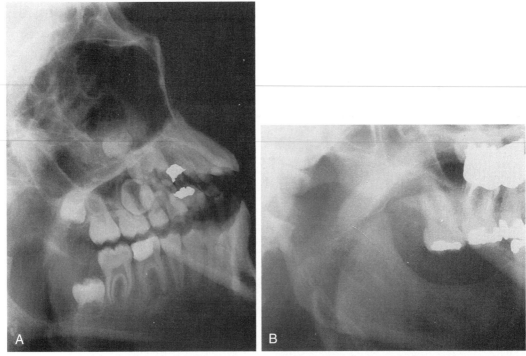

Figure 11-5 **A,** The body of the mandible is properly imaged. **B,** The ramus area is properly imaged.

cephalostats have a nasion guide that touches the patient at the bridge of the nose to ensure the correct orientation of the Frankfort plane (Fig. 11-6).

The x-ray source is 60 inches from the patient's midsagittal plane in cephalometric imaging. The central ray is directed perpendicular to the cassette, through the long axis of the ear rods. A special cephalometric radiographic unit, in which the tubehead is fixed at the correct distance and alignment, makes beam alignment and patient positioning easy to achieve.

The soft tissue outline of the patient's profile must be seen on the image to accurately assess the facial structures (Fig. 11-7). This outline can be obtained in a film-based system in one of several ways:

1. A thin lead or copper filter is placed at the x-ray source so that only part of the beam reaches the patient's face.
2. A special type of film (wide-latitude, low-contrast) that will record the soft tissue *and* bony structures of the head is used.
3. An aluminum filter strip is placed over the cassette in the area of the patient's profile.
4. A cassette with special intensifying screens containing a dye in the area of the patient's profile is used; the dye reduces the amount of light emitted from that portion of the screens, and the film will receive less exposure in the profile area.

Posteroanterior Skull View

Sometimes an additional cephalometric view taken in a different direction is needed to assess a patient's cranial and dental growth and development. A **posteroanterior projection** is taken with the patient facing the cassette, and the Frankfort plane is perpendicular to the cassette (Fig. 11-8). The central ray enters at the level of the external occipital protuberance from a distance of 60 inches. A typical image is shown in Figure 11-9. This image can also be used to look at the patient's frontal sinus,

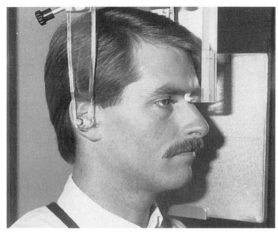

Figure 11-6 The patient is properly positioned with nasion guide in place.

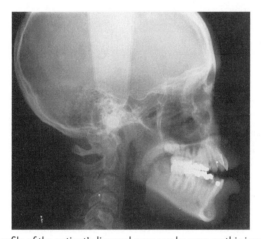

Figure 11-7 A soft tissue profile of the patient's lips and nose can be seen on this image.

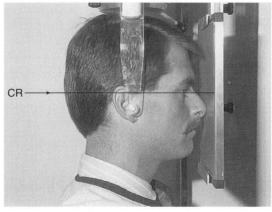

Figure 11-8 Posteroanterior position. *CR* indicates central ray.

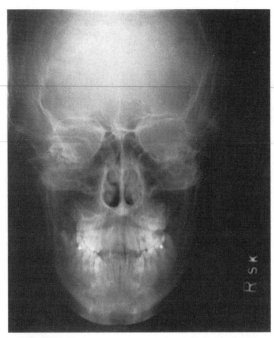

Figure 11-9 Standard posteroanterior view.

ethmoid air cells, nasal cavity, and upper portions of the mandible. Historically, this view was used as part of a "sinus series" along with a Waters view and a submentovertex view. However, it has largely been abandoned for sinus evaluation in favor of computed tomography (CT), by either conventional medical CT or cone beam volumetric imaging (CBVI).

TEMPOROMANDIBULAR JOINT VIEWS

Imaging of the TMJ is important to many practitioners, including orthodontists, prosthodontists, oral surgeons, other specialists, and many general practitioners. Advanced imaging techniques (CBVI, CT, and magnetic resonance imaging [MRI]) allow for a thorough examination of the area. Examples of these types of images are included later in the chapter.

However, there are many ways to obtain a radiographic view of the TMJ in a dental office. A standard panoramic image often shows the condyles adequately, although sometimes the glenoid fossa is obscured from view. Keep in mind that if the panoramic unit has a bitestick for patient positioning, the patient's lower jaw will be slightly forward (in protrusive position) during the exposure, and the condyles will not be seated fully in the fossae. Some panoramic x-ray machine manufacturers recommend slight changes in both patient positioning and exposure technique to achieve a better image of the TMJ (Fig. 11-10). The procedures for these variations are explained in the manuals that accompany the machines.

Transpharyngeal Projection

A transpharyngeal projection can be obtained quickly and easily, and it shows the condyle from a lateral view. However, it does not provide a reliable view of the glenoid fossa, nor is it precisely repeatable. Nevertheless, it can provide an excellent screening view of any gross changes on the condylar surfaces.

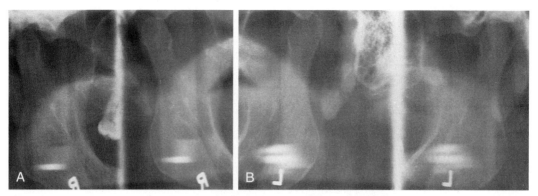

Figure 11-10 A panoramic "four-shot" series of open and closed positions. **A,** Right side closed and open. **B,** Left side open and closed.

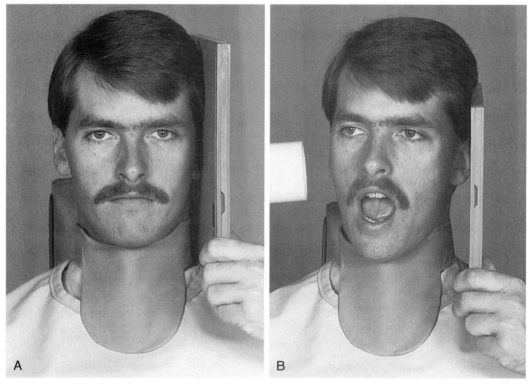

Figure 11-11 A, *Step 1 for a transpharyngeal projection:* Place the patient's midsagittal plane parallel to the cassette. **B,** *Step 2:* Rotate the patient's head 7° to 10° toward the x-ray source. Ask the patient to open the mouth 35 to 40 mm and angle the tubehead at –5° in the vertical direction.

The patient is seated with the occlusal plane parallel to the floor and the midsagittal plane perpendicular to the floor. The cassette is placed against the patient's face, in contact with the ear, on the side of the head being imaged. The patient's head is rotated slightly (7° to 10°) away from the cassette. This rotation is made to move the opposite condyle out of the way. The x-ray beam is then directed across the pharynx at a vertical angle of about –5° and at a horizontal angle of about 10° toward the back of the head. The central ray should enter beneath the zygomatic arch on the same side as the tubehead, in the direction of the condyle being imaged. The patient's jaws may be open or closed, but having the patient in an open jaw position draws the condyle out of the fossa for easier viewing. Figures 11-11 and 11-12 illustrate this technique.

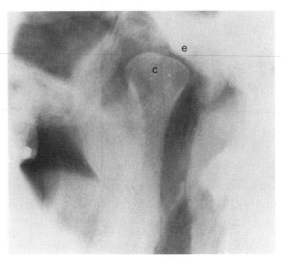

Figure 11-12 Typical transpharyngeal image: *c* is the condyle, *e* is the articular eminence.

Transorbital Projection

The transorbital projection is a frontal type of image that demonstrates the medial and lateral aspects of the condyle, the condylar neck, and sometimes the zygomatic arch. This projection allows a view that is approximately 90° to the transpharyngeal view, usually with little superimposition of other anatomic structures over the area of interest. The transorbital projection is not a precisely repeatable technique, but, like the transpharyngeal view, it is simple to obtain.

For this projection, the patient is seated with the Frankfort plane parallel to the floor and the midsagittal plane perpendicular to the floor. The cassette is placed behind the patient's head on the side to be radiographed. At this point, the cassette should be perpendicular to the patient's midsagittal plane. Without moving the cassette, rotate the patient's head approximately 20° toward the side to be imaged. Direct the x-ray beam at a vertical angulation of +30° to +35° so that the central ray passes through the floor of the orbit and TMJ (Fig. 11-13). The horizontal angulation of the beam should be perpendicular to the cassette. The patient should now open the mouth as wide as possible to move the condyle out of the glenoid fossa and onto the articular eminence. Figure 11-14 shows the resulting image.

Basilar or Submentovertex View

A basilar or submentovertex view demonstrates the condyles as if the viewer were looking directly upward from under the patient's chin (Fig. 11-15). This view allows the visualization of the condylar heads from medial to lateral poles (Fig. 11-16). Other structures that can be evaluated on this view include the mastoid air cells, the sphenoid sinus, and the lateral walls of the maxillary sinuses, and when the exposure factors are reduced, the zygomatic arches are visible.

Tomography

Tomography is a specialized imaging technique that uses motion of the x-ray source and the image receptor, but not the patient, to create the image. The details of this technique are beyond the scope of this text: it involves opposing movements of the x-ray source and image receptor to produce a "slice" through the area of interest

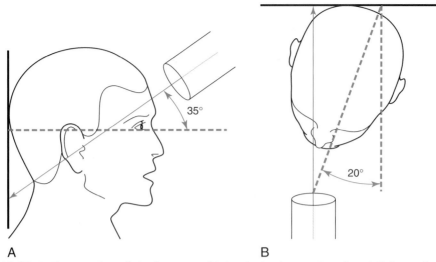

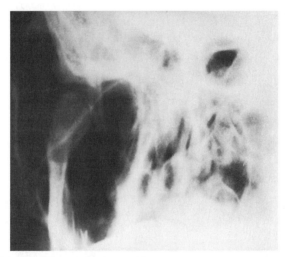

Figure 11-13   **A,** The vertical angulation for a transorbital projection is approximately +35°. **B,** Rotate the patient's head about 20° toward the condyle that is to be imaged.

Figure 11-14   Transorbital view of the mandibular condyle.

while all other areas are "blurred out" (Fig. 11-17). Special equipment is needed for tomography, and the more complex the movement of the x-ray source and image receptor, the clearer the slice becomes. Figure 11-18 shows a slice created with linear horizontal tomographic movement, whereas Figure 11-19 shows slices from a machine that moves in a more complex pattern. Note that the relationship between the condyle and the glenoid fossa is more easily visualized in the tomographs than in the other TMJ images discussed so far.

Arthrography

Before the advent of MRI, arthrography was the best way to visualize the soft tissue components of the TMJ (the articular disk and the ligaments holding it in place). In this technique, a radiopaque dye (a dye that shows up white on radiographs) is injected into the TMJ space, and images (most often tomographs) are taken. The images show the condyle; the glenoid fossa; and the joint space, which is filled with dye (Fig. 11-20).

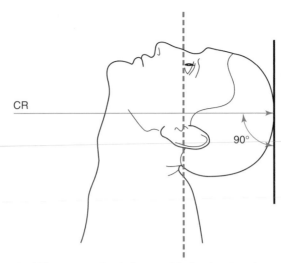

Figure 11-15 The patient should be positioned with the top of the head against the cassette for a submentovertex projection. The central ray *(CR)* should be directed at an angle of 90° to the cassette.

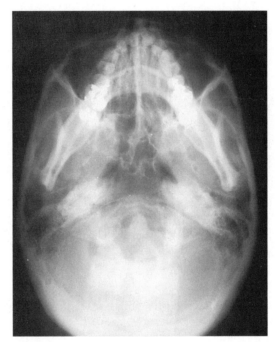

Figure 11-16 Submentovertex view.

Because of the invasive nature of this technique, it is not used much anymore, and MRI is now used when the soft tissue components of the joint need to be evaluated. Clinical arthroscopy, a procedure in which a small probe with a light source and a video camera is inserted in the joint, is also used for evaluating the TMJ components.

Computed Tomography

CT is a sophisticated imaging system in which an x-ray source rotates 360° around a patient (Fig. 11-21), imaging successive slices of a patient in small increments. The image receptor is a bank of scintillators that receives any remaining radiation

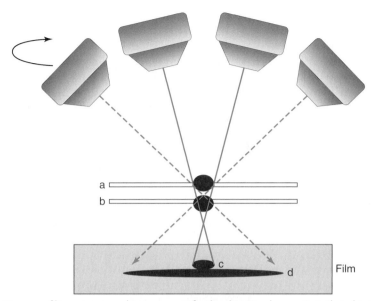

Figure 11-17 Diagram of linear tomographic movement for the object in plane *a*. Note that object *a*'s shadow *c* is representative of object *a*, while a similar object in plane *b* has been spread out and distorted (shadow *d*).

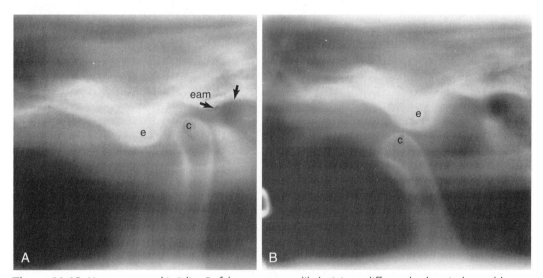

Figure 11-18 Linear tomographic "slices" of the temporomandibular joint at different depths: *c* is the condyle; *eam* is the external auditory meatus; and *e* is the articular eminence of the temporal bone. Each slice is approximately 0.5 cm thick. **A,** View with the mouth closed. **B,** View with the mouth open.

after it passes through the patient. The scintillators send a signal to a computer, the information is digitized, and a mathematical formula is applied to the data. Each bit of image is called a **pixel** (recall Chapter 7), and a number corresponding to a level of black, white, or gray (or even color) is assigned to each pixel. The data are then reconstructed as the image that the operator sees.

CT allows a clinician to view an area of interest in virtually any plane, provided that sufficient numbers of sections have been imaged (Fig. 11-22). Because of its capacity to image the TMJ in several different views, including three-dimensional reconstruction (Fig. 11-23), CT is the image of choice for thorough evaluation of the

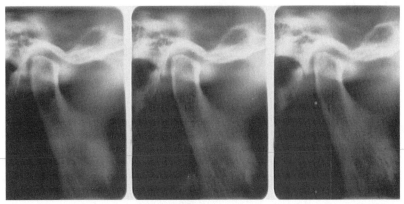

Figure 11-19 Closed views of the mandibular condyle taken with a tomographic unit. Three views are taken at different depths, or cuts, from the lateral to the medial poles of the condyle.

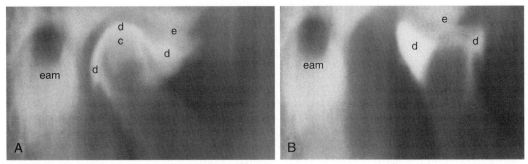

Figure 11-20 Arthrogram of the temporomandibular joint: *c* is the condyle; *d* is the dye; *e* is the articular eminence; and *eam* is the external auditory meatus. **A,** View with the mouth closed. **B,** View with mouth open.

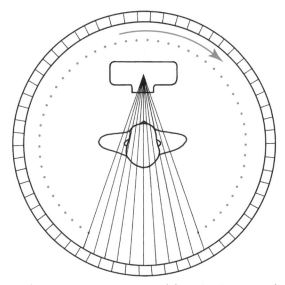

Figure 11-21 X-ray source and image receptors rotate around the patient in computed tomographic imaging. *(From White SC, Pharoah MJ: Oral radiology: principles and interpretation, ed 6, St Louis, 2009, Mosby.)*

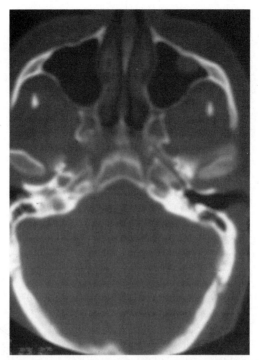

Figure 11-22   Computed tomographic image in the axial plane at the level of the condylar heads.

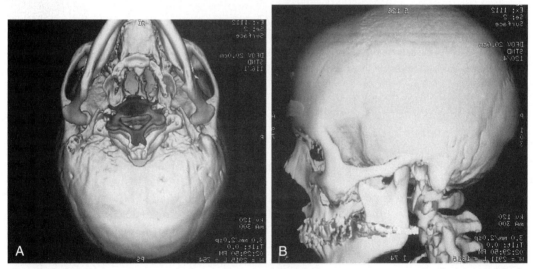

Figure 11-23   **A,** Three-dimensional reconstruction simulating a submentovertex view. Can you find the condylar heads? **B,** Three-dimensional reconstruction from a lateral perspective. Note the relationship between the condyle and the glenoid fossa.

bony components of the joint (the condyle and the glenoid fossa). However, CT does not adequately demonstrate the soft tissues in the joint.

Today, the best imaging modality for the bony portions of the TMJ and related structures is CBVI. Three-dimensional color images of the condyles and multiplanar gray-scale images can characterize joint changes more precisely and accurately with much less of a radiation dose to the patient compared with conventional CT (Fig. 11-24).

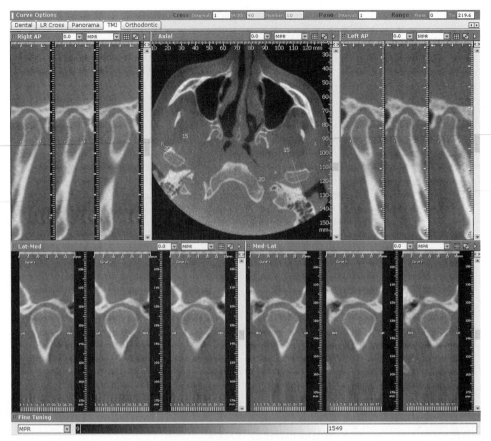

Figure 11-24 Multiplanar reformatted gray-scale images of the temporomandibular joint region. The center image is an axial view, which is flanked by lateral views of both condyles. Coronal views are seen along the bottom.

Magnetic Resonance Imaging

MRI is unique among imaging systems in that it does not utilize ionizing radiation to make the image; rather, a strong magnetic field and radio frequency signals are used. The patient is placed in a large magnet, which causes the nuclei of the atoms in the body to align themselves in the magnetic field. A radio signal is applied, disturbing the alignment of the nuclei, in particular the nuclei of the hydrogen atoms. When the radio signal is turned off, the hydrogen atom nuclei realign themselves with the magnetic field and energy is released. This energy release is detected and sent to a computer, where the image is reconstructed. Because mature bone has little water in it and therefore a low concentration of hydrogen atoms, it gives a weak signal and is black on the image. Tissues with higher water content such as fat or muscle give brighter (whiter) signals. MRI is able to determine subtle differences in soft tissues and display them with high contrast sensitivity. Therefore, MRI is the standard imaging modality for examining the soft tissue components of the TMJ (Fig. 11-25).

Cone Beam Volumetric Imaging

CBVI may also be referred to as cone beam computed tomography or cone beam volumetric tomography. We prefer the phrase *volumetric imaging* because the image acquisition is unlike conventional CT. The imaging system is complex, but

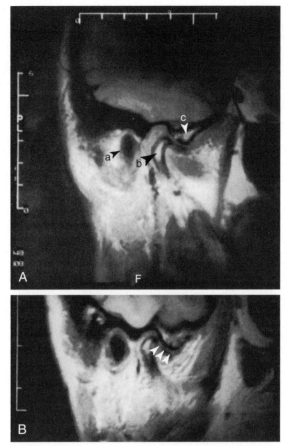

Figure 11-25   A, Magnetic resonance image of the temporomandibular joint complex: *a,* external auditory meatus; *b,* the marrow in the condylar head; and *c,* the marrow in the articular eminence. The cortical bone of both the condylar head and articular eminence is seen as thin black lines surrounding these bright signals of the marrow within. **B,** This patient's attempt to open is prevented by this displaced temporomandibular joint disk or meniscus, seen as the thin grayish band in front of the condyle *(arrows). (From Miles DA, Van Dis ML, Razmus TF:* Basic principles of oral and maxillofacial radiology, *ed 1, Philadelphia, 1992, Saunders.)*

the machines are generally rather small compared with conventional CT or MRI (Fig. 11-26), often not much larger than a panoramic unit. CBVI is available in many dentists' offices, especially orthodontists, oral surgeons, and oral and maxillofacial radiologists. CBVI data are acquired in only one 360° rotation around the patient's head, unlike a conventional CT machine in which several 360° rotations are required. The image receptor is a flat panel detector or an image intensifier coupled to a solid-state detector or a set of detectors like a charge-coupled device (recall Chapter 7). Detector sizes in CBVI machines vary greatly, from arrays as small as 4.0 cm × 4.0 cm up to 22 cm.

Spatial resolution in CBVI is expressed in **voxels** (volume elements) rather than pixels (picture elements), and the image can be reconstructed and displayed in either a two-dimensional or a three-dimensional format, with color added, in several orientations (Fig. 11-27). It is easy to understand why this imaging technique would be useful for evaluation of the TMJ!

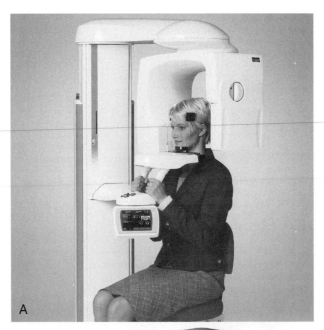

A

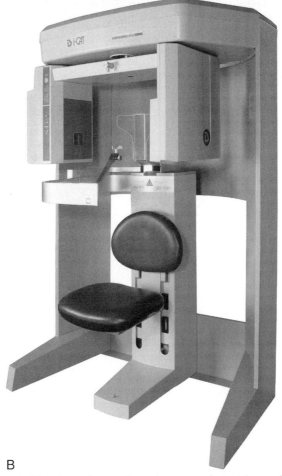

B

Figure 11-26 A, Planmeca ProMax 3D cone beam volumetric tomography imaging machine. Note that the patient may also stand in the ProMax machine. This unit allows the operator to perform a digital panoramic view just by exchanging the flat panel detector. **B,** Imaging Sciences International's i-CAT Cone Beam 3-D Dental Imaging System. *(A: Courtesy of Planmeca Oy, Helsinki, Finland. B: Courtesy of Imaging Sciences International, Hatfield, Pa.)*

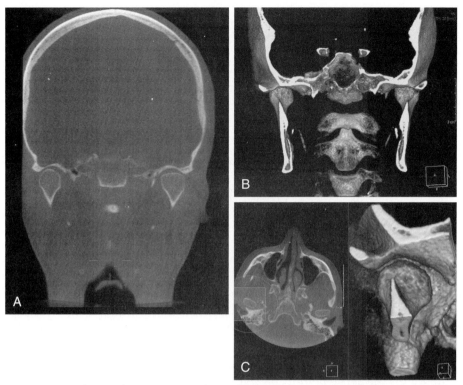

Figure 11-27 A, Cone beam volumetric image with a small volume region capture. **B,** Large volume region capture showing both condyles in a coronal plane of section. **C,** Same patient with condyle reconstructed in three-dimensional color at a thickness of 20 mm.

MAXILLARY SINUSES

Because the maxillary sinuses are in such close proximity to the maxillary posterior teeth, the inferior portions of them are visible in the maxillary posterior periapical images. A great deal of the maxillary sinuses can be seen in a panoramic image. When an unusual finding is seen in the maxillary sinus on a periapical or panoramic image or if the patient has a complaint in the area of the sinus, further imaging may be required to better assess the patient. Conventional CT and now CBVI are considered to be the gold standard for evaluation of the paranasal sinuses, including the maxillary sinus. One of these scans can essentially replace all other views mentioned here, because the CBVI data can be used to create *any* view, at higher resolution and with thinner slices.

Waters View

The radiographic view that is commonly prescribed for evaluation of the maxillary sinuses is the **Waters projection** (or occipitomental). This projection was specifically developed for visualizing the maxillary sinuses, named for one of the people who developed the technique. However, the frontal and ethmoid sinuses and the nasal cavity are also clearly seen on this view.

For this projection, the patient faces the cassette with the midsagittal plane perpendicular to the image receptor. The patient's chin is raised so that the Frankfort plane makes a 37° to 45° angle with the original horizontal position. The patient's nose should be about 1 to 2 inches away from the cassette (Fig. 11-28). Elevating the

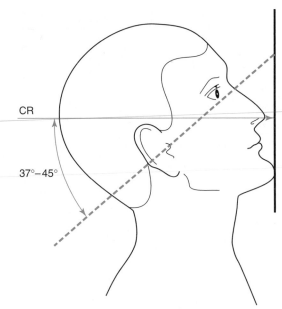

CR

37°–45°

Figure 11-28 For a Waters projection, the patient faces the image receptor and elevates the chin approximately 37° to 45°. The central ray *(CR)* is directed at an angle of 90° to the cassette.

chin moves the dense petrous portion of the temporal bone inferiorly on the image, away from the area of interest. Some clinicians prefer to ask the patient to open the mouth during the exposure to avoid superimposing any mandibular dental work over the sinuses. The x-ray beam is directed at 90° to the cassette, and the central ray enters the back of the skull. The resulting image is seen in Figure 11-29.

Advanced Images

Because the CT image can be reconstructed in virtually any plane, CT is frequently used to evaluate maxillary sinuses. The integrity of the sinus walls can be evaluated, and a general assessment of the soft tissue lining the sinus can be made in an axial and/or a coronal view (Fig. 11-30). MRI is particularly useful when evaluating fluids or lesions containing fluids within the sinuses (Fig. 11-31) because a watery exudate will show up as a very bright signal. CBVI also readily demonstrates the maxillary sinuses (Fig. 11-32) and, as mentioned previously, can give thin-slice, high-resolution images in gray scale or color.

IMPLANTS

Implant procedures are now commonplace in the dental office. Preoperative planning, including presurgical radiographic evaluation of endosseous, or root form, implants, is central to the success of the implant procedure. The single biggest fear that dentists have when placing implants is erroneously placing a fixture in an anatomic space or encroaching on the inferior alveolar nerve resulting in implant failure and an unhappy (and potentially litigious) patient. Case selection involves both clinical assessment of the site(s) by both visual examination and *appropriate* imaging. Other factors include patient education, patient preparation, and risk estimation for the procedure.

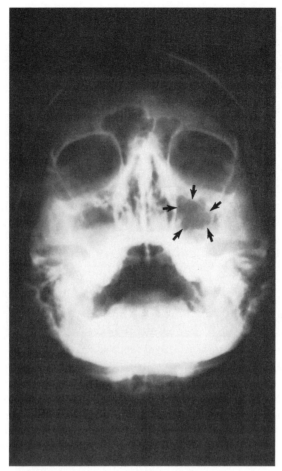

Figure 11-29 Open-mouth Waters view. The *arrows* mark the maxillary sinus.

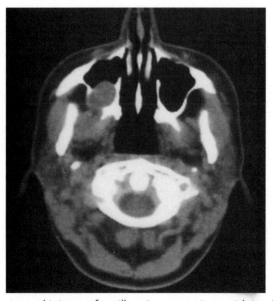

Figure 11-30 Computed tomographic image of maxillary sinuses seen in an axial view. Note the mass in the posterior aspect of the right maxillary sinus.

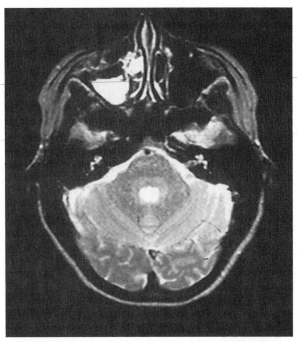

Figure 11-31 Magnetic resonance image of maxillary and ethmoid sinuses that have bright *(white)* signals indicating the presence of watery or mucinous material.

Presurgical radiographic evaluation of implant sites should help the dentist determine (1) the quantity of bone present, (2) the quality of bone present, and (3) the location of critical anatomic structures. Generally it is sound practice to obtain multiple views of the proposed site to adequately assess the height and width of the alveolar bone. This assessment may require several imaging techniques.

Periapical, Occlusal, and Panoramic Evaluation for Implants

Conventional, two-dimensional images like periapicals or panoramics do not adequately allow for assessment of alveolar ridge width. Additionally, the potential projection geometry errors (foreshortening, elongation, magnification) inherent in both periapicals and panoramics do not allow for precise calculations. The most information that panoramic images, together with intraoral images, can reveal is about bone quality, such as density and trabecular pattern, or the presence of anomalies in the proposed region.

Panoramic and intraoral images may provide for a *preliminary* evaluation of multiple implant sites because the operator can compare contralateral structures. *Nevertheless, periapical and panoramic imaging as the* sole *means of radiographic presurgical implant assessment is inappropriate because the techniques are extremely sensitive to errors, image distortion, and magnification.* Unless clinicians have sufficient training to fully understand the limitations of a panoramic image, they risk initiating an unsuccessful implant procedure and potential litigation problems owing to inadequate radiographic assessment.

Tomographic Techniques

For fewer than three proposed implant sites, plain (not computerized) tomography as discussed for viewing the TMJs can be used for showing bone shape and the location of anatomic structures (Fig. 11-33). However, because of the

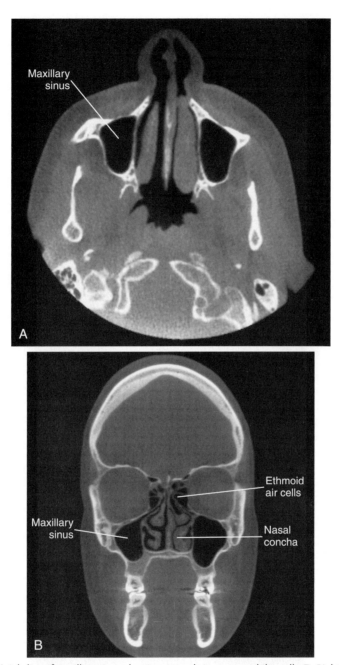

Figure 11-32   **A,** Axial slice of maxillary sinus showing normal sinus spaces bilaterally. **B,** Right coronal plane of section showing maxillary sinuses, ethmoid air cells, and related nasal cavity structures.

preliminary "scout" film, calculations, and measurements that the clinician must make, this is a time-consuming technique and is not efficient for just a few sites. CT, with its two-dimensional and three-dimensional reconstruction capabilities, is often prescribed for assessment of multiple implant sites. Software specifically designed for implants allows for rapid, detailed image processing and visualization of proposed sites at a 1:1, that is, life-sized, ratio (Figs. 11-34 through 11-36).

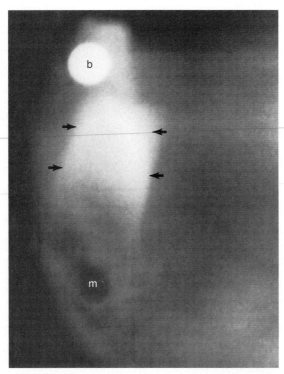

Figure 11-33 Plain film tomography showing a proposed implant site in the mandible. The patient is wearing an appliance in which metal balls have been placed where the clinician wants the implants *(b)*. The width of the alveolus is indicated by the *arrows*, and the mental foramen is marked with *m*. There appears to be adequate width and height for an implant in this location.

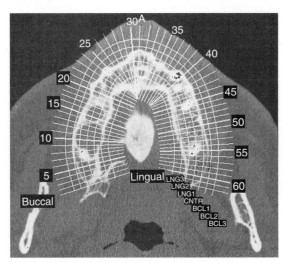

Figure 11-34 Axial view of a section of the maxilla at the level of the mid-palate. The large opacity in the middle of the palate is a maxillary torus. The grid is a reference for implant placement sites.

Cone Beam Volumetric Imaging

The current state of the art for implant assessment is with CBVI. The multiplanar and three-dimensional reconstruction of images plus the software enhancements provide a detailed, accurate presurgical assessment of the patient (Figs. 11-37 and 11-38).

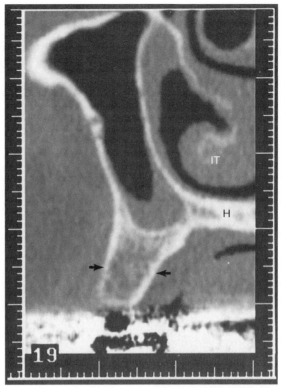

Figure 11-35 Close-up view of the maxilla in the premolar region as seen in a coronal section (patient "sliced" through the face from ear to ear). The bone width available for an implant lies between the *arrows,* and the dark area above the alveolus is the maxillary sinus. You can see the soft tissue lining the sinus floor. *IT* is the inferior turbinate bone in the nasal cavity; *H* is the hard palate.

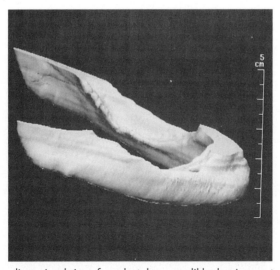

Figure 11-36 Partial three-dimensional view of an edentulous mandible showing greater height in the anterior region than in the posterior areas. Can you find the mental foramen?

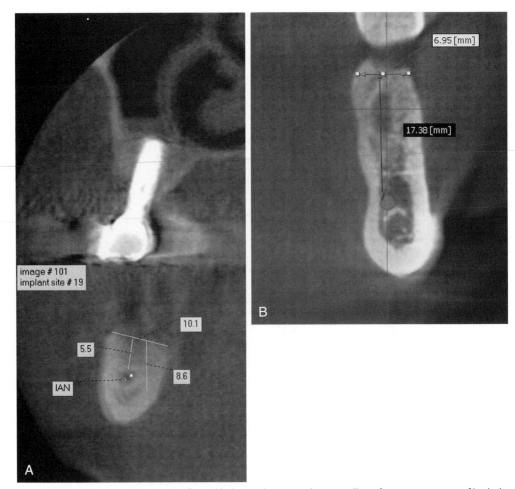

Figure 11-37   A, Cross-sectional view of mandibular implant site. This view allows for measurements of both the width and height of the alveolus, plus the location of the inferior alveolar canal. Note the implant in close proximity to the maxillary sinus and nasal cavity. **B,** Cross-sectional view of a maxillary implant site. Note the close proximity of the implant to the maxillary sinus and the nasal cavity.

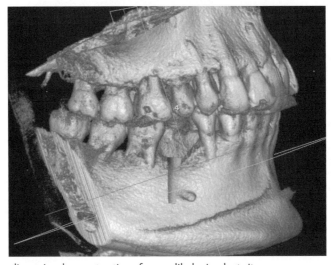

Figure 11-38   Three-dimensional reconstruction of a mandibular implant site.

This is especially true when this technique is used in conjunction with an x-ray marker that allows the operator to determine the exact location of the proposed implant site. The marker material should be easily identifiable and should not produce an imaging artifact. Gutta percha is an ideal material for this purpose. It is nonmetallic, radiopaque, and readily available. Because the most appropriate approach to a successful implant procedure is multidisciplinary, the coordinated team efforts of an oral and maxillofacial radiologist and the surgeon placing the implants will provide the best care for the patient, including assessment of patient problems or conditions other than those directly associated with implant placement.

STUDY QUESTIONS

1. A lateral cephalometric image
   A. Is often used to measure changes and predict growth patterns
   B. Contains a soft tissue outline
   C. Is commonly used by orthodontists
   D. All of the above

2. The bony anatomic structures of primary importance in TMJ projections are the
   A. Condyle and coronoid process
   B. Condyle and maxillary tuberosity
   C. Condyle and glenoid fossa
   D. Coronoid process and glenoid fossa

3. The technique of imaging a body joint such as the TMJ with radiopaque dye is called
   A. Arthrography
   B. Tomography
   C. Topography
   D. Cephalometry

4. The TMJ view that allows you to see the medial and lateral aspects of the condyle is the
   A. Waters projection
   B. Transorbital projection
   C. Transpharyngeal projection
   D. Lateral oblique jaw projection

5. The radiographic view for evaluation of the maxillary sinuses is the
   A. Waters projection
   B. Submentovertex projection
   C. Transpharyngeal projection
   D. Transorbital projection

6. Which of the following specialized techniques does not employ ionizing radiation?
   A. Computed tomography
   B. Cone beam volumetric imaging
   C. Magnetic resonance imaging
   D. Arthrography

7. Presurgical implant images are taken for each of the following reasons except one. Which one is the exception?
   A. Determine bone quality
   B. Locate anatomic structures
   C. Assess bone quantity
   D. Locate the densest bone

8. Which of the following techniques provides the *least* accurate information for assessing the jaws for implant placement?
   A. Panoramic and periapical images
   B. Plain film tomography
   C. Computed tomography
   D. Cone beam volumetric imaging

9. Which of the following is a disadvantage of using computed tomography for implant assessment?
   A. It provides information in only two dimensions
   B. There is a high dose of radiation to the patient
   C. Accurate measurements cannot be obtained
   D. It cannot be used to assess the maxilla

10. Three-dimensional imaging can be obtained with which of the following techniques?
    A. Plain film tomography
    B. Computed tomography
    C. Cone beam volumetric imaging
    D. B and C

12

Basics of Interpretation: Normal versus Abnormal and Common Radiographic Presentation of Lesions

DETECTION OF DISEASE OR OTHER ABNORMAL CONDITIONS

Diagnoses are not made from images alone; the radiographic image is only one tool for the clinician. For many disorders, such as dental caries, periodontal disease, or trauma, the image is a *sensitive* detector: it readily shows changes in the patient's mouth. With these disorders, it is also quite *specific:* the radiographic features are specific to certain conditions. In other disorders, such as the periapical infection or dental cysts and tumors, although one can detect the disease by means of radiography, one cannot precisely name the specific tumor or cysts by studying the radiographic features alone. With these disorders, the image is less specific. Nevertheless, the intraoral image is an indispensable diagnostic tool when properly used.

Dental auxiliaries can play a significant role in disease detection. As a dental team member, the well-trained auxiliary should be able to differentiate abnormal from normal radiographic features. Armed with a sound knowledge of normal anatomy, the dental assistant or dental hygienist becomes an additional detector of disease processes in the patient. In this way, the quality of the patient's care is enhanced.

This chapter illustrates radiographic features of common dental diseases and anomalies that may be visualized on dental images. In a comparative approach, examples of abnormal processes are illustrated together with normal anatomic structures.

BASIC VIEWING PRINCIPLES

Detecting differences between normal and abnormal structures involves more than just a casual glance at the images. Certain viewing strategies maximize the information garnered from a radiographic survey.

Viewing Conditions

1. You must begin with good quality images, that is, those that are properly positioned, exposed, processed, and for film, mounted.

2. The viewing conditions should be quiet and free from distractions. If films are being viewed, they should be placed on a view box and the room should have subdued ambient light. If images are being viewed on a monitor, it should be positioned so that the viewer is comfortable and no glare is on the screen.

3. A magnifying glass is useful for films. Enlarging or otherwise enhancing a digital image (adjusting contrast or brightness) with appropriate software may prove helpful.

4. You should look at multiple views of an area, if possible.

Viewing Technique

Keep these basic factors in minds as you view your images:
1. Follow a consistent pattern. For example,
   a. Take an overview of the patient's images. Sit back and look at the survey as a whole to see whether anything strikes you as unusual.
   b. Start left to right, viewing the maxilla first (the equivalent of starting with tooth no. 1).
   c. Begin surveying the supporting structures of the teeth: the alveolar bone, the periodontal ligament space, and the lamina dura.
   d. Finally, move your gaze to the structures of the teeth, from the outer surfaces to the internal pulp chamber and root canals.
2. Use constant eye movement. Do not stare at the images. You will not be able to detect subtle shades of gray if you stare.
3. Watch for possible indicators of abnormality, such as
   a. *Breaks in continuity.* Does the lamina dura have a break in it, or does the surface of the dental enamel have a dark area?
   b. *Asymmetry.* Are obvious differences seen from one side of the patient to the other? If you see a radiolucent or radiopaque area, does the contralateral side have a similar appearance?
   c. *Change in size.* Are there any dimensional changes, expansion of the bone, or changes in the shape of the teeth, jaws, or temporomandibular joint?

DESCRIBING ABNORMAL CONDITIONS

Although a definitive diagnosis of an abnormal condition in the jaws may require more diagnostic tests than a radiographic image alone, describing the changes seen in the abnormality may prove extremely useful in narrowing the diagnostic possibilities for the clinician. Therefore being able to use radiographic descriptors that are universally understood by anyone reading the patient record or radiographic report is a key skill for all dental personnel to acquire.

Description of an abnormal condition seen on an image of the jaws should include the following elements:
1. The type of image being viewed (e.g., periapical image or panoramic image)
2. The location of the abnormality (right, left, maxillary, mandibular)
   a. Single or isolated
      i. Associated with teeth (pericoronal, periapical)
      ii. Not associated with teeth
   b. Multiple areas involved
   c. Generalized throughout one or more quadrants or an entire jaw

3. The general shape of the lesion (round, ovoid, scalloped, irregular)
   a. Unilocular (single compartment)
   b. Multilocular (multiple compartments)
4. Density of the lesion
   a. Radiolucent (dark)
   b. Radiopaque (light)
   c. Mixed (dark and light areas within the same lesion)
5. Size (usually measured in millimeters or centimeters; example, 2 mm × 4 mm)
   a. Small (a subjective descriptor but usually <1 cm)
   b. Medium (also subjective but usually 1 cm to 3 cm)
   c. Large (another subjective descriptor but usually >3 cm)
6. Borders of the lesion
   a. Sharply demarcated
      i. Corticated (white outline)
      ii. Noncorticated (no white border, appears "punched out")
   b. Ill-defined (not distinct, hard to tell where lesion starts and stops)
7. Effects on adjacent structures
   a. Displacement (lesion moves a structure; often teeth are displaced)
   b. Expansion (often the outer cortex of the jaw may show a bulge)
   c. Resorption (resorption of tooth structure)
   d. Destruction (destruction of normal anatomic structures)
   e. Perforation (perforation of cortex)

An example of a radiographic description of the abnormality depicted in Figure 12-1 would be as follows:

This panoramic image shows a single, medium-sized, ovoid radiolucency in the posterior aspect of the left side of the mandible. The lesion measures approximately 2 cm × 3 cm, is well-defined, and has corticated borders. There are no teeth in the area. The lesion is located superior to the mandibular canal and may have displaced the canal inferiorly.

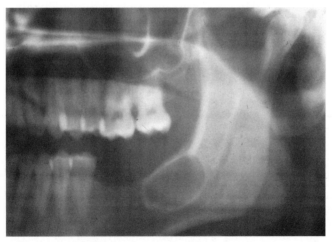

Figure 12-1 Example of a pathologic lesion seen on a radiograph.

INTERPRETATION OF ABNORMALITIES

This chapter is not meant to be an exhaustive review of oral pathology or radiographic interpretation. It is designed to sensitize the student to common dental abnormalities. We hope that by comparing normal and abnormal structures, you will reinforce your knowledge of normal radiographic anatomic landmarks and will become competent at detecting abnormal features that might affect patient care.

At the end of this chapter, a series of line drawings outlines typical radiographic presentations of pathologic lesions. These diagrams are followed by multiple examples of images of odontogenic cysts and tumors to compare with the line drawings. A thorough discussion of the etiology, clinical characteristics, and histologic features of these lesions is beyond the scope of this textbook. The reader can find such information in other oral and maxillofacial radiology or oral and maxillofacial pathology textbooks.

RADIOGRAPHIC CHANGES RESULTING FROM DENTAL CARIES

The dental auxiliary is often the first person to view the images after they are processed. If carious lesions are detected as the images are mounted or digitally saved, they can be pointed out to the dentist. The dentist holds the ultimate responsibility for caries diagnosis and treatment decisions, but the dental auxiliary should help with caries detection.

Where to Look for Dental Caries

Dental carious lesions that occur interproximally (between the teeth) are best detected on bitewing radiographs. The point of the carious attachment on this part of the tooth is at or just apical to the contact point (where the teeth touch). Figure 12-2, A, shows the typical radiographic classes of interproximal carious lesions. Figure 12-2, B, illustrates root surface caries as seen interproximally. Root surface decay may occur in patients who have lost alveolar bone support for the teeth because of periodontal disease.

Caries may spread along the junction of the dentin and enamel in a linear fashion, whether they are interproximal or occlusal lesions. An occlusal carious lesion

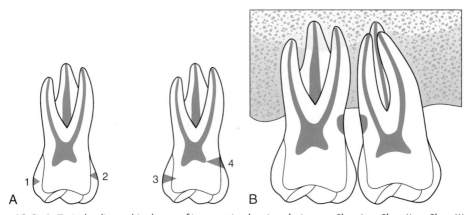

Figure 12-2 **A,** Typical radiographic classes of interproximal carious lesions. *1,* Class I; *2,* Class II; *3,* Class III; *4,* Class IV. **B,** Root caries apical to the cementoenamel junction as a result of bone loss and different locations of bacteria and food debris. Lesions are usually rounded and somewhat indistinct.

is one that starts on the biting surface of a posterior tooth in the developmental pit and fissure areas. Early occlusal caries is best detected clinically because lesions that are still contained within enamel are not readily demonstrated on intraoral images.

Radiographic Classification of Interproximal Caries

Class I: Caries that is less than halfway through the enamel.
Class II: Caries that is more than halfway through the enamel.
Class III: Caries that extends to and through the dentinoenamel junction (DEJ) but less than half the distance to the pulp chamber.
Class IV: Caries that extends more than half the distance to the pulp chamber.

Compare the illustrated carious lesions in Figure 12-2 with the dental caries on the image in Figure 12-3, a bitewing of a young patient (7 to 8 years old). Two classifications of caries are seen. All the lesions involve the DEJ. The lesion on the distal part of the first maxillary primary molar *(d)* has destroyed a large portion of the tooth and extends more than halfway to the pulp chamber; therefore, it is a Class IV lesion. The lesions in the second maxillary primary molar and the first and second mandibular primary molars all extend through the enamel, just into the dentin. Therefore, they are Class III lesions.

A classic interproximal carious lesion appears on the distal surface of the mandibular right second premolar in Figure 12-4. It is a triangular defect, and its point is toward the dentin. It has not yet reached the DEJ, but it is more than halfway through the enamel. It is therefore a Class II carious lesion. A similar lesion is seen on the tooth's mesial surface; however, its shape is less well-defined. Some interproximal lesions are less conspicuous because of variance in enamel thickness, thickness of the patient's overlying soft tissue, degree of enamel destruction, or variability in technique (e.g., angulation or exposure factors). Carious lesions of all types, marked with arrows, appear in Figure 12-5. Note how much less conspicuous the lesions on the second premolar and second molar are than the large lesion on the first molar is.

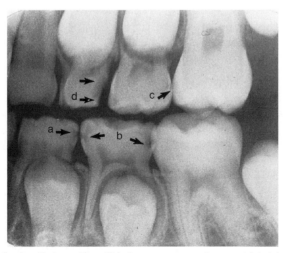

Figure 12-3 Two types of carious lesions: Class III lesions appear on primary teeth L *(a)*, K *(b)*, and J *(c)*; a Class IV lesion is seen on tooth I *(d)*.

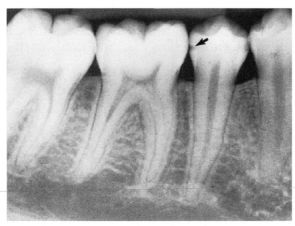

Figure 12-4 Classic interproximal carious lesion *(arrow)* on the distal surface of the mandibular right second premolar.

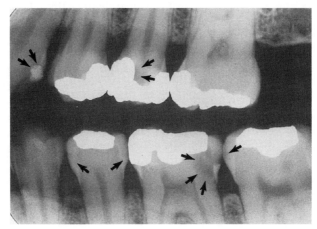

Figure 12-5 Carious lesions on tooth no. 11 distal, recurrent; tooth no. 13 mesial, recurrent; tooth no. 18 mesial; tooth no. 19 distal; tooth no. 20 distal and mesial.

Facial/Lingual Caries

On what surface of the second molar is the cavity marked *a* in Figure 12-6 (seen here as a circular radiolucency)? It may be on either the buccal (facial) or the lingual surface. Remember that a radiographic image is just a two-dimensional representation of an object. One cannot tell from the single image alone on which side—buccal or lingual—the lesion is located. This can, however, be confirmed clinically.

Occlusal Caries

In Figure 12-7, the letter *a* shows the radiographic appearance of a typical occlusal carious lesion; a darker, more radiolucent area is just beneath the enamel. A smaller, more subtle occlusal lesion is seen at the DEJ on the second premolar as a radiolucency marked *b*. Occlusal lesions as seen on intraoral images are those that have already reached the dentin, and they are usually associated with the developmental pits in the biting surfaces of teeth.

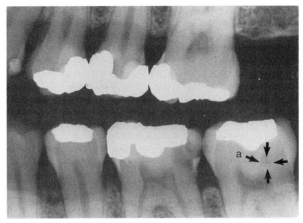

Figure 12-6 Facial (buccal) or lingual caries *(a)*. This is the same radiograph as in Fig. 12-5. Find the same lesion on Fig. 12-5 without the arrows to guide you.

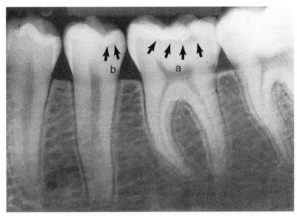

Figure 12-7 Carious lesion *(a)* on the occlusal surface of the molar. The cavity marked *b* began in the occlusal distal pit of this premolar.

Recurrent or Secondary Caries

Caries may also recur, or begin anew, under margins of existing restorations. These recurrent lesions are also called secondary caries. In Figure 12-8, two examples of rather large recurrent or secondary lesions, both interproximal, appear around and beneath existing amalgam restorations. Anterior teeth that have been restored with tooth-colored restoration may demonstrate radiolucent rims around the internal aspect of the filling. These generally do not represent secondary caries, but are related to the primer material or bonding agent that is placed into the cavity preparation before the final filling material. These primers are often radiolucent, whereas the filling material itself is opaque. Figure 12-9 illustrates this appearance.

Dental caries, if left untreated, can destroy large amounts of tooth structure. Figure 12-10 reveals many extensive and advanced carious lesions. Only root stumps are left for the maxillary premolars and maxillary second molar. Similarly, only root tips remain of the mandibular first molar. Such destructive decay is sometimes referred to as gross decay.

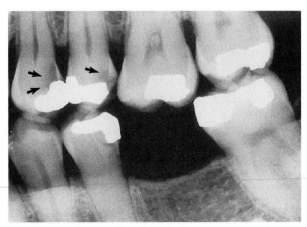

Figure 12-8 Two examples of large interproximal carious lesions *(arrows)* around or beneath existing amalgam restorations.

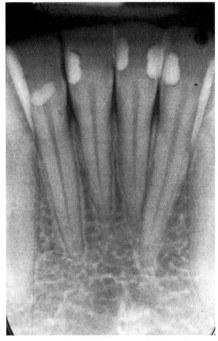

Figure 12-9 Radiopaque resin restorations with a radiolucent rim along the internal cavity walls. This most likely represents the primer material that is placed in the cavity preparation before the placement of the resin.

This type of rampant dental decay is not limited to the adult dentition. Figure 12-11 shows a bitewing image of an 8-year-old patient with a gross carious lesion on the maxillary first primary molar *(arrows)*. The maxillary second primary molar has been restored conservatively with amalgam. The mandibular primary molars have had pulpotomies (removal of diseased pulp tissue), and temporary stainless steel crowns have been placed on the primary molars. The stainless steel crown on the second primary molar has fallen off; the image was taken to determine why. The radiolucent area beneath the crown of the tooth and between the roots is a large area of bone destruction caused by a dental abscess.

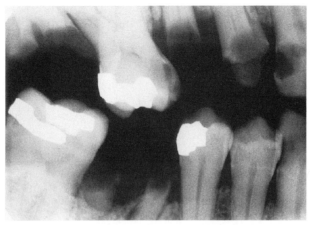

Figure 12-10 Tooth structure destruction as a result of untreated dental caries.

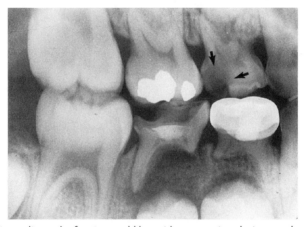

Figure 12-11 A bitewing radiograph of an 8-year-old boy with gross carious lesions on the maxillary first primary molar *(arrows)*.

Root Caries

The final type of dental caries to discuss is root caries. Root caries occurs apical to the cementoenamel junction (CEJ). Usually it is preceded by exposure of the root surface to the oral environment owing to the bony destruction of alveolar crestal bone in periodontal disease. With this decreased level of bone, plaque develops more apically on the tooth, not just at the contact point. The accumulation of plaque and its bacteria in this region leads to cervical or root decay. Compared with caries that starts in enamel, root surface lesions are not usually triangular in shape but appear rounded or cupped out. Because the caries progresses rapidly on the unprotected root surface, the lesions are often well advanced when detected on images. A typical lesion appears in Figure 12-12 on the maxillary second premolar *a.* A less obvious and somewhat smaller lesion is seen on the molar *b.* Figure 12-13 shows a well-advanced lesion that is encroaching on the pulp space of the maxillary canine. Such a lesion often results in pulp death (see the section on periapical disease).

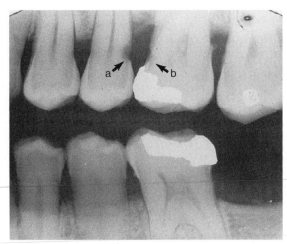

Figure 12-12 Typical root caries *(a)* on the maxillary second premolar. A less distinct lesion *(b)* is seen on the molar.

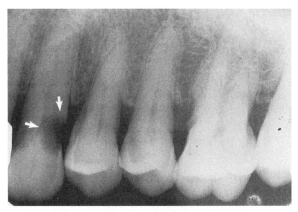

Figure 12-13 Well-advanced carious lesion *(arrows)* encroaching on the pulp.

RADIOGRAPHIC CHANGES RESULTING FROM PERIODONTAL DISEASE

Healthy alveolar bone has an intact crestal lamina dura at right angles to the teeth and is located about 1 mm apical to the CEJs of the teeth (Fig. 12-14). In the anterior area, the alveolar crestal bone may have sharp points or crests between the incisors but will still have intact lamina dura (Fig. 12-15). The inflammation associated with periodontal disease will lead to alveolar bone loss if left untreated. Local factors such as plaque and calculus contribute to and complicate the injury to tissues. Chronic inflammation, toxins, and enzymes cause breakdown of the periodontium (the gingiva and bone). The ravages of these processes are reflected radiographically by these bony defects. Both horizontal bone loss and vertical bone defects may be present. The radiographic changes may be localized to one area or generalized throughout the dentition. Factors other than plaque and calculus may affect the nature of the bone involvement. Systemic diseases such as diabetes or other immunologic problems may impair the patient's ability to mount a defense against infection. Classification and discussion of the various types of periodontal diseases are available in other dental textbooks and are beyond the scope of this text.

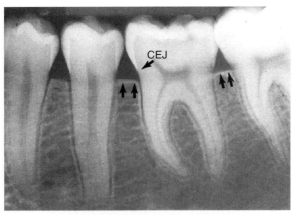

Figure 12-14   Healthy alveolar bone with an intact crestal margin; *CEJ* marks the cementoenamel junction.

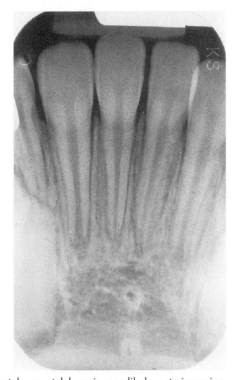

Figure 12-15   Healthy interdental, or septal, bone in mandibular anterior region.

The images reflect only the changes that have occurred in the past, not whether the process is currently active. Periodontitis with associated bone change is a chronic, recurring disease with periods of inactivity and periods of active inflammation.

An early sign of chronic inflammation is "blunting" of the alveolar crests *(a)* in the anterior area (Fig. 12-16). Note that the lamina dura is still present at the crest, which suggests that the blunting occurred in the past and that the inflammation is currently inactive. Calculus deposits (spurs) seen as *b* suggest that local factors are contributing to these bone changes. More severe bone loss and large calculus deposits are also seen in Figure 12-17. Figures 12-16 and 12-17 reveal calculus spurs

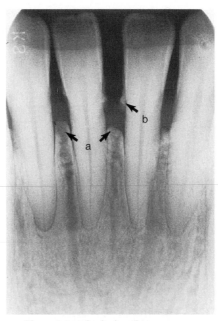

Figure 12-16 Mild blunting of crestal bone *(a)* and calculus *(b)*.

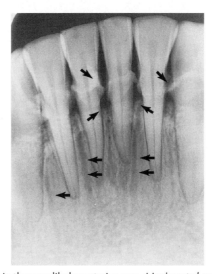

Figure 12-17 Calculus deposits in the mandibular anterior area. *Horizontal arrows* mark vascular channels.

in one of their most common locations: the mandibular central incisor region. Note that the bone loss is horizontal. Also note the multiple vertical radiolucent lines marked with arrows in Figure 12-17. These are vascular channels (passageways for blood vessels), also referred to as nutrient canals. These canals are also seen in Figure 12-16. They are another sign of chronic inflammatory changes associated with periodontal disease. Figure 12-18 shows calculus deposits in the posterior areas, both in the mandible and maxilla, yet there is little bone loss.

Figure 12-19 reveals advanced, localized bone loss in the posterior maxilla. Note that the defect is primarily in the second premolar region. Figures 12-20 and 12-21 show extensive localized bone loss in a 20-year-old patient with a rapidly progressive

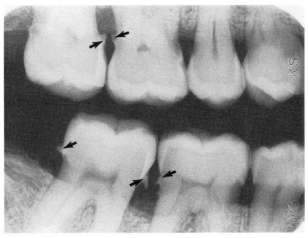

Figure 12-18 Examples of calculus deposits *(arrows)* in the posterior dentition in both the mandible and the maxilla.

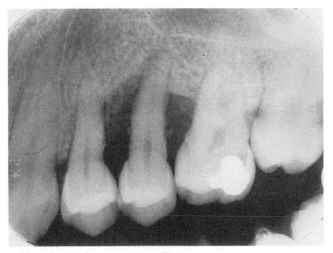

Figure 12-19 Advanced bone loss in the posterior maxilla.

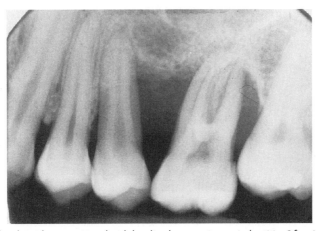

Figure 12-20 Maxillary bone loss associated with localized aggressive periodontitis. Often it is the posterior areas that are affected by this type of periodontitis.

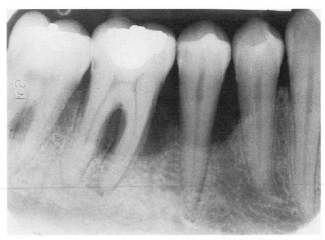

Figure 12-21 Mandibular bone loss associated with localized aggressive periodontitis.

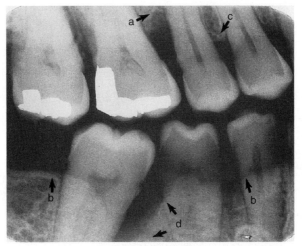

Figure 12-22 Vertical bone defect *(a)*, maxillary alveolar crest at near-normal height *(c)*, alveolar crest *(b)*, and severe vertical defect *(d)*.

type of periodontal disease that occurs in young patients. The patient seen in Figure 12-22 has a more generalized, chronic loss of bone but with localized severe vertical defects.

RADIOGRAPHIC CHANGES RESULTING FROM PERIAPICAL INFECTION

The most common radiographic appearance of a periapical infection is the periapical radiolucency: a dark hole at the apex of a tooth, representing loss of alveolar bone in this localized area. The source of this bone loss may be of pulpal origin or periodontal origin. If a dental pulp dies as a consequence of deep caries or perhaps trauma, inflammation at the apex of the tooth where the pulp tissues communicate with the periodontal ligament space causes a localized loss of bone in this area. In cases of severe periodontal disease, the loss of alveolar bone may reach the apex of the tooth, exposing the pulp tissue to the oral cavity, often resulting in its death.

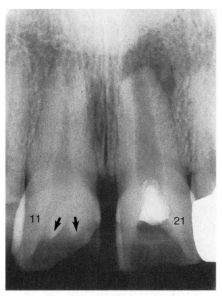

Figure 12-23 Pulp death of tooth no. 9 probably resulted from a carious lesion in the developmental pit on the lingual aspect of the tooth. Note the talons or extra cusps on tooth no. 8 *(arrows)*. Endodontic treatment has been started on no. 9.

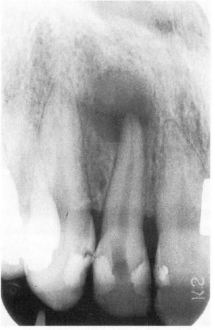

Figure 12-24 Restored carious lesions on several anterior teeth. The pulp death and apical problem could have resulted from either the initial decay or the recurrent decay seen around the restorations.

Figures 12-23 through 12-25 show various radiographic appearances of periapical radiolucency produced by deep carious lesions. Note that two anatomic structures in the jaws can mimic periapical radiolucency: the *incisive foramen* and the *mental foramen*. Care must be taken to carefully examine periapical radiolucency in the area of the maxillary central incisors and mandibular premolars to make sure that normal anatomy is not mistaken for pathology.

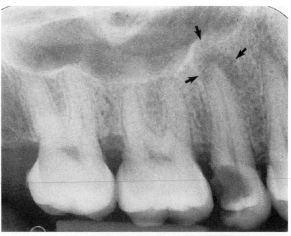

Figure 12-25 Periapical radiolucency *(arrows)* approaching the floor of the maxillary sinus.

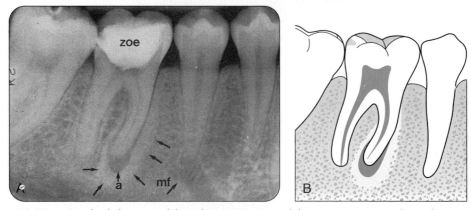

Figure 12-26 **A,** Apical radiolucency and dense bone pattern around these apices suggest a chronic long-standing pulpal inflammation that the patient's defenses tried to wall off. The temporary pulp capping procedure has failed. The structure labeled *mf* is the mental foramen (recall Chapter 3); *a* is the widened periodontal ligament space; *zoe* is the zinc oxide and eugenol base; and *arrows* indicate the proliferation of reactive bone. **B,** Diagram of apical radiolucency with surrounding dense bone.

The mental foramen is labeled *mf* in Figure 12-26, A. The second premolar has neither a carious lesion or periodontal bone loss. Consequently, no reason exists for the radiolucency to be pathologic. If you look carefully, you can see that the periapical radiolucency associated with the second premolar communicates with the inferior alveolar canal. In contrast, the area at the apex of the mesial root of the first molar, labeled *a,* shows a widened periodontal ligament space (the first sign of apical inflammation) and opaque, reactive bone *(arrows)*. Alveolar bone occasionally appears more opaque and dense around an area of inflammation, as if the body were trying to wall off the infection. The molar also has a deep cavity preparation, "temporized" by a sedative material, zinc oxide and eugenol *(zoe)*. Therefore adequate reason exists for the molar to have an inflamed pulp.

Compare the appearance of Figure 12-27 with Figure 12-23. Note that the incisive foramen *a* is centered between the two central incisors; neither tooth has any caries or alveolar bone loss. In Figure 12-23, the apical radiolucency is associated with the apex of the left central incisor and is not centered between the teeth. Again, the left central incisor has a deep cavity preparation (an access opening for root canal treatment), so ample reason exists for the apical change.

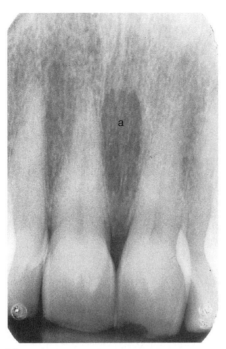

Figure 12-27 Incisive foramen *(a)*.

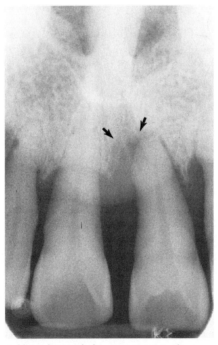

Figure 12-28 Advanced periodontal bone loss with direct extension to the apex of tooth no. 9. *Arrows* indicate the greatest vertical defect.

Periodontal involvement of the apex of a tooth is usually by direct extension of inflammation in cases of advanced periodontal disease with deep bony defects. Figures 12-28 and 12-29 show examples of this type of periapical disease. These defects should be easily recognized on intraoral images.

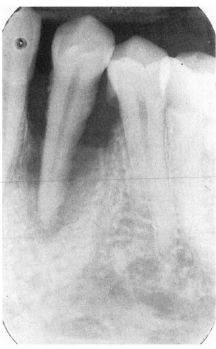

Figure 12-29 Periapical radiolucency of periodontal origin. Note the large deposits of calculus.

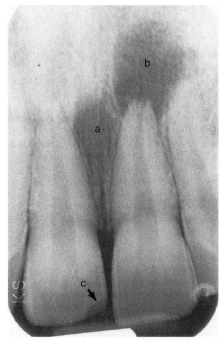

Figure 12-30 Incisive foramen *(a)*, periapical lesion *(b)*, incisal fracture *(c)*.

RADIOGRAPHIC CHANGES RESULTING FROM TRAUMA

The area labeled *c* in Figure 12-30 is an incisal edge fracture. One can assume that some sort of trauma to the anterior maxilla produced this fracture. The left central incisor has a large apical radiolucency marked *b*, suggesting that the pulp tissue

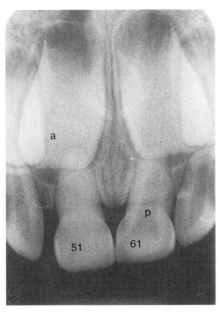

Figure 12-31 The right primary central incisor *(51)* shows no radiographic evidence of a pulp chamber or canal. Compare this with the left primary central incisor *(61)*, which has a pulp chamber *(p)*. The developing right permanent central incisor is marked *a*.

in this tooth has died, leading to local bone destruction in the periapical area. This radiolucency is *not* the incisive foramen because of the following:

1. Its location (apical rather than centered between the teeth)
2. Its size (it is quite large)
3. Its shape (the foramen is often ovoid in shape)
4. The evidence of trauma in the area

Both children and adults often sustain trauma to their teeth. The pulp may degenerate or die, which produces an apical lesion such as the one in Figure 12-30. Another consequence of trauma may be atrophy of the pulp and subsequent calcification of the pulp chamber and canal(s), as seen in the right primary central incisor in Figure 12-31. Despite the fact that the tooth appears to have "done its own root canal treatment," such a tooth must be closely watched by the dentist because an infection may develop at a later date. An apical infection in a primary tooth might compromise the developing permanent tooth, marked *a* in Figure 12-31.

In Figure 12-32, fracture lines *a* and *c* are seen after a blow to the maxillary incisors. A similar line *b* crosses several teeth. This line, however, represents the outline of the soft tissue of the nose and must not be mistaken for evidence of trauma. The outline of the nose is often a smooth, uninterrupted line, whereas a fracture line is often jagged in appearance and may be noncontinuous. Figure 12-33 demonstrates a clearer view of the soft tissue outline of the nose that crosses the roots of several anterior teeth.

Another consequence of trauma to a tooth can be termination of normal apical development. Figure 12-34 shows a central incisor with an open apex and wide pulp chamber and canal. Figure 12-35 shows a similar appearance. However, in Figure 12-34, the lateral incisor's apex is closed and its pulp spaces look normal. In Figure 12-35, all of the incisors' apices are open, which is a normal finding when pulps are still developing in young patients. The central incisor apex in Figure 12-34 failed to fully develop

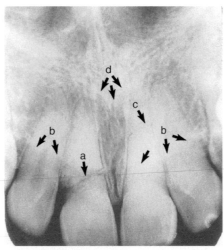

Figure 12-32 Fracture in tooth no. 8 *(a)*, shadow of the nose *(b)*, fracture in root of tooth no. 9 *(c)*, anterior nasal spine *(d)*.

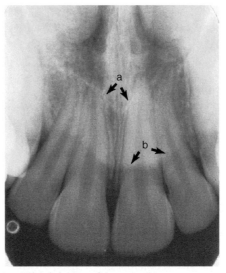

Figure 12-33 Anterior nasal spine *(a)* and shadow of the nose *(b)*.

and close normally because of an injury. Its pulp chamber has remained large, unlike the pulp of the lateral incisor. Therefore comparing the apices and pulp tissues of surrounding teeth will assist the clinician in evaluating the health of those teeth.

Root resorption (erosion or blunting of a root apex) may also be the consequence of trauma. Figure 12-36 shows a short, blunted root on the right central incisor. This may have been the result of earlier trauma, or it is possible that the orthodontic movement (the patient is wearing a retainer) may have caused root resorption. As teeth move through bone during orthodontic treatment, the cells that resorb the bone (osteoclasts) sometimes act on the tooth roots. This is most common if the orthodontic forces are excessive. Figure 12-37 demonstrates severe root resorption in an orthodontic patient.

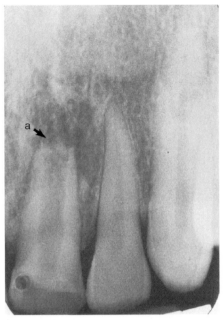

Figure 12-34 Apex of left central incisor *(a)*.

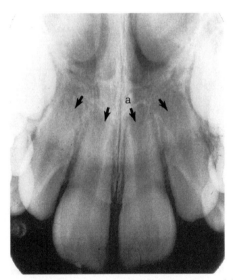

Figure 12-35 Apex of left central incisor *(a)*. Other arrows indicate the apices of the other incisors.

RADIOGRAPHIC FEATURES OF DENTAL ANOMALIES

Considering that 52 tooth buds undergo a complex sequence of maturation and growth in close proximity to each other, it is not surprising that anomalies occasionally occur. Most of these anomalies require no active treatment, although a few exceptions exist: dens in dente may require a prophylactic restoration, and the presence of taurodonts, multiple supernumerary teeth, or multiple congenitally missing teeth may be signs of a systemic syndrome that requires further investigation.

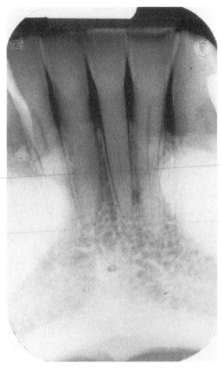

Figure 12-36 Sometimes root resorption is associated with orthodontic tooth movement as seen on the right central incisor in this patient.

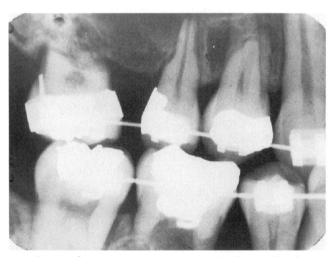

Figure 12-37 This patient has significant root resorption on several teeth. Note that the patient is undergoing orthodontic tooth movement.

Numbers of Teeth

The small toothlike structure labeled *a* in Figure 12-38 is a *mesiodens,* which is a supernumerary (extra) toothlike structure *(dens)* that occurs in the midline area *(mesio).* These anomalies are often smaller than normal teeth and are frequently conical in shape. If you look closely, you can distinguish enamel-like material at its superior surface. The mesiodens also has a radiolucent rim, or border, which appears similar to a normal dental follicle. Figure 12-39 also demonstrates a mesiodens.

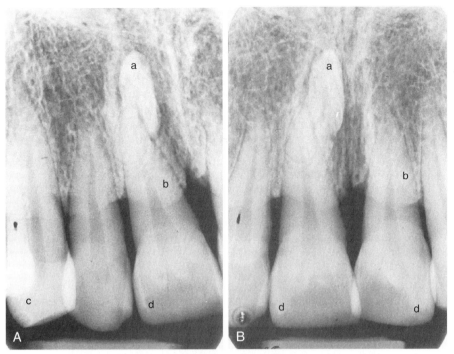

Figure 12-38 Mesiodens *(a)*, alveolar bone level *(b)*, maxillary right canine *(c)*, central incisors *(d)*.

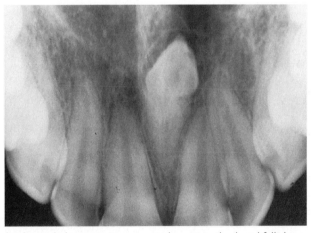

Figure 12-39 Occlusal radiograph demonstrating a mesiodens. Note the dental follicle around the "crown" of the mesiodens.

The mesiodens in Figure 12-38 can be seen in both the lateral incisor image and the central incisor image. This gives us an opportunity to use the buccal object rule (Clark's rule or SLOB rule) discussed in Chapter 10 to help us determine where the mesiodens lies in relation to the normal teeth. As the tubehead is shifted mesially from the lateral incisor view to the central incisor view, the mesiodens also appears to move mesially. Recall that SLOB stands for *same/lingual-opposite/buccal*. Because the mesiodens appears to be moving in the *same* direction that the tubehead shifts, it is located on the *lingual* aspect of the central incisor.

Supernumerary teeth can occur in areas other than the maxillary midline. Other common locations are the lateral incisor area, third molar regions, and the premolar regions. Figure 12-40 shows a supernumerary tooth in the mandibular premolar area, and Figure 12-41 illustrates a "fourth molar" in the right maxilla. It has prevented the eruption of the normal third molar. A supernumerary third molar is sometimes called a *paramolar* or *distodens*. Bilateral supernumerary lateral incisors are seen in Figure 12-42. This is a rare finding, especially because the incisors are well formed and symmetrical. It would be easy to miss them clinically! The condition of having supernumerary teeth is called *hyperdontia*. Just as you would in the clinical examination, you should count the teeth present on images to identify which are present and which are missing.

Just as hyperdontia (too many teeth) is possible, so is *hypodontia* (too few teeth). Usually there is a familial, or genetic, component to these conditions; thus discovery of a condition in one family member should raise suspicion that other family members may be similarly affected. Areas of congenitally missing teeth mirror the areas where extra teeth are often found: lateral incisors, second premolars, and third molars.

Figure 12-43 shows a relatively common finding in mixed dentition. A developing dental follicle beneath the mandibular second primary molar is not evident. Hence, this person will not have a permanent second premolar. In contrast, the patient seen

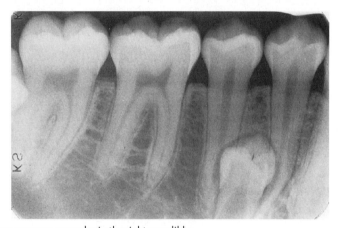

Figure 12-40 Supernumerary premolar in the right mandible.

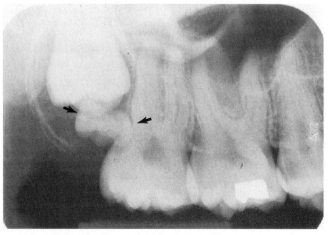

Figure 12-41 Supernumerary third molar *(arrows)* in the right maxilla.

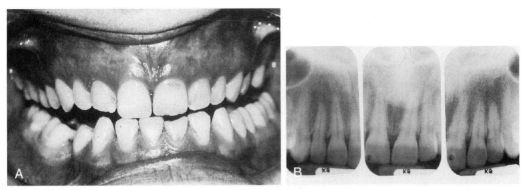

Figure 12-42 Example of bilateral supernumerary lateral incisors. **A,** Clinical photo of patient. **B,** Maxillary anterior periapical radiographs show the extra lateral incisors.

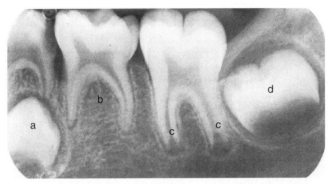

Figure 12-43 Developing first premolar *(a)*, lack of follicle for a second premolar *(b)*, developing apices of permanent first molar *(c)*, and developing permanent second molar *(d)*.

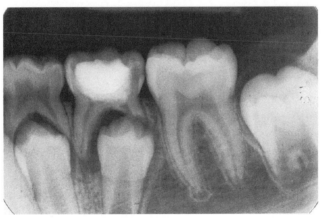

Figure 12-44 Normally developing dentition.

in Figure 12-44 has both developing mandibular premolars. Note the resorption of the distal root of the primary second molar. Succeeding permanent teeth force the primary teeth to exfoliate by resorbing their roots. This is a normal physiologic process.

Sometimes the tooth buds split abnormally as they are developing. A tooth bud that splits only partially produces *gemination,* in which the clinical crown of the tooth is larger than normal and may be split while the root shape remains unchanged. If the tooth bud splits completely, it is called *twinning,* and two separate teeth form.

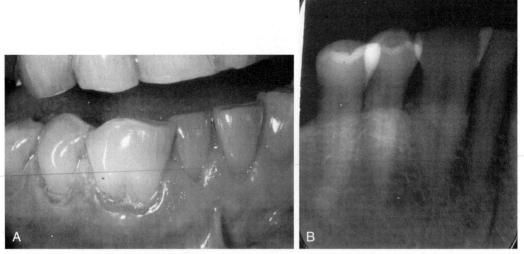

Figure 12-45 **A,** Fusion between a mandibular canine and lateral incisor results in an abnormally large crown. **B,** Radiograph shows the large pulp chamber and canal.

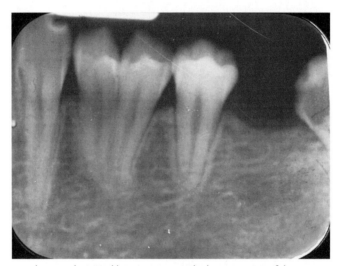

Figure 12-46 Two premolars may be joined by cementum at the lower portion of the roots.

This may have been the cause of the extra lateral incisors in Figure 12-42. The cause of gemination and twinning is unknown.

In contrast, two tooth buds may fuse to form an unusually large tooth. The teeth seen in Figure 12-45 demonstrate *fusion*. Again, the cause for this phenomenon is unknown.

If two teeth are united only by cementum, the outer layer of material on tooth roots, it is called *concrescence*. Concrescence is sometimes considered an incomplete form of fusion. Figure 12-46 shows two teeth that appear to have a cementum union.

Resorption of Structures

By contrast to the normal resorptive process in Figure 12-44, the root resorption seen in Figure 12-47 is not normal. Unerupted teeth may cause external root resorption on adjacent teeth, especially if the unerupted teeth are not in their normal position.

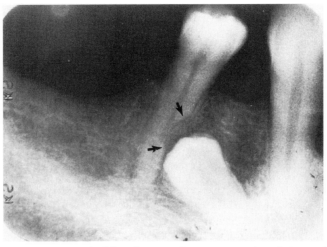

Figure 12-47 Root resorption as a result of force from an adjacent unerupted tooth *(arrows)*.

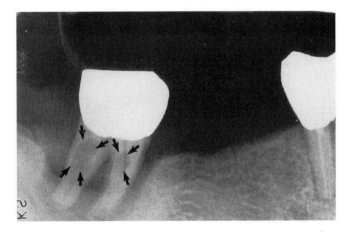

Figure 12-48 Internal resorption of both roots. These roots show isolated enlargement of the pulp canals *(arrows)*.

Resorption originating from the outside of a tooth is called *external resorption*. External root resorption may result in the loss of both teeth.

Figure 12-48 shows a tooth in serious trouble. Evidence of bone loss and inflammation that is periradicular (all around the roots) exists. The tips of the roots show blunting or external resorption from the inflammation. Additionally, the internal aspect of the root canals show localized widening, a sign of *internal resorption*. A tooth with internal resorption may be treated endodontically to remove all the pulp tissue and stop the internal resorption process. However, in this case, too many problems are present to save this tooth. Similarly, the molar seen in Figure 12-49 shows severe resorption, and it is difficult to tell at this point whether the resorption started on the outside and worked its way in or whether it started as internal resorption and perforated the outside of the tooth.

Teeth that have been impacted for many years sometimes become ankylosed (fused to the bone). The follicle around the tooth breaks down and resorbs, and cells called osteoclasts may attack the bone and dental enamel to cause another type of

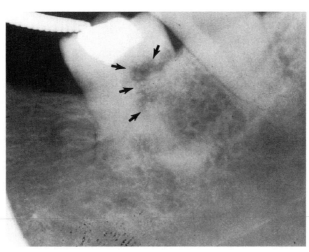

Figure 12-49   Idiopathic external resorption *(arrows)*.

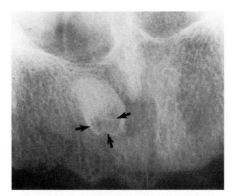

Figure 12-50   External resorption of an impacted tooth *(arrows)* that has become ankylosed.

resorption. This process is seen in Figure 12-50. Note the absence of any follicular space around the remnants of the tooth structure. The reason for such resorption is unknown, or *idiopathic*.

Shapes of Dental Structures

Roots

Teeth that show excessive root curvature or angulation demonstrate *dilaceration*. Root dilacerations make extraction of teeth and root canal treatment difficult. Trauma has been proposed to be the cause of dilacerations, but it is unlikely to be the cause in all cases. Other theories include lack of space in the dental arch or obstruction during eruption of the developing tooth. Figures 12-51 and 12-52 show teeth with unusual root curvatures.

Multiple and Bifurcated Roots

Canines, premolars, and molars can sometimes have more roots than normal and, consequently, more pulp canals. The molar in Figure 12-53 has at least three roots. The arrows point to a periodontal ligament space that appears to be within the mesial root; this suggests that the mesial root may also be divided.

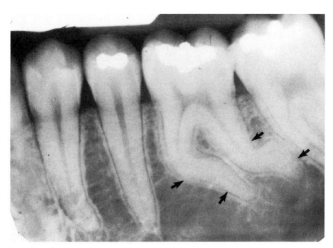

Figure 12-51 Dilacerated molar roots (arrows).

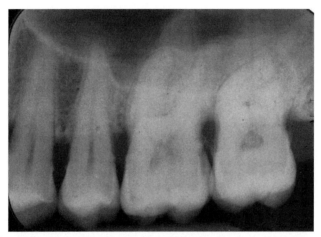

Figure 12-52 The distal dilaceration of the buccal roots of the second molar would make extraction or root canal treatment very difficult. Note that the palatal root is straight.

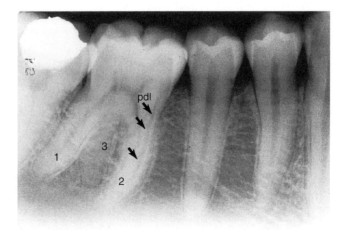

Figure 12-53 Multiple roots on the molar (*1*, *2*, and *3*). The arrows point to a periodontal ligament space *(pdl)* that appears to be within the mesial. This suggests that the mesial root may be divided or have a large concavity (indentation).

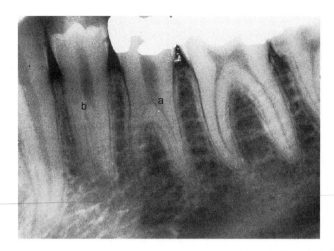

Figure 12-54 Bifurcated root canals *(a)*. Note how the pulp chamber in the first premolar *(b)* seems to stop halfway down the root. This is a sign of a split in the root canal.

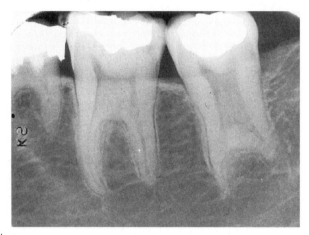

Figure 12-55 Taurodonts.

If the pulp chamber in a tooth appears to end abruptly part way down the root (Fig. 12-54), the canal is likely to be *bifurcated*, or split in two. The bifurcation may indicate that another root is present or, sometimes, that the canal splits within a single root. This is highly significant if the tooth requires endodontic treatment. The second premolar seen in Figure 12-7 earlier in this chapter also demonstrates this phenomenon.

Taurodontism

Sometimes a tooth will have an elongated, large pulp chamber and very short roots (Fig. 12-55), a condition referred to as *taurodontism* (*tauro* means *bull;* the roots resemble bull horns). Taurodonts can occur in either the primary or permanent dentition (Fig. 12-56). The exact cause is unknown but appears to be linked to a malfunction of a portion of the dental epithelium during development. Taurodontism can occur as an isolated finding of no consequence, or it may be a sign of a syndrome such as ectodermal dysplasia or Down syndrome. Occasionally, a syndrome has been initially diagnosed in a patient because of a dentist's recognition of taurodontism.

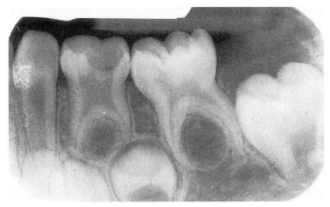

Figure 12-56 Taurodontism in the primary molar.

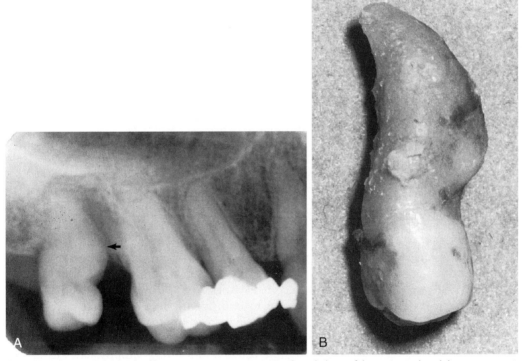

Figure 12-57 **A,** Radiograph of hypercementosis *(arrow)*. **B,** Clinical photo of the same tooth with hypercementosis. *(Courtesy of Dr. John Lovas, Dalhousie University, Halifax, Nova Scotia, Canada.)*

Hypercementosis

An overproduction of cementum is called *hypercementosis* and is frequently seen as an alteration in root shape. Most commonly, inflammation is the cause of this reaction; however, a tooth with an opposing "partner" with which to occlude may show hypercementosis. Hypercementosis may also be seen in patients with Paget's disease of bone. Figure 12-57, A, shows an image of a tooth with hypercementosis caused by inflammation from periodontal disease. Figure 12-57, B shows the

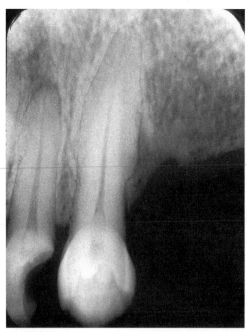

Figure 12-58 Hypercementosis. Note that the periodontal ligament space is seen around the outer surface of the extra cementum.

extracted tooth. Figure 12-58 demonstrates another example of hypercementosis where the difference in the density between the cementum and dentin can be seen.

Shape of Dental Structures in the Area of the Pulp Chamber

Dens in Dente

Dens in dente is a "tooth within a tooth." The term *dens invaginatus* is more appropriate, but dens in dente remains a commonly used descriptor. This anomaly is characterized by an invagination of the outer covering of a tooth into the normal dental structure. An enamel layer can be seen extending into the area of the pulp chamber, most often on a maxillary lateral incisor where a lingual pit is normally present (Figs. 12-59 and 12-60). The depth of the invagination ranges from a barely perceptible pit to a direct pulp exposure. The cause is unknown. Prophylactic restoration of the lingual pit is recommended because the enamel covering is usually very thin, and the tooth is predisposed to develop caries in this area.

Enamel Pearl

The enamel pearl is a circular mass of calcified material attached to the external surface of a tooth, most often in the area just apical to the pulp chamber where roots are bifurcating. It is thought to arise from Hertwig's epithelial root sheath before it loses its enamel-forming potential. Figure 12-61 shows enamel pearls on both the first and second maxillary molars.

It is easy to misinterpret the overlapping of root structures in molars for enamel pearls. The apparent circular opacity between the roots of the molar in Figure 12-62, A, "miraculously" disappears in the bitewing view of the same patient (Fig. 12-62, B).

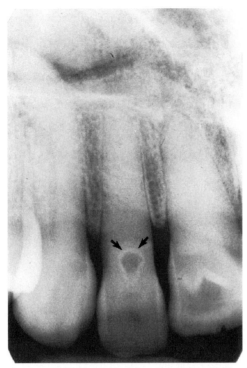

Figure 12-59 Dens in dente. The inverted teardrop-shaped pit *(arrows)* is lined with thin enamel, which can easily become decayed.

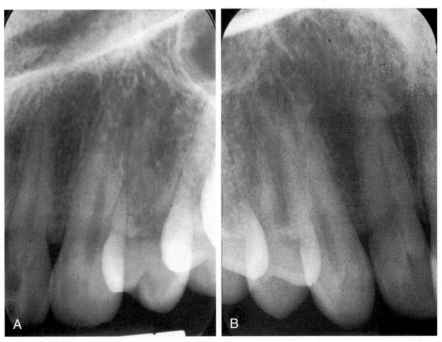

Figure 12-60 Dens in dente in the lateral incisors.

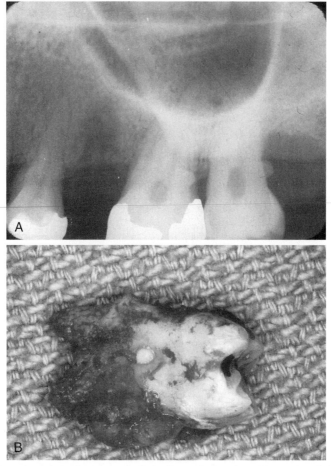

Figure 12-61 **A,** Enamel pearls can be seen on both the first and second maxillary molars; it is much more obvious on the second molar. **B,** Clinical photo of an enamel pearl.

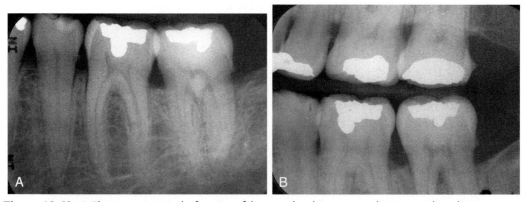

Figure 12-62 **A,** The opaque area in the furcation of the second molar appears to be an enamel pearl. However, this is due to overlapping of the mesial and distal roots. Note that the interproximal contact is also overlapped. **B,** Bitewing radiograph of the same patient. Note that the overlapping in the furcation of the molar and overlapped mandibular interproximal contacts have disappeared with a change in horizontal angulation.

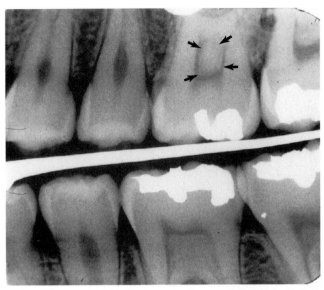

Figure 12-63 Dystrophic pulpal calcification *(arrows)*. Note the more diffuse pulpal calcification in the mandibular first molar.

Note that the horizontal angulation is different in each view: overlapping of the interproximal contacts is seen on the periapical view but not on the bitewing. This overlapping also occurs in the furcation area of the molar in the periapical view. The horizontal angulation is such that the mesial root overlaps on the distal root near the furcation, creating the false enamel pearl.

Pulp Stones

Dystrophic pulpal calcifications are sometimes referred to as *pulp stones.* They may appear as distinct opacifications as seen in the maxillary first molar in Figure 12-63, or they may be more diffuse as seen in the mandibular first molar in the same image. This phenomenon occurs primarily in molar teeth, but many other teeth in the dentition can show calcifications in pulp chambers and canals. It is of no consequence to the patient unless root canal treatment is needed. Such calcifications may interfere with endodontic therapies.

Common Radiopacities in the Jaws

Impacted Teeth

Unerupted teeth are commonly seen in the alveolar bone of the jaws. Teeth that are fully developed, including the roots, but that have not erupted are considered to be impacted. Teeth that are commonly impacted are maxillary canines (Fig. 12-64) and third molars (Figs. 12-65 and 12-66).

Remnants of Teeth

Root tips are occasionally left behind after an extraction. They are easy to identify on images because they look like roots! They are conical and found in former tooth locations (Fig. 12-67). These fragments do not need to be removed unless they become problematic. They should, however, be examined periodically for any changes.

Sometimes root fragments of mandibular primary molars are left behind in the alveolar bone. The succeeding permanent premolar may not resorb all of the

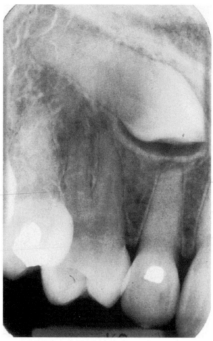

Figure 12-64 Maxillary right permanent canine impaction.

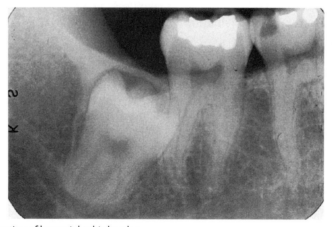

Figure 12-65 Impaction of lower right third molar.

divergent root tips. Thin, vertical opacities seen in the mandibular premolar area are often remnants of the primary molars or "tracks" of where these roots used to be (Fig. 12-68).

Exostoses

An *exostosis* is a dense outgrowth of normal bone. These are commonly seen in the oral cavity as a *palatal torus* or a *mandibular torus* (Fig. 12-69). Often the lingual mandibular projections occur bilaterally and are referred to as mandibular *tori* (*tori* is the plural form of *torus*). These bony projections are seen as diffuse radiopacity in the midroot area of the mandibular lateral incisors, canines, and/or premolars,

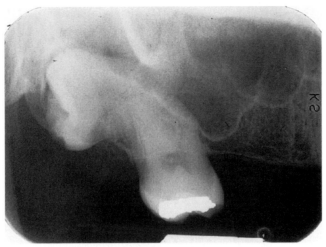

Figure 12-66 Horizontal impaction of maxillary right third molar.

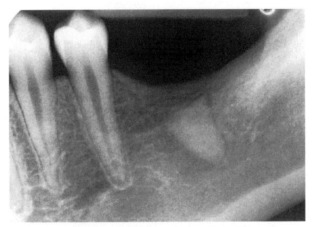

Figure 12-67 Retained root tip, probably from the permanent mandibular first molar.

depending on how large the torus is (Figs. 12-70 and 12-71). Large tori, whether palatal or mandibular, can make image-receptor placement a challenge.

Condensing Osteitis

Condensing osteitis is a term widely used to describe a denser (more opaque) area of bone surrounding a periapical radiolucency of pulpal origin (Fig. 12-72). It is considered to be a proliferative bony response to chronic inflammation. It is most commonly seen in young adults. It itself is not a condition that requires treatment, but the offending tooth invariably needs treatment in the form of endodontic therapy or possibly extraction.

Osteosclerosis (Sclerotic Bone or Dense Bone Island)

There is a great deal of similarity between osteosclerosis and condensing osteitis. In fact, the terms are often used interchangeably. The dense area of bone may have been a response to trauma or some other insult, or it may occur for no apparent

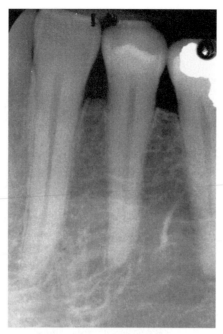

Figure 12-68 Vertical opacity between the premolars representing the area where the primary molar root was resorbed.

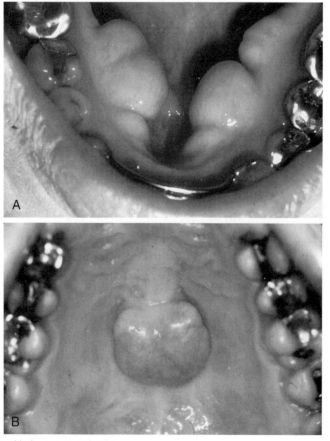

Figure 12-69 A, Mandibular tori. **B,** Palatal torus.

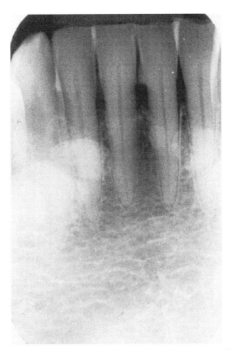

Figure 12-70 Mandibular tori appear as rounded opacities in the midroot area of the anterior teeth.

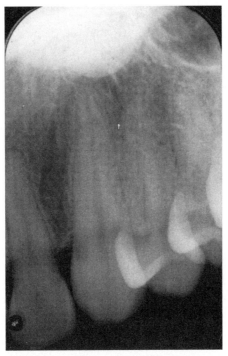

Figure 12-71 The rounded opacity at the top of this image is a palatal torus.

reason at all (idiopathic osteosclerosis). It is seen most often in the mandible, from the canine to the molar area (Figs. 12-73 and 12-74). The lesion will appear to blend in with the trabecular bone pattern and will not be separated from the surrounding bone by a radiolucent rim.

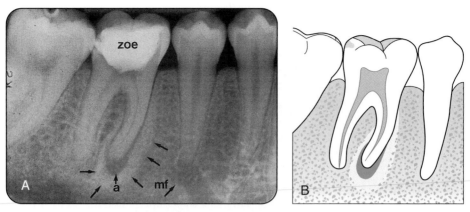

Figure 12-72 **A,** The proliferation of dense bone around the root *(arrows)* and apical radiolucency *(a)* suggests a chronic, long-standing pulpal inflammation that the host's defenses tried to wall off. A temporary restoration is marked *zoe; mf* indicates the mental foramen. **B,** Diagram of apical radiolucency with surrounding dense bone.

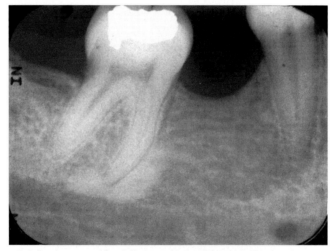

Figure 12-73 This well-defined opacity around the mesial root of the molar has no obvious cause and can be considered idiopathic osteosclerosis.

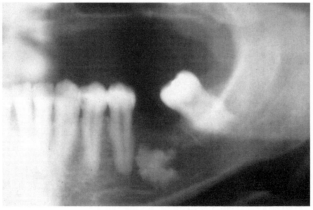

Figure 12-74 This irregularly shaped opacity distal to the premolar is most likely idiopathic osteosclerosis, also known as a dense bone island or sclerotic bone.

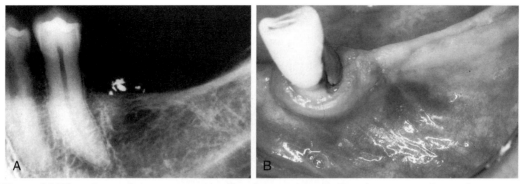

Figure 12-75 **A,** Opaque fragments suggestive of amalgam particles. **B,** Clinical appearance of an amalgam tattoo.

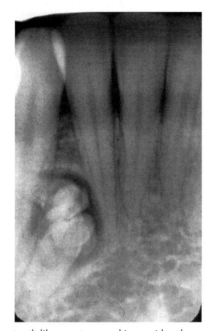

Figure 12-76 This lesion contains tooth-like structures and is considered a compound odontoma.

Foreign Objects

If a foreign material that has a high density is found in the jaws, it will appear as a radiopacity. The most common foreign material seen is amalgam. Sometimes during an extraction, a portion of an amalgam restoration will chip off and be left behind in the extraction site. These remnants of amalgam, if large enough, will be seen on images (Fig. 12-75). Sometimes the amalgam fragments are embedded close to the overlying gingiva and occasionally leave a bluish mark on the gums. When this is seen clinically, it is referred to as an "amalgam tattoo."

Odontomas

An odontoma is a common odontogenic tumor. *Compound odontomas* look similar to small teeth (Fig. 12-76), whereas *complex odontomas* are less organized and appear more like a jumbled mass of enamel and/or dentin (Fig. 12-77). The opacities have a radiolucent rim around them, similar to a dental follicle. These abnormalities are usually found in young patients in either jaw, most often in the anterior portion.

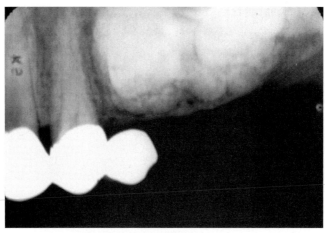

Figure 12-77 A complex odontoma. Note the radiolucent rim around the opaque mass.

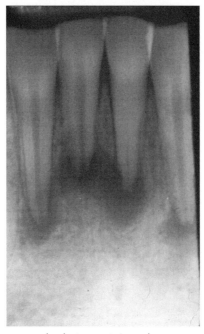

Figure 12-78 Periapical cemento-osseous dysplasia seen in its early stage as multiple radiolucencies at the apices of the mandibular incisors. The teeth remain vital.

These lesions are usually surgically removed because it is possible that a cyst or tumor could occur in the follicle that surrounds the hard tissues.

Periapical Cemento-Osseous Dysplasia

This is a relatively commonly occurring lesion that starts out as a periapical radiolucency, but as the lesion matures, it acquires a radiopaque component (Figs. 12-78 and 12-79). This opaque content resembles bone and cementum when examined under a microscope. It is an asymptomatic lesion (causes no symptoms), and blacks and women in their fourth and fifth decades are predisposed to it. The

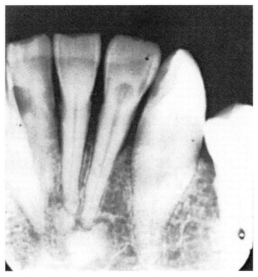

Figure 12-79 Periapical cemento-osseous dysplasia, mature form (more opaque).

lesions frequently occur in groups rather than as a single lesion, and they are most often seen in the anterior of the mandible. Even though these lesions resemble periapical inflammation associated with a dead pulp, especially when the lesions are in their radiolucent stage, the teeth in this condition remain vital. Periapical cemento-osseous dysplasia requires no treatment, so careful clinical examination that includes pulp testing is key to a correct diagnosis.

Common Radiolucencies in the Jaws

Periapical Periodontitis

The fact that deep caries or trauma might cause pulp death has been discussed previously. The end result of that pulp death is an inflammatory reaction in the bone at the apex of the affected tooth (see Fig. 12-30). The actual lesion at the root apex might be one of three conditions: an abscess, a granuloma, or a cyst. An *abscess* is a circumscribed area of pus (dead white blood cells) and is the result of the dental infection. A *granuloma* is accumulation of inflammatory cells but does not contain actual pus. A *cyst* is a fluid-filled cavity, lined by epithelium. The fluid is not pus. Any of these three conditions may be the result of pulp death, and all three appear similar on a radiographic image. It is impossible to tell which is which just from the image alone (Fig. 12-80). So that all three conditions do not have to be listed as a possible diagnosis, the term *periapical periodontitis* is used to describe the radiolucency at the apex. It certainly is periapical, and *periodontitis* refers to the fact that it is an inflammatory condition *(-itis)* stemming from the periodontal ligament space. Any nonvital tooth with such a lesion requires treatment.

Incisive Canal Cyst (Nasopalatine Duct Cyst)

Remember that a cyst is a fluid-filled cavity, lined by epithelium. The *incisive canal cyst* (nasopalatine duct cyst) is a developmental cyst arising from the epithelium of nasal ducts as the nose and palate were developing. The anterior portion of the palate may be slightly swollen in the area of the incisive papilla, or the patient may

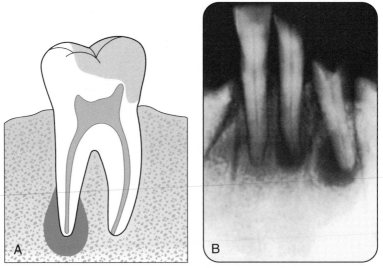

Figure 12-80 A, Periapical periodontitis appears as an apical radiolucency. The lesion could be an abscess, granuloma, or cyst. It arises after the death of the pulp. Waste products from the necrotic pulp escape through the apex into the alveolar bone. **B,** Well-defined radiolucent areas secondary to severe dental caries. Both lesions could be termed *periapical periodontitis.*

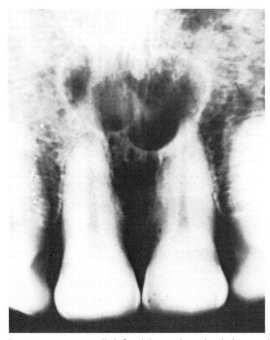

Figure 12-81 Incisive canal cyst appears as a well-defined, heart-shaped radiolucency between the maxillary central incisors. Note the corticated (opaque) border around the lesion.

have no symptoms at all. The lesion is seen as an ovoid, circular, or heart-shaped radiolucency between the maxillary central incisors (Figs. 12-81 and 12-82). The radiolucency will have distinct radiopaque borders. The teeth will remain vital. Treatment of the lesion is surgical removal.

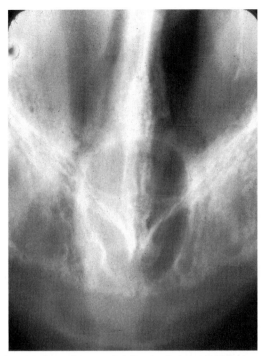

Figure 12-82 Incisive canal cyst seen as a large, well-defined radiolucency with opaque borders in the anterior midline of an edentulous patient.

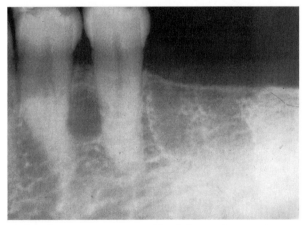

Figure 12-83 Lateral periodontal cyst appears as an ovoid radiolucency between the roots of the premolars. Both teeth remain vital.

Lateral Periodontal Cyst

This cyst arises from remnants of the dental lamina as teeth develop. It is seen as a round or ovoid radiolucency with radiopaque borders and usually occurs in the mandibular canine-premolar area (Fig. 12-83). The cysts tend to be no more than about a centimeter in diameter, and the teeth remain vital. Treatment is surgical removal.

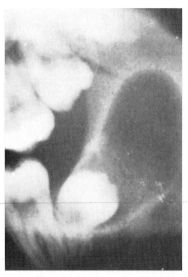

Figure 12-84 Dentigerous cyst seen as a large radiolucency around the crown of an unerupted third molar. Note that the lesion is well-defined and has an opaque (corticated) border.

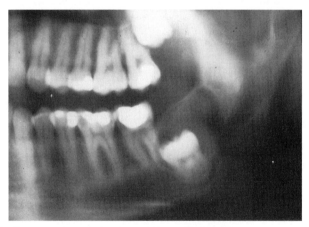

Figure 12-85 Large dentigerous cyst around an impacted mandibular molar.

Dentigerous Cyst (Follicular Cyst)

A dentigerous or follicular cyst develops from the reduced enamel epithelium of the follicle surrounding an unerupted (often impacted) tooth. The cyst is seen on an image as a radiolucency with radiopaque borders surrounding the crown of the impacted tooth (Figs. 12-84 and 12-85). Although the cysts are often asymptomatic, they can become quite large and locally destructive. In addition, they may give rise to more serious lesions such as an odontogenic keratocyst, ameloblastoma, or even carcinoma. Therefore, treatment is surgical removal.

Submandibular Salivary Gland Defect (Stafne Cyst)

The mandible normally indents or is thinner below the ridge where the mylohyoid muscle attaches. This is referred to as the submandibular fossa because the submandibular salivary gland lies there. Sometimes the mandible will have an

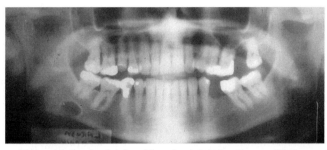

Figure 12-86 Submandibular salivary gland defect. Note that it is below the mandibular canal and has a thick cortical outline.

extradeep indentation, like a little pouch or pocket in this area, and sometimes a small lobe of the submandibular salivary gland extends into the indentation. This is referred to as a submandibular salivary gland defect, even though nothing is really defective about it; it is a developmental anomaly. An older term for it is a *Stafne cyst*, which is a misnomer because it is not a cyst at all. On a radiographic image, this indentation will be radiolucent and have a thick radiopaque outline (Fig. 12-86). This appearance is different from the cysts and apical lesions described previously in this chapter because it will always be *below* the level of the inferior alveolar canal in the posterior part of the mandible. No treatment is required.

RADIOGRAPHIC SIGNS OF DISEASE

Multilocular Radiolucency

A radiolucency that has several different compartments or locules is referred to as *multilocular* (Fig. 12-87, A). You can think of it as multiple soap bubbles sticking together. Often a lesion must be quite large to be multilocular (Fig. 12-87, B). Lesions that appear multilocular include cysts of odontogenic origin, odontogenic tumors, and vascular lesions. Here is a partial list of such lesions:
- Odontogenic keratocyst
- Ameloblastoma
- Odontogenic myxoma
- Central giant cell granuloma
- Aneurysmal bone cyst
- Central hemangioma

Mixed Radiolucent–Radiopaque Lesions

Many times lesions in the jaws will contain some sort of radiopaque product. They are often radiolucent lesions with scattered opacities within the lesions (Figs. 12-88). The product may represent toothlike (cementum) or bonelike (osseous) material. This may be reflected in the name of the lesion. Some lesions contain a lot of opacification, and some contain only little bits. These lesions can be odontogenic cysts or tumors, or they may represent lesions referred to as fibro-osseous lesions. Examples of these types of lesions include
- Florid osseous dysplasia
- Cemento-osseous fibroma
- Benign cementoblastoma
- Calcifying odontogenic cyst

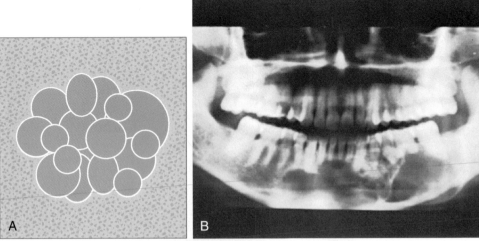

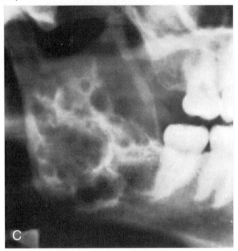

Multilocular (soap bubble)

Figure 12-87 **A,** Schematic diagram of a multilocular lesion. **B,** Large, expansile, multilocular lesion in the anterior mandible. It has a cortical outline and has displaced teeth and resorbed roots. Because it has crossed the midline, a central giant cell granuloma should be considered in the differential diagnosis. **C,** A multilocular lesion in the right ramus of the mandible.

- Calcifying epithelial odontogenic tumor
- Adenomatoid odontogenic tumor
- Ameloblastic fibro-odontoma

Ill-Defined Lesions

Most of the lesions discussed so far have been distinct lesions; that is, it is easy to identify the borders of the lesions. Lesions are *ill-defined* if it is difficult to determine exactly where they start and stop. This appearance is often caused by one of two conditions: inflammation or malignancy. In inflammatory conditions such as osteomyelitis (*osteo* meaning bone; *myel* meaning marrow; *itis* meaning inflammation), the bone may take on the appearance of interspersed areas of radiolucency and radiopacity (Fig 12-89) or it may appear chewed on or eroded. Various

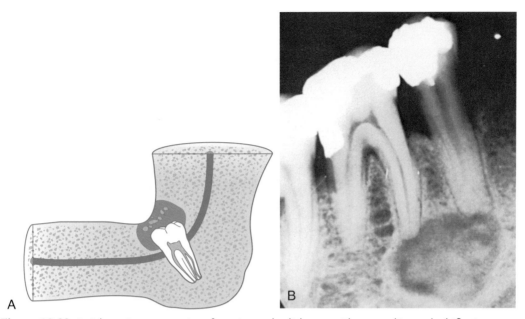

Figure 12-88 **A,** Schematic representation of a pericoronal radiolucency with scattered internal calcifications. **B,** Mixed radiolucent–radiopaque lesion at the apices of the premolar and molar. This lesion was a cemento-ossifying fibroma.

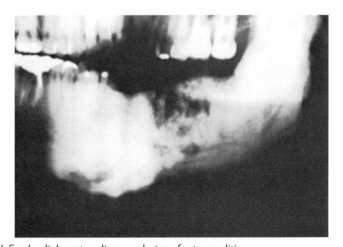

Figure 12-89 Ill-defined radiolucent–radiopaque lesion of osteomyelitis.

malignancies of the jaws also demonstrate a chewed-on or moth-eaten appearance (Fig. 12-90). In some instances, enough bone is lost such that a tooth appears to float in the air (Fig. 12-91). Additionally, some neoplastic lesions such as an osteosarcoma or vascular lesions such as a hemangioma produce a "sun ray" appearance in which bony spicules radiate from the lesion (Fig. 12-92). In any event, lesions that are ill-defined are decidedly in need of proper diagnosis and treatment (Box 12-1).

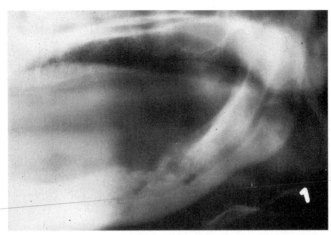

Figure 12-90 This cupped-out, ill-defined radiolucency is characteristic of osteomyelitis or invasive squamous cell carcinoma.

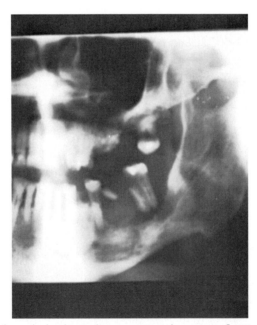

Figure 12-91 The mandibular molar has lost its bony support and appears to float in space. The bone was destroyed by a squamous cell carcinoma.

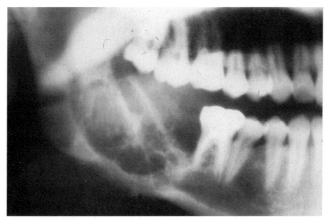

Figure 12-92 This large, expansile, multicompartmented lesion shows evidence of radiating spokes or a "sun ray" appearance. This suggests that a vascular lesion such as a central hemangioma should be considered in the differential diagnosis, as should osteosarcoma.

Box **12-1** Ill-Defined Lesions

Ill-Defined

- Chronic osteomyelitis
- Osteoradionecrosis
- Osteosarcoma/chondrosarcoma
- Squamous cell carcinoma
- Metastatic tumors

"Floating Tooth"

- Langerhans cell granuloma
- Osteosarcoma/fibrosarcoma
- Lymphoma

"Sun Ray"

- Osteosarcoma/chondrosarcoma
- Hemangioma

STUDY QUESTIONS

1. Which of the following viewing strategies maximizes your ability to detect and interpret abnormal conditions?
   A. Continuous eye movement
   B. Standardized sequence for viewing multiple images
   C. Quiet surroundings free of distractions
   D. All of the above

2. All of these characteristics would signal that an abnormal condition is present except one. Which one is the exception?
   A. Symmetry of anatomic structures
   B. Breaks in continuity
   C. Changes in size
   D. Changes in shape

3. A carious lesion on a proximal surface of a tooth often appears as a(n)
   A. Radiopaque extension or spur
   B. Radiolucent line all along the outer edge of the enamel
   C. Triangular or wedge-shaped radiolucency in the enamel
   D. Indistinct radiolucency between the CEJ and the alveolar crest

4. Interproximal caries is most often seen in which of the following locations?
   A. Slightly coronal to the pulp chamber
   B. At or slightly apical to the contact point
   C. At or slightly coronal to the contact point
   D. Slightly apical to the central occlusal pit

5. In which of the following ways does root caries differ from interproximal caries?
   A. Location on the tooth
   B. The shape of the lesion
   C. Rapidity of progression
   D. All of the above

6. Which of the following is an early sign of bone loss associated with periodontal disease?
   A. Blunting of the alveolar crests
   B. Presence of periapical radiolucencies
   C. Presence of calculus spurs
   D. All of the above

7. Which of the following anatomic structures might be confused with a periapical radio-lucency?
   A. Genial tubercles
   B. Zygomatic process
   C. Mental foramen
   D. Maxillary sinus

8. Which of the following is frequently seen as a rounded opacity over the midroot area of mandibular teeth?
   A. Mandibular torus
   B. Lateral periodontal cyst
   C. Mental foramen
   D. Odontoma

9. Which of the following is most likely to be seen in a pericoronal (around the crown of a tooth) location?
   A. Palatal torus
   B. Dentigerous cyst
   C. Periapical abscess
   D. Incisive canal cyst

10. The term *multilocular* can be described by which of the following phrases?
    A. The rays of the sun
    B. A piece of cotton
    C. A group of soap bubbles
    D. Like a bull's head

Glossary of Radiologic Terms*

Absorb To take into the skin or body tissue.

Absorbed Dose The amount of energy imparted by ionizing radiation to a unit mass of irradiated material at a place of interest. The unit of absorbed dose in the traditional system is the *rad* (100 ergs/g). The currently accepted unit of absorbed dose is the *gray* (Gy). (1 Gy = 1 joule/kg). *See also* Dose (Dosage of Radiation).

Absorption A process whereby the intensity of a beam of radiation is reduced because some (or all) of the particles (or photons) or the incident beam are eliminated or reduced in energy by interactions with matter.

Accelerator, Developer *See* Developer.

Acid A solution containing more hydrogen ions than water. Its pH is less than 7. The hydrogen ions can be replaced by a base to form salts.

Actual Focal Spot The area of the target (tungsten) that is always larger than the effective focal size. It is the area of the anode on which the electrons strike. *See also* Effective Focal Spot.

Acute Exposure Radiation exposure of short duration; usually refers to radiation of relatively high intensity.

ALARA As Low As Reasonably Achievable; a concept emphasizing that exposure to radiation must be kept to a minimum.

Alpha Particle Positively charged particulate radiation containing two protons and two neutrons emitted from the nucleus of a heavy metal.

Aluminum Filter Any of various thicknesses of aluminum used as filtration in an x-ray beam to absorb the longer-wavelength, less-penetrating radiation.

Alveolar Bone Bone that surrounds and supports the roots of the teeth.

Alveolar Crest The most coronal portion of alveolar bone.

Ammonium Thiosulfate *See* Fixer.

Ampere (A) The unit of intensity of an electrical current produced by 1 volt acting through a resistance of 1 ohm.

Anatomic Landmark An anatomic structure that serves as an aid in the localization and identification of regions to be radiographed.

Angulation The direction of the primary beam of radiation in relation to object and film. There is a horizontal and vertical angulation to the beam.

Anion An ion carrying a negative charge.

Anode The positive terminal of an x-ray tube; a tungsten block embedded in a copper stem and set at an angle to the cathode *(q.v.)*. The anode emits x rays from the point of impact of the electron stream from the cathode. A *rotating anode* is one that rotates constantly during x-ray production to present a changing focal spot to the electron stream and to permit use of smaller focal spots or higher tube voltages or currents without overheating.

Anteroposterior Projection (AP) An examination in which the film is placed at the posterior location (for example, the back of the head), with the x rays passing from the anterior to the posterior direction.

Artifact Either (1) a substance or structure not naturally present in living tissues but that produces an authentic image in a radiograph or (2) a blemish or unintended radiographic image resulting from faulty manufacture, manipulation, exposure, or processing of an x-ray film.

Adapted from Schiff T, Nummikoski P: Glossary of maxillofacial radiology, *ed 3, Jackson, Miss., 1990, American Academy of Oral and Maxillofacial Radiology.*

Atom The smallest part of an element that is capable of entering into a chemical reaction. It consists of a positively charged nucleus and an extranuclear portion composed of electrons equal in number to the nuclear protons.

Atomic Number The number of electrons outside the nucleus of a neutral atom. It is also the number of protons in the nucleus.

Background Density The density of a processed film due to factors other than the radiation exposure received through the recorded objects or structures. *See also* Density (Photographic or Film).

Background (Radiation) Background implies radioactivity arising from nature. This includes cosmic rays *(q.v.)* and radioactive elements in the earth and air.

Backscatter Radiation deflected by scattering processes at angles greater than 90° to the original direction of the beam of radiation. *See also* Scattered Radiation.

Barrier, Infection Control Protective material that is impervious to fluids (plastic) placed on surfaces that could potentially be contaminated with body fluids such as saliva.

Barrier, Protective A barrier of radiation-absorbing material, such as lead, concrete, or plaster, used to reduce radiation hazards. *See also* Primary Protective Barrier, Secondary Protective Barrier.

Base A solution containing fewer hydrogen ions than water. Its pH is greater than 7. Bases can react with acids to form salts.

Beam An emission of electromagnetic radiation or particles. A *central beam* is the center of the beam of x rays emitted from an x-ray tube, usually called the *central ray*. A *useful beam* is the part of the primary radiation that is permitted to emerge from the tubehead assembly of an x-ray machine, as limited by the tubehead port and accessory collimating devices.

Beam-Guiding Instrument Instrument used during radiography to facilitate correct alignment of the central ray. *See also* Position-Indicating Device (PID).

Beta Particle Electron emitted from the nucleus of a radioactive atom.

Binding Energy The energy needed to eject an electron from the atom.

Bisecting-Angle Technique A technique for the radiographic exposure of intraoral films whereby the central axis or central ray of the x-ray beam is directed at right angles to a plane determined by bisecting the angle formed by (1) the long axis of the tooth or teeth being radiographed and (2) the plane in which the film is positioned behind the teeth.

Bite-Pin A positioner used in panoramic imaging on which the patient bites to assist in correct patient positioning within the image layer.

Bite Block An intraoral image-receptor holder on which the patient bites to provide stable retention of the image receptor.

Bitewing Radiograph The x-ray shadow images of the crowns, necks, and coronal third of the roots of both upper and lower teeth, so called because the patient bites on a cardboard tab, or wing, placed in the center of the film packet. A special type of intraoral radiograph for depicting interproximal features of the teeth and interdental bone crests, made on a film positioned by special (bitewing) tabs on which the patient's teeth are closed. *See also* Interproximal Radiograph.

Block In intraoral radiography, a block is a film holder that the patient bites on to provide stable retention of the film packet or orientation of tooth position. In panoramic radiography, a block is a tooth positioner that provides correct orientation of the dentition within the image layer.

"Boiling Off" Electrons Heat or incandescence of the filament of the x-ray tube, which produces a source of free electrons by thermionic emission.

Bound Electron An electron that is close to the nucleus: for example, the K shell electron.

Bremsstrahlung Radiation A spectral distribution of x rays ranging from very low-energy photons to those produced by the peak kilovoltage applied across an x-ray tube.

Bremsstrahlung means *braking radiation,* referring to the sudden deceleration of electrons as they interact with highly positively charged nuclei.

Buccal The surface of a tooth that rests against the buccal mucosa (lining of the cheek).

Buccal Object Rule A method for determining the buccal/lingual relationship of an object using two images taken at different angles.

Calcium Tungstate A chemical substance in crystal form used to coat radiographic intensifying screens; the screens fluoresce when struck by x rays.

Carcinogen A substance having the ability to produce cancer.

Caries Dental decay.

Cassette A light-tight container in which x-ray films are placed for exposure to x radiation; usually backed with lead to reduce the effect of backscattered radiation *(q.v.)*. A *screen-type cassette* is a film holder, usually made of metal, with the exposure side made of a low-atomic-number material such as Bakelite, aluminum, or magnesium; the cassette contains intensifying screens between which a screen-type film is placed for exposure.

Cathode A negative electrode from which electrons are emitted. In x-ray tubes, the cathode usually consists of a helical tungsten filament behind which a molybdenum reflector cup is located to focus the electron emission toward the target of the anode.

Cathode Ray A stream of electrons passing from the hot filament of the cathode to the target, or anode, in an x-ray tube.

Cathode Ray Tube A tube cathode containing a spirally wound filament that becomes incandescent, producing electrons when a low-voltage electrical current is passed through it.

Cation A positively charged ion.

Cell A minute protoplasmic mass that, in the aggregate, makes up organized tissue. The cell consists of a circumscribed mass that contains a nucleus and a surrounding cytoplasm. *Germ cells* have the function of reproducing an entity similar to the organism from which the germ cells originate. They are characteristically haploid, that is, have a single set of chromosomes. *Somatic cells* are body cells (any cells that are not germ cells); they are characteristically diploid, that is, have two set of chromosomes.

Centigrade (° C) The metric temperature scale on which the freezing point of water is 0 and the boiling point of water is 100. The formula for the conversion of degrees centigrade to degrees Fahrenheit is $° F = \frac{9}{5} ° C + 32$.

Central Ray The theoretical center of the x-ray beam. The term is used to designate the direction of the x rays in a given projection; the central ray may be considered to extend from the focal spot of the x-ray tube to the x-ray film.

Cephalometric Projection Examination by means of film placed to obtain lateral and Caldwell posteroanterior views of the head. Used in orthodontics, maxillofacial surgery, and to some degree, prosthodontics to measure and study maxillofacial growth and maxillary and mandibular relationships. The head is held in position by means of a holding device called a cephalostat.

Cervical Pertaining to (1) the neck, or cervical vertebrae, and (2) the cementoenamel junction (CEJ) area of a tooth.

Characteristic (Discrete) Radiation Electromagnetic radiation produced by electron transitions from higher-energy orbitals to replace ejected electrons of inner-electron orbitals. The energy of the electromagnetic radiation emitted is unique to and characteristic of the emitting atom (element).

Charge-Coupled Device (CCD) A solid-state image detector found in some intraoral digital radiography sensors.

Chromosome Aberration Any rearrangement of chromosome parts as a result of breakage by radiation or other means.

Chronic Exposure Radiation exposure of long duration, either continuous (protracted exposure) or intermittent (fractionation exposure); usually refers to exposure of relatively low intensity.

Clearing Agent Agent in the fixer used to remove nonactivated silver halide crystals.

Coherent Scattering Sometimes called *unmodified scattering*. One of the four interactions that occur when photons (x rays) and atoms collide with each other. The low-energy x-ray photon collides with an inner-orbital electron, but its low energy cannot dislodge the electron. The electron may absorb the photon, which then sets the photon into vibration. This causes an electromagnetic wave that is the same as the incident (incoming) photon but that travels in a different direction. This type of interaction is below the energy range useful in clinical radiology.

Collimation Any device used for the elimination of the peripheral divergent portion of the useful x-ray beam, such as metal tubes, "cones," or diaphragms interposed in the path of the beam.

Collimator A lead disk with an aperture of various sizes and shapes. The diaphragm limits the size of the primary beam to the area of interest, thereby minimizing patient exposure to the primary beam.

Complete Mouth Radiographic Survey (CMRS) A series of intraoral dental images that show all tooth-bearing areas of both the upper and lower jaws; also knows as a *full mouth series*.

Compton Scatter Radiation Commonly called *scatter radiation*. The incident radiation has sufficient energy to dislodge a bound electron; when it attacks a loosely bound electron and dislodges it, the remaining radiation energy proceeds in a different direction as scatter radiation.

Cone A device on a dental x-ray machine that is designed to indicate the direction of the central ray and to serve as a guide in establishing a desired source-to-film distance. A *short cone* establishes an anode-to-skin distance of up to approximately 18 cm. A *long cone* establishes an extended anode-to-skin distance, usually within the range of 27 cm to 36 cm.

Cone Beam Volumetric Imaging A three-dimensional digital imaging method employing a cone-shaped beam of radiation that rotates around the patient.

Cone Cutting Failure to cover or expose the entire area of a radiograph with the useful beam, thereby only partially exposing the film.

Cone Length The distance between the focal spot and the end of the cone, usually expressed in inches or centimeters.

Constant Potential Kilovoltage *See* Kilovoltage.

Continuous Spectrum For electromagnetic radiation, a spectrum that exhibits a gradual variation of wavelength. Examples include the spectrum of light from an incandescent solid and an x-ray spectrum.

Contrast The difference in image density appearing on a radiograph, representing various degrees of beam attenuation. *See also* Film Contrast, Long-Scale Contrast, Short-Scale Contrast, Subject Contrast.

Coolidge Tube A vacuum tube in which x rays are generated when the target (integral with the anode) is bombarded by electrons emitted from a heated filament and accelerated toward the anode across a high potential difference. *See also* X-Ray Tube.

Cortical Bone The outermost layer of bone.

Cosmic Rays Radiation of extremely short wavelengths that originates outside the earth's atmosphere.

Coulomb The amount of electrical charge transferred by 1 ampere in 1 second.

Coulombs per Kilogram The number of ion pairs in 1 kilogram of air.

Critical Organs (Tissues) Those tissues that either react unfavorably to radiation or, by their nature, attract and absorb specific radiochemicals.

Crookes' Tube A vacuum discharge tube developed by Sir William Crookes in early experimental work with cathode rays. Wilhelm Roentgen first discovered that, in addition to the production of cathode rays, x rays were emitted during the operation of these tubes. *See also* X-Ray Tube.

Cumulative Dose The total dose resulting from repeated exposures to radiation of the same region or the whole body. *See also* Dose (Dosage of Radiation).

Cumulative Radiation Effects Additive biologic effects of repeated exposure to radiation.

Current, Alternating An electrical current in which electrons alternately flow in opposite directions.

Current, Direct An electrical current in which electrons flow in one direction.

Darkroom A room that can be completely darkened so that photographic or x-ray film may be processed.

Daylight Loading System A method of loading, unloading, and feeding films into the processor in normal room light. This system entails the use of special equipment, with no need for a darkroom.

Definition (Image) The property of images pertaining to their sharpness, distinctness, or clarity.

Density (Photographic or Film) The degree of darkening of exposed and processed photographic or x-ray film. *See also* Background Density, Inherent (Film) Density, Object (Tissue) Density.

Depth Dose The radiation delivered to a particular depth beneath the surface of the body; it is usually expressed as a percentage of surface doses. *See also* Dose (Dosage of Radiation).

Detail A visual quality that depends on sharpness (definition). Factors that influence detail include (1) the size of the tube focal spot, (2) the source-to-film distance, (3) the distance of the object from the film, (4) the motion of the object or x-ray source, (5) the type of intensifying screens, and (6) the image contrast.

Developer A chemical (potassium bromide) used in a developer to check the development of the unexposed silver bromide and to control the working speed of the developer with respect to the exposed silver bromide. The developer also contains a reducing agent.

Development The first step in film processing in which the halides in the film emulsion are reduced to black metallic silver.

Digital Imaging A filmless method of capturing an image and displaying it by using an electronic sensor, electronic signals, and a computer to process and store the image.

Direct Effects of Radiation Biologic damage that occurs when ionizing radiation interacts directly with a component of a cell.

Direct-Exposure Film Highly sensitive to the direct action of x rays but with low sensitivity to screen fluorescence (e.g., intraoral dental film). *See also* Film.

Direct Imaging The method in which an electronic sensor is directly exposed to radiation and the image is generated electronically on a computer.

Distal Remote; farther from any point of reference (e.g., midline).

Distortion An inaccuracy in the size or shape of an object as it is displayed in the radiograph. *Magnification distortion* is the proportional enlargement of a radiographic image. It is always present to some degree in oral radiography but is minimized with increased source-to-film distance or decreased object-to-film distance. *Vertical distortion* is the disproportional change in size, either elongation or foreshortening, due to incorrect vertical angulation or improper film placement.

Dose (Dosage of Radiation) The amount of energy absorbed per unit mass of tissue at a site of interest. *See also* Absorbed Dose, Cumulative Dose, Depth Dose, Doubling Dose, Entrance Dose, Erythema Dose, Exit Dose, Threshold Dose, Tissue Dose.

Dose Equivalent The product of absorbed dose and modifying factors (i.e., the quality factor, distribution factor, and any other necessary factors). The traditional unit of dose equivalence is the *rem* (rad × qualifying factors). The international system (SI) unit of dose equivalence is the sievert (Sv) (grays × qualifying factors).

Dosimeter An instrument used to detect and measure an accumulated dosage of radiation.

Double Exposure Two superimposed exposures on the same radiographic or photographic film.

Doubling Dose The amount of ionizing radiation absorbed by the gonads of the average person in a population over a period of several generations that will result in a doubling of the current rate of spontaneous mutations. *See also* Dose (Dosage of Radiation).

Effective Focal Spot The apparent size and shape of the focal spot when viewed from a position in the useful beam; with the use of a suitable inclined anode face, it is smaller than the actual focal spot size. *See also* Line Focus.

Electrode Either of the two terminals of an electrical source, an anode or a cathode (*qq.v.*).

Electromagnetic Radiation The forms of energy propagated by wave motion as photons or discrete quanta. The forms of radiation have no matter associated with them. They differ widely in wavelength, frequency, and photon energy and have strikingly different properties. Covering an enormous range of wavelengths (from 10^{17} to 10^{-6} angstroms), they include radio waves, infrared waves, visible light, ultraviolet radiation, x rays, gamma rays, and cosmic radiation.

Electron A negatively charged elementary particle.

Electron Stream Electrons moving from the cathode to the anode across a potential difference in a low-pressure gas tube or a vacuum tube.

Electron Volt The kinetic energy gained by an electron falling through a potential difference of 1 volt.

Element A pure substance consisting of atoms of the same atomic number that cannot be decomposed by ordinary chemical means.

Elon *See* Developer.

Elongation A form of radiographic distortion in which the image is longer than the object radiographed.

Entrance Dose Dose measured at the surface of an irradiated object. It includes both primary radiation and backscatter from materials beneath the surface. *See also* Dose (Dosage of Radiation).

Epithelium The cells lining all canals and body surfaces, including those cells that are specialized for secretion.

Equivalent The thickness of pure aluminum, concrete, or lead that would afford the same radiation attenuation, under specified conditions, as any given material being considered.

Erythema Dose Antiquated measurement based on the amount of radiation that will cause erythema (redness) of the skin. *See also* Dose (Dosage of Radiation).

Excitation The addition of energy to a system, thereby transferring it from its ground state to an excited state.

Exit Dose The absorbed dose delivered by a beam of radiation to the surface through which the beam emerges from an object. *See also* Dose (Dosage of Radiation).

Exposure A measure of the ionization produced in air by x radiation or gamma radiation. It is the sum of the electrical charges on all of the ions of one sign produced in air when all of the electrons liberated by the photons in a volume element of air are completely stopped in air, divided by the mass of the air in the volume element.

Exposure Factors Radiographic kilovoltage, exposure time, milliamperage, and source-to-film distance: the primary radiographic factors considered when making an exposure.

Extraoral Radiograph An examination of the teeth and bones made by placing the film or cassette against the side of the head or face and projecting the x rays from the opposite side.

Filament Coiled tungsten wire that emits electrons when heated to incandescence.

Film A thin, transparent sheet of cellulose acetate or similar material coated on one or both sides with an emulsion sensitive to radiation and light. *See also* Direct-Exposure Film, Screen Film, X-Ray Film.

Film Badge A metal container of radiographic film used for the detection and measurement of radiation exposure of personnel.

Film Base The thin, transparent sheet of cellulose acetate or similar material that carries the radiation- and light-sensitive emulsion of x-ray films.

Film Contrast A characteristic inherent in the type of film used. *See also* Contrast, Long-Scale Contrast, Short-Scale Contrast, Subject Contrast.

Film Emulsion A coating on a film base consisting of a mixture of gelatin and halide crystals with which the radiation interacts.

Film Holder A device used to hold a film packet or image receptor in a patient's mouth; most also assist in x-ray beam alignment.

Film Mount A device used to hold and arrange intraoral radiographs in an appropriate way for interpretation.

Film Packet A lightproof, moisture-resistant, sealed paper or plastic envelope containing x-ray film, used in making radiographs.

Film Processing The process of converting a latent image to a visible image by immersion in developer and fixer, followed by rinsing in water and drying.

Film Speed The amount of exposure to light or x rays (the latter in roentgens) required to produce a given image density. Film speed is expressed as the reciprocal of the exposure in roentgens necessary to produce a density of 1.0 above base and fog. Films are classified on this basis in six speed groups, from A through F. *See* Speed.

Filter The material (usually aluminum) placed in the useful beam to absorb preferentially the less energetic (less penetrating) forms of radiation.

Filtration The use of absorbers or filters for the preferential attenuation of radiation of certain wavelengths from a useful primary beam of x radiation.

Fixation *See* Fixer.

Fixer (Film or Hypo-) The solution (primarily ammonium thiosulfate) in which the manifest image is fixed and hardened, removing the silver halide crystals from the exposed film that was unexposed to or unaffected by the action of the x radiation.

Fluorescence The emission of radiation of a particular wavelength by certain substances as the result of absorption of radiation of a shorter wavelength. The emission occurs essentially only during the period of irradiation.

Fluorescent Screen A sheet of material coated with a substance (e.g., calcium tungstate or zinc sulfide) that emits visible light when irradiated with x radiation.

Focal Spot The part of the target on the anode of an x-ray tube that is bombarded by the focused electron stream when the tube is energized.

Focal Trough In panoramic radiography, a three-dimensional horseshoe-shaped zone or image layer in which structures are reasonably well-defined.

Focusing Cup Along with the filament, the focusing cup determines the size and shape of the target (focal) spot. The cup is constructed of molybdenum.

Fog A darkening of the whole or part of a radiograph by sources other than the radiation of the primary beam to which the film was exposed. *Chemical fog* is film darkening due to imbalance or deterioration of processing solutions. *Light fog* is darkening due to unintentional exposure to light (to which the emulsion is sensitive), either before or during processing. *Radiation fog* is darkening due to radiation from sources other than intentional exposure to the primary beam (e.g., scatter radiation) or exposure of film during unprotected storage.

Foreshortening A form of distortion in which the image is shorter than the object radiographed. In the angle-bisecting technique it is caused by misdirecting the x-ray beam perpendicular to the plane of the film instead of to the plane of the bisector (i.e., the vertical angulation is too steep).

Frankfort Plane An imaginary line that connects the floor of the orbit and the external auditory meatus (ear opening).

Free Radical An uncharged but highly reactive molecule with an unpaired electron in the outermost shell.

Gamma Radiation Short-wavelength electromagnetic radiation of nuclear origin, within a range of wavelengths from about 10^{-8} cm to 10^{-11} cm.

Gas Tube An early type of x-ray tube in which electrons were derived from residual gases within the tube. *See also* X-Ray Tube.

Gelatin A protein obtained from animal skin and hooves by boiling; used in x-ray film manufacture as a means of suspending the silver halide crystals in the film emulsion.

Gene The fundamental unit of inheritance that determines and controls transmissible characteristics.

Genetic Effects (Radiation) Changes produced in the genes and chromosomes of all nucleated body cells. In customary usage, the term relates to the effect produced in the reproductive cells.

Geometric Unsharpness Impairment of image definition due to the penumbra (shadow).

Ghost Image In panoramic radiography, a blurred, radiopaque artifact produced by a dense object.

Gonad An ovary or a testis; the site of origin of oocytes or spermatozoa.

Gray (Gy) A unit of radiation measurement established in 1974 by the International Commission on Radiation Units and Measurements. One gray (Gy) = 1 joule/kg = 100 rad. The gray is a unit of absorbed dose and replaces the rad.

Grid A device used to prevent as much scattered radiation as possible from reaching an x-ray film during the exposure of a radiograph.

Half Value Layer The thickness of a particular material that will reduce an x-ray exposure by one half.

Halides Compounds of metals with halogen elements: bromine, chlorine, and iodine.

"Hard" Radiation A slang term for x rays of short wavelengths and high-penetrating power. In usage, the shorter the wavelength is, the "harder" the radiation.

Horizontal Angulation *See* Angulation.

Identification Dot A small raised area on the corner of an intraoral film packet used to determine correct image orientation.

Image Receptor A recording medium for an image, normally either film or a digital sensor.

Impulse The burst of radiation generated during a half cycle of alternating current.

Indirect Effects Biologic damage that occurs as a result of the formation of highly reactive chemical compounds by the interaction of radiation and cellular components.

Indirect Imaging The method in which an existing image is scanned and converted to digital form.

Inherent (Film) Density The density of a processed film due to such intrinsic factors in the film as the density of the film base and the emulsion gelatin. *See also* Density (Photographic or Film).

Intensifying Screen Material contained in an extraoral cassette that emits light when exposed to x radiation; the emitted light exposes the film, thereby intensifying the action of the x-ray beam.

Intensity (Beam) The total qualitative and quantitative energy of an x-ray beam.

Interpretation (of X-Ray Film) The study of a radiograph; the interpretation of that which is seen; and the integration of the findings with the case history, laboratory, and clinical examinations to arrive at a diagnosis.

Interproximal Between two adjacent tooth surfaces.

Interproximal Radiograph *See* Bitewing Radiograph.

Intraoral Radiograph Radiograph produced on a film placed intraorally to the teeth.

Inverse Square Law of Radiation The intensity or exposure rate of radiation at a given distance from the source inversely proportional to the square of the distance.

Ion An atomic particle, atom, or chemical radical bearing an electrical charge, either negative or positive.

Ionization The process or the result of a process by which a neutral atom or molecule acquires either a positive or a negative charge.

Ionizing Radiation Electromagnetic radiation (x rays or gamma rays) or particulate radiation (electrons, neutrons, and protons) capable of ionizing air directly or indirectly.

K Electron An electron having an orbit in the K shell, which is the first shell of electrons surrounding the atom's nucleus.

Kilo (k) A prefix representing 1000.

Kiloelectron Volt (keV) The symbol for 1000 electron volts.

Kilovolt (kV) Equal to 1000 volts.

Kilovoltage (in X-Ray Machines) The potential difference between the anode and the cathode of an x-ray tube. *Constant-potential kilovoltage* is the potential formed by a constant-voltage generator expressed as constant-potential kilovolts (kVcp).

Kilovoltage Peak (kVp) The crest value (in kilovolts) of the potential difference of a pulsating-potential generator. When only half of the wave is used, the value refers to the useful half of the cycle.

Lamina Dura The thin plate of dense, or compact, bone that lines the tooth sockets; it appears on a radiograph as a fine radiopaque line passing around the tooth.

Latent Image The invisible change produced in a photographic or x-ray film emulsion by the action of x radiation or light, from which the visible image is subsequently developed and fixed chemically.

Latent Period The period between the time of exposure of tissue to an injurious agent (e.g., radiation) and the clinical manifestation of a particular response.

Lateral Cephalometric Projection An extraoral radiographic image depicting the skull as seen from the side, used to determine growth and development of the face and jaws; frequently used in orthodontic evaluations.

Lateral Jaw Projection An examination in which the film is placed adjacent to the patient's ramus, or the body of the mandible, with the rays directed obliquely upward from the opposite side and the central beam directed at the point of interest. The vertical angulation is such that it casts the image of the near mandible superior or anterior to the area of interest.

Lateral Skull Projection An examination in which the film is placed parallel to the sagittal plane of the patient's head with the rays directed at right angles to the plane of the film and the sagittal plane; the entire skill is shown.

Latitude, Film Exposure The range between the minimum and maximum radiation exposures that yield diagnostically useful images of structures.

Latitude, Object The range between the maximum and minimum object densities recorded on a radiograph.

Leaded Apron A lead-impregnated rubber apron that provides protection for patients and auxiliary personnel from radiation.

Light-Tight A term used to describe darkroom conditions in which all white light has been excluded.

Line Pairs per Millimeter (lp/mm) A measure of image resolution or detail.

Lingual The surface of a tooth that rests against the tongue.

Localization The making of a radiograph for the purpose of identifying a site in relation to surrounding tissues.

Long Cone *See* Cone.

Long-Scale Contrast An increased range of grays between the blacks and whites on a radiograph. Higher kilovoltages increase this range. *See also* Contrast.

Long-Term Radiation Effects Biologic effects of radiation that appear long after exposure to the radiation.

mA *See* Milliampere (mA).

mAs *See* Milliampere-Seconds (mAs).

Magnification, Radiographic The enlargement or distortion of a radiographic image recorded on film emulsion, minimized by reducing the object-to-film distance and increasing the focal-film distance.

Magnification Distortion *See* Distortion.

Maximum Permissible Dose (MPD) The MPD is the maximum dose of radiation that, in view of present knowledge, is not expected to produce significant radiation effects. For radiation workers, 50 mSv per year is permissible.

Mesial Toward the center of the dental arch.

Metal Housing The metal body of an x-ray tubehead that surrounds the x-ray tube and the transformers.

Midsagittal Plane An imaginary line passing through the center of the body, dividing it into right and left halves.

Milli Prefix meaning one thousandth (1/1000).

Milliampere (mA) Electrically, the milliampere is 1/1000 of an ampere (*q.v.*). In radiography, milliamperage refers to the current flow from the cathode to the anode, which in turn regulates the intensity of radiation emitted by the x-ray tube, hence directly influencing the radiographic density.

Milliampere-Seconds (mAs) The product of the x-ray tube operating amperage and exposure time in seconds.

Molecule The smallest quantity of matter that can exist by itself and retain its chemical properties; it is composed of one or more atoms.

Monochromatic Radiation Electromagnetic radiation of a single wavelength.

Multilocular Having multiple compartments or locules.

Mutation A departure from the parent type, as when an organism differs from its parents in one or more heritable characteristics as a result of genetic change.

Nano Prefix meaning one billionth (1/1,000,000,000).

Neutron An elementary particle having no electrical charge. The neutron is a constituent of the nucleus of all atoms except hydrogen.

Nucleus, Atomic The small central part of an atom containing the protons and neutrons; most of the atomic mass is concentrated here.

Object (Tissue) Density The resistance of an object to the passage of x rays. *See also* Density (Photographic or Film).

Object-to-Film Distance Distance between the object or skin and the cassette or film.

Oblique An angular view of a surface or object.

Occlusal Relating to the chewing surfaces of teeth.

Occlusal Plane The plane of the masticating surfaces of the molar and bicuspid teeth when the maxilla and mandible are closed.

Occlusal Radiograph A radiograph made with a film designed for placement between the occlusal surfaces of the teeth, with the x-ray beam directed caudad or cephalad.

Orbital Electron An electron that is moving in an orbit around the nucleus of an atom.

Overdevelopment Permitting the film to remain in the developer beyond the normal or pre-set time. This decreases radiographic contrast and increases radiographic density.

Overexposed Condition of a radiographic image in which the image displays an overall darkness, indicating that too much radiation reached the image receptor.

Oxidation A chemical reaction in which an electron is removed from an atom.

Panoramic Image An image obtained by rotation of an x-ray source about the patient to produce a continuous image of both jaws and related structures.

Pantomograph *See* Panoramic Radiograph.

Paralleling Technique The production of a radiographic exposure of intraoral film whereby the plane of the film packet is made parallel to the long axis of the tooth being radiographed. The central beam axis, or central ray of the x ray, is directed at right angles to both.

Paranasal Sinuses The collection of sinuses in the head that surround the nasal cavity; they include the maxillary, sphenoid, and frontal sinuses plus the ethmoid air cells.

Penetrability The ability of a beam of x radiation to pass through matter; kilovoltage and filtration determine the degree of penetrability.

Penumbra The secondary shadow that surrounds the periphery of the primary shadow; the term pertains to the shadow proper. A penumbra is the ill-defined margin or shadow produced by light. In radiography, it is the blurred margin of an image detail, also called *geometric unsharpness*.

Periapical Radiograph A radiograph made by intraoral placement of film for recording shadow images of the outline, position, and mesiodistal extent of the teeth and surrounding tissue.

Phosphors Types of crystals in intensifying screens that fluoresce when exposed to x rays.

Photoelectric Effect The ejection of bound electrons by an incident photon such that the whole energy of the photon is absorbed and transitional or characteristic x-ray emissions are produced.

Photoelectron An electron emitted from a substance under a stimulus or other radiation of appropriate wavelength. *See* Photoelectric Effect.

Photon A quantum of electromagnetic radiation.

Pixel Picture element; a minute piece of electronic information in a digital image.

Position-Indicating Device (PID) A device usually composed of a plastic ring through which a metal rod can be placed to assist in properly aligning the cone and film (see Chapter 1).

Posteroanterior Projection A radiographic examination of the skull in which the image receptor is placed near the patient's face and the x-ray beam enters the posterior aspect of the head.

Potassium Bromide *See* Developer.

Preservative A chemical that inhibits oxidation of the reducing agents by air. Sodium sulfite is the chemical usually used as a preservative.

Primary Beam of Radiation The radiation that is produced at the target of the anode and exits the tubehead.

Primary Protective Barrier A barrier sufficient to reduce the useful beam to the permissible dose rate. *See also* Barrier, Protective.

Projection A term for the position of a part of the patient's anatomy with relation to the x-ray film and the x-ray beam.

Proton An elementary nuclear particle with a positive electrical charge.

Proximal Nearest; closest to a point of reference.

Quality Assurance Maintaining continuously optimal functioning of both technical and operational aspects of radiologic procedures so that maximal diagnostic information is produced while minimizing patient exposure to radiation.

Quality Factor (QF) The linear-energy-transfer–dependent factor by which absorbed doses are multiplied to obtain (for radiation protection purposes) a quantity that expresses the effect of the absorbed dose on a common scale for all forms of ionizing radiation.

Radiation The emission and propagation of energy in the form of waves or particles through space or a material medium. *See also* Magnification, Radiographic; Monochromatic Radiation.

Radiation Absorbed Dose (rad) A unit of measurement for the absorbed dose of any type of ionizing radiation in any medium. One rad is the energy absorption of 100 ergs (*q.v.* Gray).

Radiation Sickness A syndrome associated with exposure to ionizing radiation that may result in nausea, vomiting, and diarrhea; later symptoms include malaise, depression, epilation, purpura, hemorrhage, fever, and emaciation.

Radiobiology That branch of biology dealing with radiation effects on biologic systems.

Radiograph A visible image on a radiation-sensitive film emulsion produced by chemical processing after exposure of the film emulsion to ionizing radiation that has passed through an area, region, or substance of interest.

Radiographer Someone who exposes and processes radiographic images.

Radiographic Survey A series of radiographic projections constituting a study.

Radiography The technical process of positioning, exposing, and processing radiographs.

Radiologic Health The art and science of protecting humans from injury by radiation, as well as promoting better health through beneficial applications of radiation.

Radiolucency The appearance of dark images on film caused by the greater amount of radiation that penetrates the structures and reaches the film.

Radiolucent Permitting the passage of x rays with relatively little attenuation by absorption.

Radiopacity The appearance of light images on film caused by the lesser amount of radiation that penetrates the structures and reaches the film.

Radiopaque Strongly inhibiting the passage of x rays.

Radioresistant Demonstrating low amounts of biologic damage after exposure to radiation.

Radiosensitivity Relative susceptibility of cells, tissues, organs, organisms, or any substances to the injurious action of radiation.

Rare Earth Commonly used to refer to intensifying screens that contain one or more of the rare-earth elements and that use the absorption and conversion features of these elements in x-ray imaging. May also refer to a screen-film system used for x-ray imaging. These systems are considered fast exposure systems.

Rectification Conversion of alternating current to direct current. *Full-wave rectification* is conversion of the entire wave of an alternating current to a direct current. *Half-wave rectification* is conversion of half of the sine wave of an alternating current to a direct current. *Self-rectification* is rectification of half of the sine wave of the alternating current across an x-ray tube as a result of the absence of electron emission at the anode.

Reducing Agent *See* Developer.

Relative Biologic Effectiveness (RBE) A factor used to compare the biologic effects of absorbed dosages of differing types of ionizing radiation in a particular organism or tissue. The standard of comparison is medium-voltage x rays delivered at about 10 rads per minute. The unit of RBE is the *rem (q.v.).*

Relative Risk The ratio of the risk of biologic harm: in those exposed, to the risk; in those not exposed, to radiation.

Replenisher Concentrated processing solution added to compensate for volume reduction and oxidation that takes place during normal processing steps.

Resolution (Image) The discernible separation of closely adjacent image details. In optics, to separate and make visible the parts of an image.

Reticulation A network of corrugations in the emulsion of a radiograph as a result of too great a difference in temperature between any two of the three darkroom solutions.

Right-Angle Technique *See* Paralleling Technique.

Roentgen (R) An international unit of exposure based on the ability of radiation to ionize air; an exposure to gamma or x radiation such that the associated corpuscular emission per 0.0001293 grams of air produces, in air, ions carrying 1 electrostatic unit of quantity of either positive or negative electricity (2.083 billion ion pairs).

Roentgen-Equivalent-Man (rem) A unit of dose of any radiation to body tissue, expressed in terms of its estimated biologic effects relative to an exposure of 1 roentgen of gamma or x radiation.

Rollers A component of an automatic processor that moves the film through the processing compartments.

Safelight Special lighting used in the darkroom that permits film to be transferred from cassette to processor without fogging.

Safelight Filter A colored filter placed over a safelight bulb designed to remove portions of the visible light spectrum that will expose radiographic film.

Same/Lingual-Opposite/Buccal (SLOB) Rule *See* Buccal Object Rule.

Scattered Radiation Radiation that, during passage through a substance, has been deviated in direction. It may also have been modified by an increase in wavelengths. Scattered radiation is one form of secondary radiation *(q.v.)*.

Screen Film Sensitive to the fluorescent light of intensifying screens but not as sensitive to the direct action of x rays (e.g., panoramic film). *See also* Film.

Secondary Ionization Particles, usually electrons, ejected by recoil when a primary ionizing particle passes through matter.

Secondary Protective Barrier A barrier sufficient to reduce the secondary, or scatter, radiation to the permissible dose rate. *See also* Barrier, Protective.

Secondary Radiation Particles or photons produced by the interaction of primary radiation with matter.

Sensor, Image A detector used in digital radiography to capture an image.

Sharpness (Image) The ability of an image to demonstrate an interface line as one-dimensional.

Short-Scale Contrast A reduced range of grays between the blacks and whites on a radiograph. Lower kilovoltages decrease this range. *See also* Contrast, Film Contrast, Long-Scale Contrast, Subject Contrast.

Short-Term Effects of Radiation Biologic effects of radiation that are displayed within a relatively short amount of time (e.g., minutes, days, or weeks).

Sievert (Sv) A unit of radiation measurement of dose equivalence; 1 Sv = 100 rem.

"Soft" Radiation X rays of relatively long wavelength with relatively little penetrating ability.

Somatic Effects Biologic effects of radiation that affect cells and tissues of the body, excluding the gonads.

Source The point of emanation of gamma or x rays when used as an origin of radiation.

Spatial Resolution The smallest distance between two points in an object that can be distinguished as separate detail in the image; generally indicated as a number of black and white line pairs per millimeter.

Speed, Film Speed in radiography refers to the relative amount of darkening produced on a film (with reference to film or screen characteristics) from a given amount of radiation. Speed and sensitivity may be used interchangeably. Officially, the speed of a film system is defined as the reciprocal of the exposure in roentgens required to produce a density of 1.0 above base-plus-fog density. The measurement unit of film speed is R^{-1}.

$$Speed = \frac{1}{Roentgens\,(R)}$$

Speed of Light Light travels 186,000 miles per second. All electromagnetic radiation travels at the speed of light.

Speed of X rays X rays travel at the speed of light, 186,000 miles per second, or at 3×10^8 meters per second in a vacuum.

Static Electricity Marks on a radiograph resembling small streaks of lightning; they result from static electricity that occurs when the film is removed from the wrapper paper or when films are separated after being piled on top of one another.

Step-Down Transformer This transformer produces a lower voltage output by stepping down the input voltage. Stepping down the voltage results in a step up in amperage because the power input is equal to the power output. The filament transformer of the x-ray circuit is a step-down transformer.

Step-Up Transformer This transformer produces a higher voltage output than the input by stepping up the input voltage. Stepping up the voltage results in a step down in amperage because the power input is equal to the power output. The high-voltage transformer of the x-ray circuit is a step-up transformer.

Stepwedge A device with varying layers of material used to demonstrate a scale of density and contrast.

Stop Bath A solution of water and acetic acid used between the developer and the fixer that stops the development of the film.

Storage Phosphor Imaging A method of digital imaging in which the image is captured on phosphor-coated plates that are subsequently scanned by a laser to produce the visible image on a computer.

Subject Contrast The relative difference in density and thickness of the components of the radiographed subject, as evidenced by the varied radiographic densities caused by the difference in absorbing power of the different kinds of material traversed by an x-ray beam. See also *Contrast, Film Contrast, Long-Scale Contrast, Short-Scale Contrast.*

Subject Thickness The relative thickness of hard and soft patient tissues.

Submentovertex Projection An extraoral radiographic examination used to demonstrate positions of the condyles, zygomatic arches, and some of the paranasal sinuses.

Tank, Processing Metal tanks used to hold processing solutions. These tanks are constructed of stainless steel to resist corrosion and permit rapid equalization of temperature control. The outside walls of the tanks are insulated to prevent condensation of moisture and to maintain temperature control.

Target The area on the anode subject to electron bombardment, usually consisting of a tungsten insert on the end face of a solid copper anode.

Target-Film Distance (TFD) This is the same as focal-film distance (FFD), in that it is the distance from the focal spot of the x-ray tube to the x-ray film.

Thermionic Emission The release of electrons from the cathode filament by heating.

Threshold Dose The minimum dose that will produce a detectable degree of any given effect. See also *Dose (Dosage of Radiation).*

Thyroid Collar A leaded shield used to protect the thyroid gland from radiation exposure.

Timer A switch mechanism used to complete the electrical circuit to produce x rays for a predetermined time. An *electronic timer* is a timer that functions through a mechanical clock mechanism. A *hand timer* is an attachment to or part of a timer that requires thumb or finger pressure to actuate the timing device. A *mechanical timer* is a timer operated by a spring mechanism.

Tissue An aggregation of similarly specialized cells united in the performance of a particular function.

Tissue Dose The radiation dose received by a tissue. In the case of x rays and gamma rays, tissue doses are expressed in *rads*. The *rem* is the generally accepted unit of tissue dose for other ionizing radiations. See also *Dose (Dosage of Radiation).*

Tomography A method of imaging using movement of the x-ray source and receptor, resulting in a selected plane that is in focus but has remaining structures blurred out.

Transcranial Projection An extraoral radiographic examination used to demonstrate the mandibular condyle and the glenoid fossa.

Transorbital Projection An anteroposterior radiographic examination that demonstrates the head and neck of the mandibular condyle.

Transpharyngeal Projection A lateral extraoral radiographic examination that demonstrates the mandibular condyle.

Tubehead The component of an x-ray machine that includes the metal housing, x-ray tube, insulating oil, transformers, filter, collimator, and cone or cylinder.

Tumor Either (1) a swelling or a morbid enlargement of tissue or (2) a neoplasm; that is, a mass of new tissue that persists and grows independently of its surrounding structure and that has no physiologic function.

Tungsten A metal with a high melting point that is used in the filament and target of an x-ray tube.

Umbra A complete shadow produced by light, with sharply demarcated margins. In radiography, a sharply delineated image detail.

Underexposed A condition of a radiograph in which the image displays insufficient silver deposits.

Vertical Angulation *See* Angulation.

View Box A light source used to view and interpret radiographs.

Volt (V) The unit of electrical pressure or electromotive force necessary to produce a current of 1 ampere through a resistance of 1 ohm. An electrical volt is the kinetic energy gained by an electron in falling through a potential difference of 1 volt: 1.6×10^{-12} ergs.

Voxel Volume element; essentially a three-dimensional pixel.

Waters Projection An extraoral radiographic examination designed to demonstrate the maxillary sinuses.

Wave, Electromagnetic Energy manifested by movements in an advancing series of alternating elevations and depressions.

Wavelength The distance between the peaks of waves in any waveform, such as light, x rays, and other electromotive forms; also the distance from any point on a wave to the identical point on an adjacent wave. In electromagnetic radiation, the wavelength is equal to the velocity of light divided by the frequency of the wave.

Wetting Agent A solution used in film processing; it follows the washing process to accelerate the flow of water from both film surfaces and to hasten the drying of radiographs.

X Radiation A high-energy portion of the electromagnetic spectrum that is capable of ionizing matter.

X Ray A type of electromagnetic radiation characterized by wavelengths of 100 angstroms or less.

X-Ray Beam The radiation emerging from an x-ray generator or source.

X-Ray Film (1) Film manufactured for use in radiography or (2) a radiograph. See also *Film.*

X-Ray Tube An electronic tube in which x rays are generated. *See also* Crookes' Tube, Gas Tube.

Index

Page numbers followed by *f* indicate figures; *t*, tables; *b*, boxes.

L

Lamina dura, radiographic appearance of, 75-76, 76f,
Latent image formation, 49, 93
Latent period in radiation effects, 111
Lateral oblique jaw projection, 226, 227f, 228f
Lead barrier, 2, 3f
Leaded apron, 2
  in panoramic imaging, 158, 161
    improper placement of, 168f
Lead-lined cylinders, 112, 119
Legal accountability, 121
Lens of eye, effects of radiation on, 115
Lesions, interpretation of. *See* Interpretation
Leukemia, due to radiation exposure, 116
Liability, 121
Light films, 195-196, 196f
Lighting in darkroom, 58-59
  coin test and, 58-59
Linear array, 141, 142f
Lingual caries, 256, 257f
Localization technique, 217f, 216-218, 218f
Locator ring, 12, 14f, 21, 22f
Long-scale contrast, 130, 131f
Lymphocyte, effects of radiation on, 111

M

Magnetic resonance imaging (MRI)
  of maxillary sinuses, 242, 244f
  of temporomandibular joint, 238, 239f
Maintenance of automatic processors, 60
Mandible
  anatomic landmarks of, 77-90
    canine view, 83f, 89f
    incisor view, 81f, 82f, 87f, 89f
    molar bitewing, 86f
    molar view, 85f, 90f
    occlusal, 82f
    premolar view, 83f, 84f, 87f
  film placement, 42
    horizontal, 19
    incorrect, 18, 18f, 19f
    vertical, 16-19
  lateral oblique jaw projection of, 226, 226f, 227f, 228f
  occlusal imaging, 208, 208b, 209b, 208f, 209f, 210f
  paralleling periapical imaging of teeth in, 12, 13f
Mandibular torus, 221, 286-287, 288f, 289f
Manual film processing, 51f, 50-52
  check film in, 54-55, 56f
  checklist for, 52, 53b
  chemicals in, 52, 54t
    changing of, 56-57
    preparation and mixing of, 55-56
    quality assurance and daily care of, 52-53, 54b
  control film in, 54-55, 55f
  darkroom in, 57b, 57-59
  developing in, 50-51, 51f
  fixing in, 51

Manual film processing *(Continued)*
  rinsing in, 51
  stepwedge in, 53-54, 55f
  washing and drying in, 52
mAs. *See* Milliampere-seconds (mAs)
Maxilla
  anatomic landmarks of, 77b, 77-90
    canine view, 78f
    incisor view, 77f, 78f, 87f
    molar view, 79f, 80f, 88f
    premolar view, 79f, 87f
  film placement in, 41-42, 42f
    horizontal, 19
    vertical, 16, 17f
  occlusal imaging, 206b, 206f, 207b, 207f, 205-208
  tilting of teeth in, 12, 13f
Maxillary sinuses
  extraoral radiography of, 241-242, 242f, 243f, 244f, 245f
  radiographic appearance of, 86
Maximum permissible dose (MPD), 120
Medical history, 43
Mental foramen, periapical radiolucency *versus*, 265, 266, 266f
Mesiodens, 272, 273, 273f
Metal objects, panoramic imaging and, 161, 167f
Midsagittal plane in panoramic imaging, 158, 158f, 166f
Miller'(tm)s technique, 216
Milliamperage, 98, 99f
Milliampere-seconds (mAs), 128
Misaligned teeth, 223
Molar view
  bitewing, 21, 86f
  mandibular, 85f, 90, 90f
  maxillary, 79f, 80f, 88f
Molecule, radiation effects on, 107-110
  classic scattering in, 107-108, 108f
  Compton effect in, 108f, 109
  direct, 108f, 107-109
  indirect, 109-110
  photoelectric effect in, 108, 108f
Mounting of film. *See* Film mounting
Movement
  of film or image-receptor, 189f, 188-190
  of patient, 188, 189f
MPD. *See* Maximum permissible dose (MPD)
MRI. *See* Magnetic resonance imaging (MRI)
Multilocular radiolucency, 297, 298f
Multiple roots, 279f, 278-280

N

Nasion guide, 227-228, 229f
Nasopalatine duct cyst, 294f, 295f, 293-295
National Council on Radiation Protection and Measurement Report No. 145, 52
Nucleus, effects of radiation on, 98
Nutrient canal, 261-262